100 Case Reviews
in Neurosurgery

100 Case Reviews in Neurosurgery

RAHUL JANDIAL, MD, PhD

Associate Professor
Division of Neurosurgery, Department of Surgery
City of Hope Cancer Center & Beckman Research Institute
Los Angeles, CA, USA

MICHELE R. AIZENBERG, MD

Associate Professor of Neurological Surgery and Oncology,
Director, Brain and Spine Cancer Center
University of Nebraska Medical Center
Omaha, NE, USA

MIKE Y. CHEN, MD, PhD

Associate Professor
Division of Neurosurgery, Department of Surgery
City of Hope Cancer Center & Beckman Research Institute
Los Angeles, CA, USA

SECTION EDITORS
Henry E. Aryan, MD
Ramsis Benjamin, MD
Justin Brown, MD
Joseph D. Ciacci, MD
Griffith R. Harsh IV, MD
Adam S. Kanter, MD
Aasim S. Kazmi, MD
Alexander A. Khalessi, MD
Paul S. Larson, MD
Michael L. Levy, MD, PhD
Neal Prakash, MD, PhD
J. Dawn Waters, MD

For additional online content visit http://expertconsult.inkling.com

ELSEVIER

Edinburgh   London   New York   Oxford   Philadelphia   St Louis   Sydney   Toronto   2017

ELSEVIER

ISBN: 978-0-323-35637-4

Content Strategist: Charlotta Kryhl
Content Development Specialist: Alexandra Mortimer
Content Coordinator: Devika Ponnambalam
Project Manager: Louisa Talbott
Design: Christian Bilbow
Illustration Manager: Amy Naylor
Marketing Manager: Rachael Pignotti

Printed in China

Last digit is the print number: 9   8   7   6   5   4   3   2   1

Contents

SECTION I
Vascular Neurosurgery
Section Editor: Alexander A. Khalessi, MD

SECTION II
Nontraumatic Cranial Lesions
Section Editor: Griffith R. Harsh IV, MD • J. Dawn Waters, MD

SECTION III
Neurosurgical Trauma
Section Editor: Joseph D. Ciacci, MD

SECTION VI
Stereotactic and Functional Neurosurgery
Section Editor: Paul S. Larson, MD

SECTION VII
Peripheral Nerve Neurosurgery
Section Editor: Justin Brown, MD

SECTION VIII
Neurology
Section Editors: Neal Prakash, MD, PhD • Ramsis Benjamin, MD

Preface

As the most challenging discipline, Neurosurgery rebuffs any single text's attempt at revealing its intricacies and complexities. Accordingly, this text and its individual chapters aim for a more humble goal. Together, they aspire to serve as a primer of essential material often reviewed during certification examinations and a framework into which deeper knowledge can be contextualized.

From the perspective of didactic utility, the standard, time-tested neurosurgical textbooks offer a distillation of the most useful art and schemata. Therefore, figures from these familiar texts have been incorporated into this book, along with new art and imaging, in the hope that the aggregate will constitute a robust visual fabric within *100 Case Reviews in Neurosurgery*.

The book is divided into intuitive sections. The information provided and the questions posed follow the experience of a neurosurgeon being consulted in the hospital or seeing a new patient in clinic that has come to them for care. The vascular section covers surgical and nonsurgical elements that are key elements of essential vascular cases. The peripheral nerve section is particularly detailed since this is a specialized field most general neurosurgeons have limited exposure to in daily practice. The appendices provide information that is vital yet cumbersome to include in the flow of the chapters. The layout and presentation of information follows the formats of common grand rounds and examinations most readers have experienced from the beginning of their neurosurgical training through their current continuing education.

The most challenging part of constructing the book you now read has been to find that elusive balance invaluable to the modern pedagogical text between comprehensiveness and concision, between textual explanation and visual illustration, between esoteric specificity and simple intelligibility. My hope is that the content presented here has been insightfully and incisively curated for your purposes.

Rahul Jandial

List of Contributors

Salman Abbasifard, MD
International Pediatric Neurosurgery
Fellow
Rady Children's Hospital
University of California – San Diego
San Diego, CA, USA

Michele R. Aizenberg, MD
Associate Professor of Neurological
Surgery and Oncology
Director, Brain and Spine Cancer Center
University of Nebraska Medical Center
Omaha, NE, USA

Abdulrazag Ajlan, MD
Clinical Instructor
Department of Neurosurgery
Stanford Hospitals and Clinics
Stanford, CA, USA

Ali H. A. Muhammad Altameemi, MD
International Fellow of Neurosurgery
Rady Children's Hospital San Diego
Division of Pediatric Neurosurgery
University of California – San Diego
San Diego, CA, USA

Henry E. Aryan, MD
Clinical Professor of Neurosurgery, UC
San Francisco
Chief, Spine Center
Sierra Pacific Orthopedic & Spine Center
Fresno, CA, USA

Nicholas Barbaro, MD
Chairman
Department of Neurosurgery
Indiana University School of Medicine
Indianapolis, IN, USA

Thomas L. Beaumont, MD, PhD
Senior Resident
Department of Neurological Surgery
Washington University School of
Medicine
St. Louis, MO, USA

Ramsis Benjamin, MD
City of Hope National Medical Center
Duarte, CA, USA

Daniel M. Birk, MD
Resident
Department of Neurosurgery
University of Illinois at Chicago
Chicago, IL, USA

Michael Bohl, MD
Resident Physician
Division of Neurological Surgery
Barrow Neurological Institute
St. Joseph's Hospital and Medical Center
Phoenix, AZ, USA

Justin Brown, MD
Associate Professor
Department of Neurosurgery
University of California
San Diego School of Medicine
San Diego, CA, USA
  Section Editor for Section 7
  Peripheral Nerve Neurosurgery
  Case 82: Thoracic Outlet Syndrome
  Case 83: Peroneal Neuropathy
  Case 84: Nerve Sheath Tumor
  Case 85: Cubital Tunnel Syndrome
  Case 86: Carpal Tunnel Syndrome
  Case 87: Brachial Plexus Injury
  Case 88: Parsonage-Turner Syndrome
  Case 89: Radial Nerve Injury
  Case 90: Ulnar Nerve Injury
  Case 91: Median Nerve Injury

Kim J. Burchiel, MD
John Raaf Professor and Chairman
Department of Neurological Surgery
Oregon Health and Science University
Portland, OR, USA
  Case 72: Trigeminal Neuralgia

Edward F. Chang, MD
Associate Professor
Department of Neurological Surgery
University of California – San Francisco
San Francisco, CA, USA
  Case 76: Mesial Temporal Sclerosis

Mike Y. Chen, MD, PhD
Associate Professor
Division of Neurosurgery, Department of
Surgery
City of Hope Cancer Center & Beckman
Research Institure
Los Angeles, CA, USA
  Case 55: Spinal Metastases

Tsinsue Chen, MD
Neurosurgery Resident
Division of Neurological Surgery
Barrow Neurological Institute
St. Joseph's Hospital and Medical Center
Phoenix, AZ, USA
  Case 75: Progressive Spastic
  Paraparesis and Decreased Mobility in
  a Young Patient

Vincent J. Cheung, MD
Neurosurgical Resident
Division of Neurosurgery
University of California – San Diego
San Diego, CA, USA
  Case 3: Ruptured Middle Cerebral
  Artery Aneurysm
  Case 4: Unruptured Anterior
  Communicating Artery Aneurysm
  Case 36: Normal Pressure
  Hydrocephalus
  Case 38: Penetrating Head Injury
  Case 39: Intractable Intracranial
  Hypertension
  Case 40: Epidural Hematoma
  Case 44: Hangman's Fracture

Omar Choudhri, MD
Neurosurgery Chief Resident
Stanford University School of Medicine
Stanford, CA, USA
  Case 20: Sphenoid Wing Meningioma

Kevin K.H. Chow, MD, PhD
Neurosurgery Resident
Department of Neurosurgery
Stanford University School of Medicine
Palo Alto, CA, USA
  Case 26: Glioblastoma
  Case 31: Brain Metastases

Joseph D. Ciacci, MD
Program Director UCSD Neurosurgery
Residency
Academic Community Director
UCSD School of Medicine
Chief of Neurosurgery VASDHS
Professor, Division of Neurosurgery
University of California, San Diego
School of Medicine
San Diego, CA, USA
  Section Editor for Section 3
  Neurosurgical Trauma
  Case 38: Penetrating Head Injury
  Case 39: Intractable Intracranial
  Pressure
  Case 40: Epidural Hematoma
  Case 41: Chronic Subdural Hematoma
  Case 42: Subaxial Cervical Fracture
  Case 43: Odontoid Fractures
  Case 44: Hangman's Fracture
  Case 45: Thoracolumbar Burst
  Fractures
  Case 46: Chance Fractures
  Case 47: Jumped Cervical Facets

Aaron Cohen-Gadol, MD
Associate Professor
Department of Neurosurgery
Indiana University School of Medicine
Indianapolis, IN, USA
    Case 73: Hemifacial Spasm

John R. Crawford, MD, PhD
Associate Professor of Clinical
Neurosciences and Pediatrics
University of California – San Diego
Director Neuro-Oncology Rady Children's
Hospital
San Diego, CA, USA
    Case 63: Cerebellar Medulloblastoma
    Case 64: Brainstem Glioma
    Case 65: Hypothalamic Hamartoma
    Case 66: Endoscopic Third
    Ventriculostomy
    Case 67: Slit Ventricle Syndrome
    Case 71: Pilocytic Astrocytoma

Erik I. Curtis, MD
Neurosurgical Resident
Division of Neurosurgery
University of California, San Diego
School of Medicine
San Diego, CA, USA
    Case 41: Chronic Subdural Hematoma
    Case 42: Subaxial Cervical Fracture
    Case 43: Odontoid Fractures
    Case 45: Thoracolumbar Burst
    Fractures

Gehaan D'Souza, MD
Fellow in Plastic Surgery
Department of Plastic Surgery
University of California
San Diego School of Medicine
San Diego, CA, USA
    Case 89: Radial Nerve Injury

Benjamin D. Elder, MD, PhD
Resident
Department of Neurosurgery
The Johns Hopkins University School of
Medicine
Baltimore, MD, USA
    Case 79: Idiopathic Intracranial
    Hypertension (Pseudotumor Cerebri)

Nicholas Fain, MD
Resident Physician
Department of Radiology
University of Iowa
Iowa City, IA, USA
    Case 42: Subaxial Cervical Fracture

Brandon C. Gabel, MD
Neurosurgical Resident
Division of Neurosurgery
University of California, San Diego
School of Medicine
San Diego, CA, USA
    Case 15: Moyamoya Disease
    Case 16: Venous Sinus Thrombosis
    Case 38: Penetrating Head Injury
    Case 39: Intractable Intracranial
    Hypertension
    Case 40: Epidural Hematoma
    Case 41: Chronic Subdural Hematoma
    Case 42: Subaxial Cervical Fracture
    Case 43: Odontoid Fractures
    Case 44: Hangman's Fracture
    Case 45: Thoracolumbar Burst
    Fractures
    Case 46: Chance Fractures
    Case 47: Jumped Cervical Facets
    Case 70: Vein of Galen Malformations

Gurpreet S. Gandhoke, MD
Department of Neurological Surgery
University of Pittsburgh Medical Center
Pittsburgh, PA, USA
    Case 48: Atlanto-Axial Dislocation
    Case 51: Cauda Equina Syndrome

Melanie G. Hayden Gephart, MD
Assistant Professor
Department of Neurosurgery
Stanford University School of Medicine
Stanford, CA, USA
    Case 24: Pituitary Macroadenoma
    – Prolactinoma
    Case 27: Anaplastic
    Oligodendroglioma
    Case 32: Intraventricular Colloid Cyst
    Case 35: Ependymoma
    Case 61: Pineal Tumor

Thomas J. Gianaris, MD
Resident
Department of Neurosurgery
Indiana University School of Medicine
Indianapolis, IN, USA
    Case 73: Hemifacial Spasm

Gunjan Goel, MD
Neurosurgical Resident
Division of Neurosurgery
University of California – San Diego
San Diego, CA, USA
    Case 5: Intradural Internal Carotid
    Artery Fusiform Aneurysm

David D. Gonda, MD
Neurosurgery Chief Resident
Division of Neurosurgery
University of California – San Diego
San Diego, CA, USA
  Case 25: Craniopharyngioma

C. Rory Goodwin, MD, PhD
Resident
Department of Neurosurgery
The Johns Hopkins University School of
Medicine
Baltimore, MD, USA
  Case 79: Idiopathic Intracranial
  Hypertension (Pseudotumor Cerebri)

Li Gordon, MD
Assistant Professor, Department of
Neurosurgery
Stanford University School of Medicine
Stanford, CA, USA
  Case 30: CNS Lymphoma

Griffith R. Harsh IV, MD
Professor
Department of Neurosurgery
Stanford Hospital and Clinics
Stanford, CA, USA
  Section Editor for Section 2 Non-
  traumatic Cranial Lesions
  Case 21: Cerebellar Cystic
  Hemangioblastoma

Todd Harshbarger, MD
Neurosurgery Division, City of Hope
Duarte, CA, USA
  Case 55: Spinal Metastases

David S. Hong, MD
Pediatric Neurosurgery Fellow
Division of Pediatric Neurosurgery
Rady Children's Hospital San Diego
University of California – San Diego
San Diego, CA, USA
  Case 67: Slit Ventricle Syndrome

Reid Hoside, MD
Neurosurgical Resident
Division of Neurosurgery
University of California – San Diego
San Diego, CA, USA
  Case 7: Cranial Dural Arteriovenous
  Fistula
  Case 14: Cerebellar Hemorrhage

Rahul Jandial, MD, PhD
Associate Professor
Division of Neurosurgery, Department of
Surgery
City of Hope Cancer Center & Beckman
Research Institure
Los Angeles, CA, USA

Henry Jung, MD
Neurosurgery Resident
Department of Neurosurgery
Stanford Hospital and Clinics
Stanford, CA, USA
  Case 33: Cerebral Abscess
  Case 34: Chiari I Malformation

Adam S. Kanter, MD
Associate Professor
Department of Neurological Surgery
University of Pittsburgh Medical Center
Pittsburgh, PA, USA
  Section Editor for Section 4 Spinal
  Neurosurgery
  Case 48: Atlanto-Axial Dislocation
  Case 49: Basilar Invagination –
  Rheumatoid Pannus
  Case 50: Cervical Spondylotic
  Myelopathy
  Case 51: Cauda Equina Syndrome
  Case 52: Foot Drop and Far Lateral
  Disc Herniation
  Case 53: Thoracic Disc Herniation
  Case 54: Spinal Epidural Abscess
  Case 56: Spinal Intradural
  Extramedullary Mass
  Case 57: Intradural Intramedullary
  Mass
  Case 58: Cervical Ossified Posterior
  Longitudinal Ligament
  Case 59: Ankylosing Spondylitis
  Case 60: Chordoma

Michael G. Kaplitt, MD, PhD
Residency Director and Vice Chairman
for Research
Department of Neurological Surgery
Weill Cornell Medical College
New York Presbyterian Hospital
New York, NY, USA
  Case 80: Intractable Oncologic Pain

Aasim S. Kazmi, MD
Section of Neurosurgery
Meridian Health
Wall, NJ, USA
  Section Editor for Appendices

Alexander A. Khalessi, MD
Director of Endovascular Neurosurgery
Surgical Director of Neurocritical Care
Assistant Professor of Surgery and
Neurosciences
University of California – San Diego
San Diego, CA, USA
  Section Editor for Section 1 Vascular
  Neurosurgery
  Case 1: Cerebral Arteriovenous
  Malformation
  Case 2: Cavernous Malformation
  Case 3: Ruptured Middle Cerebral
  Artery Aneurysm
  Case 4: Unruptured Anterior
  Communicating Artery Aneurysm
  Case 5: Intradural Internal Carotid
  Artery Fusiform Aneurysm
  Case 6: Spinal Arteriovenous
  Malformations
  Case 7: Cranial Dural Arteriovenous
  Fistula
  Case 8: Spinal Dural Arteriovenous
  Fistulas
  Case 9: Vertebral Artery Dissection
  Case 10: Basilar Tip Aneurysm
  Case 11: Endovascular Treatment of
  Unruptured Aneurysms
  Case 12: Dominant Hemisphere
  Hemorrhagic Stroke
  Case 13: Hypertensive Thalamic
  Hemorrhage
  Case 14: Cerebellar Hemorrhage
  Case 15: Moyamoya Disease
  Case 16: Venous Sinus Thrombosis
  Case 17: Carotid Stenosis
  Case 18: Ischemic Stroke
  Management

Andrew L. Ko, MD
Fellow, Stereotactic and Functional
Neurosurgery
Department of Neurological Surgery
Oregon Health and Science University
Portland, OR, USA
  Case 72: Trigeminal Neuralgia

Audrey Kohar, DO
Physical Medicine and Rehabilitation
University of California
Irvine, CA, USA
  Case 92: Multiple Sclerosis
  Case 95: Devic's Syndrome
  Case 99: Transverse Myelitis

Thomas A. Kosztowski, MD
Resident
Department of Neurosurgery
The Johns Hopkins University School of
Medicine
Baltimore, MD, USA
  Case 79: Idiopathic Intracranial
  Hypertension (Pseudotumor Cerebri)

Christine K. Lee, MD, PhD
MD/PhD Student
Stanford University School of Medicine
Stanford, CA, USA
  Case 27: Anaplastic
  Oligodendroglioma

Paul S. Larson, MD
Professor and Vice Chair
Department of Neurological Surgery
University of California – San Francisco
San Francisco, CA, USA
  Section Editor for Section 6
  Stereotactic and Functional
  Neurosurgery

Dillon Levy
Pre-Medical Student
University of San Diego
San Diego, CA. USA
  Case 69: Craniosynostosis
  – Plagiocephaly

Michael L. Levy, MD, PhD
Professor and Chief
Division of Pediatric Neurosurgery
Rady Children's Hospital – San Diego
San Diego, CA, USA
  Section Editor for Section 5 Pediatric
  Neurosurgery
  Case 25: Craniopharyngioma
  Case 61: Pineal Tumor
  Case 62: Myelomeningocele
  Case 63: Cerebellar Medulloblastoma
  Case 64: Brainstem Glioma
  Case 65: Hypothalamic Hamartoma
  Case 66: Endoscopic Third
  Ventriculostomy
  Case 67: Slit Ventricle Syndrome
  Case 68: Neural Tube Defect–Tethered
  Cord Syndrome
  Case 69: Craniosynostosis
  – Plagiocephaly
  Case 70: Vein of Galen Malformations
  Case 71: Pilocytic Astrocytoma

Robert M. Lober, MD, PhD
Chief Resident
Department of Neurosurgery
Stanford Hospitals and Clinics
Stanford, CA, USA
    Case 19: Vestibular Schwannoma

Matthew G. MacDougall, MD
Neurosurgery Resident
Division of Neurosurgery
University of California – San Diego
San Diego, CA, USA
    Case 25: Craniopharyngioma

Mark A. Mahan, MD
Assistant Professor
Department of Neurosurgery
Clinical Neurosciences Center
University of Utah
Salt Lake City, UT, USA
    Case 82: Thoracic Outlet Syndrome
    Case 83: Peroneal Neuropathy
    Case 84: Nerve Sheath Tumor
    Case 85: Cubital Tunnel Syndrome
    Case 86: Carpal Tunnel Syndrome
    Case 87: Brachial Plexus Injury
    Case 88: Parsonage-Turner Syndrome
    Case 89: Radial Nerve Injury
    Case 90: Ulnar Nerve Injury
    Case 91: Median Nerve Injury

Joel R. Martin, MD
Neurosurgical Resident
Division of Neurosurgery
University of California-San Diego
San Diego, CA, USA
    Case 18: Ischemic Stroke
    Management

Hazem Mashaly, MD
University of Pittsburgh Medical Center
Pittsburgh, PA, USA
    Case 56: Spinal Intradural
    Extramedullary Mass
    Case 57: Spinal Intramedullary Mass
    Case 58: Cervical Ossified Posterior
    Longitudinal Ligament

Michael M. McDowell, MD
Department of Neurological Surgery
University of Pittsburgh Medical Center
Pittsburgh, PA, USA
    Case 59: Ankylosing Spondylitis
    Case 60: Chordoma

Zachary Medress
Medical Student
Stanford University School of Medicine
Stanford, CA, USA
    Case 30: CNS Lymphoma
    Case 35: Ependymoma

Hal S. Meltzer, MD
Neurosurgical Director of Craniofacial
Program
Rady Children's Hospital San Diego
Professor of Neurosurgery
University of California, San Diego
San Diego, CA, USA
    Case 68: Neural Tube Defect–Tethered
    Cord Syndrome
    Case 69: Craniosynostosis
    – Plagiocephaly

Kai Miller, MD
Resident, Department of Neurosurgery
Stanford University School of Medicine
Stanford, CA, USA
    Case 30: CNS Lymphoma

Robert A. Miller, MD
Department of Neurological Surgery
University of Pittsburgh Medical Center
Pittsburgh, PA, USA
    Case 49: Basilar Invagination –
    Rheumatoid Pannus

Nelson Moussazadeh, MD
Resident in Neurological Surgery
Weill Cornell Medical College
New York Presbyterian Hospital
New York, NY, USA
    Case 80: Intractable Oncologic Pain

Peter Nakaji, MD
Residency Program Director
Division of Neurological Surgery
Barrow Neurological Institute
St. Joseph's Hospital and Medical Center
Phoenix, AZ, USA
    Case 75: Progressive Spastic
    Paraparesis and Decreased Mobility in
    a Young Patient
    Case 78: Normal Pressure
    Hydrocephalus

Bond Nguyen
University of California – Irvine
Irvine, CA, USA
    Case 61: Pineal Tumor
    Case 62: Myelomeningocele

Scott E. Olson, MD
Assistant Professor of Surgery and
Neurosciences
Division of Neurosurgery
University of California – San Diego
San Diego, CA, USA
  Case 8: Spinal Dural Arteriovenous
  Fistulas
  Case 12: Dominant Hemisphere
  Hemorrhagic Stroke
  Case 18: Ischemic Stroke
  Management

J. Scott Pannell, MD
Endovascular Neurosurgery Fellow
Division of Neurosurgery
University of California – San Diego
San Diego, CA, USA
  Case 1: Cerebral Arteriovenous
  Malformation
  Case 2: Cavernous Malformation
  Case 3: Ruptured Middle Cerebral
  Artery Aneurysm
  Case 4: Unruptured Anterior
  Communicating Artery Aneurysm
  Case 5: Intradural Internal Carotid
  Artery Fusiform Aneurysm
  Case 6: Spinal Arteriovenous
  Malformations
  Case 7: Cranial Dural Arteriovenous
  Fistula
  Case 8: Spinal Dural Arteriovenous
  Fistulas
  Case 9: Vertebral Artery Dissection
  Case 10: Basilar Tip Aneurysm
  Case 11: Endovascular Treatment of
  Unruptured Aneurysms
  Case 12: Dominant Hemisphere
  Hemorrhagic Stroke
  Case 13: Hypertensive Thalamic
  Hemorrhage
  Case 14: Cerebellar Hemorrhage
  Case 15: Moyamoya Disease
  Case 16: Venous Sinus Thrombosis
  Case 17: Carotid Stenosis
  Case 18: Ischemic Stroke
  Management

Arjun V. Pendharkar, MD
Department of Neurosurgery
Stanford University School of Medicine
Palo Alto, CA, USA
  Case 32: Intraventricular Colloid Cyst

Neal Prakash, MD, PhD
City of Hope National Medical Center
Chief of Neurology
Associate Clinical Professor of Neurology
Director of Neurological Optical Imaging
Duarte, CA, USA
  Section Editor for Section 8
  Neurology
  Case 92: Multiple Sclerosis
  Case 95: Devic's Syndrome
  Case 97: Status Epilepticus
  Case 99: Transverse Myelitis

Robert C. Rennert, MD
Neurosurgical Resident
Division of Neurosurgery
University of California – San Diego
San Diego, CA, USA
  Case 9: Vertebral Artery Dissection
  Case 10: Basilar Tip Aneurysm
  Case 12: Dominant Hemisphere
  Hemorrhagic Stroke
  Case 36: Normal Pressure
  Hydrocephalus

Christian B. Ricks, MD
Department of Neurological Surgery
University of Pittsburgh Medical Center
Pittsburgh, PA, USA
  Case 50: Cervical Spondylotic
  Myelopathy
  Case 52: Foot Drop and Far Lateral
  Disc Herniation
  Case 54: Spinal Epidural Abscess

Daniele Rigamonti, MD
Professor
Department of Neurosurgery
The Johns Hopkins University School of
Medicine
Baltimore, MD
  Case 79: Idiopathic Intracranial
  Hypertension (Pseudotumor Cerebri)

Nathan C. Rowland, MD, PhD
Chief Resident
Department of Neurological Surgery
University of California – San Francisco
San Francisco, CA, USA
  Case 76: Mesial Temporal Sclerosis

Jayson A. Sack, MD
Neurosurgical Resident
Division of Neurosurgery
University of California – San Diego
San Diego, CA, USA
  Case 3: Ruptured Middle Cerebral
  Artery Aneurysm
  Case 4: Unruptured Anterior
  Communicating Artery Aneurysm
  Case 9: Vertebral Artery Dissection
  Case 10: Basilar Tip Aneurysm

Noriko Salamon, MD, PhD
Professor of Radiology
Chief of Neuroradiology
Section of Neuroradiology
Department of Radiological Sciences
David Geffen School of Medicine at
UCLA
Ronald Reagan Medical Center
Los Angeles, CA, USA
  Case 95: Devic's Syndrome

David R. Santiago-Dieppa, MD
Neurosurgical Resident
Division of Neurosurgery
University of California – San Diego
San Diego, CA, USA
  Case 8: Spinal Dural Arteriovenous
  Fistulas
  Case 39: Intractable Intracranial
  Hypertension

Aatman Shah, BS
Medical Student
Department of Neurosurgery
Stanford Hospital and Clinics
Stanford, CA, USA
  Case 33: Cerebral Abscess
  Case 34: Chiari I Malformation

Andrew Shetter, MD
Chair, Section of Functional Stereotactic
Neurosurgery
Division of Neurological Surgery
Barrow Neurological Institute
St. Joseph's Hospital and Medical Center
Phoenix, AZ, USA
  Case 75: Progressive Spastic
  Paraparesis and Decreased Mobility in
  a Young Patient

Jason W. Signorelli
Medical Student
Division of Neurosurgery
University of California – San Diego
San Diego, CA, USA
  Case 1: Cerebral Arteriovenous
  Malformation
  Case 13: Hypertensive Thalamic
  Hemorrhage

Konstantin V. Slavin, MD
Professor
Department of Neurosurgery
University of Illinois at Chicago
Chicago, IL, USA
  Case 81: Spinal Cord Stimulation

Alexa Smith, MD
Pediatric Neurosurgery Fellow
Rady Children's Hospital – San Diego
Division of Pediatric Neurosurgery
University of California, San Diego
San Diego, CA, USA
  Case 61: Pineal Tumor
  Case 62: Myelomeningocele
  Case 63: Cerebellar Medulloblastoma
  Case 64: Brainstem Glioma
  Case 65: Hypothalamic Hamartoma
  Case 66: Endoscopic Third
  Ventriculostomy
  Case 67: Slit Ventricle Syndrome
  Case 68: Neural Tube Defect–Tethered
  Cord Syndrome
  Case 69: Craniosynostosis
  – Plagiocephaly
  Case 71: Pilocytic Astrocytoma

Matthew D. Smyth, MD
Associate Professor of Neurosurgery and
Pediatrics
Director, Pediatric Epilepsy Program
Department of Neurological Surgery
Washington University School of
Medicine
St. Louis, MO, USA
  Case 77: Corpus Callosotomy

Philip A. Starr, MD, PhD
Professor and Co-Director, Functional
Neurosurgery Program
Department of Neurological Surgery
University of California – San Francisco
San Francisco, CA, USA
  Case 74: Parkinson's Disease

Jeffrey A. Steinberg, MD
Division of Neurosurgery
University of California – San Diego
San Diego, CA, USA
Case 2: Cavernous Malformation
Case 17: Carotid Stenosis
Case 70: Vein of Galen Malformations

YouRong Sophie Su
Medical Student
Stanford University School of Medicine
Stanford, CA, USA
Case 24: Pituitary Macroadenoma
– Prolactinoma

Zachary J. Tempel, MD
Department of Neurological Surgery
University of Pittsburgh Medical Center
Pittsburgh, PA, USA
Case 49: Basilar Invagination –
Rheumatoid Pannus
Case 53: Thoracic Disc Herniation
Case 56: Spinal Intradural
Extramedullary Mass
Case 57: Intradural Intramedullary
Mass
Case 59: Ankylosing Spondylitis
Case 60: Chordoma

Doris D. Wang, MD, PhD
Resident Physician
Department of Neurological Surgery
University of California – San Francisco
San Francisco, CA, USA
Case 74: Parkinson's Disease

J. Dawn Waters, MD
Clinical Instructor
Department of Neurosurgery
Stanford Hospital and Clinics
Stanford, CA, USA
Section Editor for Section 2 Non-
traumatic Cranial Lesions
Case 21: Cerebellar Cystic
Hemangioblastoma
Case 23: Cushing's Microadenoma
Case 29: Radiation Necrosis versus
Tumor Recurrence
Case 36: Normal Pressure
Hydrocephalus
Case 37: Arachnoid Cyst

Christina Huang Wright, MD
Resident Physician
Department of Neurological Surgery
University of Southern California School
of Medicine
Los Angeles, CA, USA
Case 22: Pituitary Apoplexy
Case 28: Low-Grade Glioma

James Wright, MD
Resident Physician
Department of Neurological Surgery
Case Western Reserve University School
of Medicine
Cleveland, OH, USA
Case 22: Pituitary Apoplexy
Case 28: Low-Grade Glioma

David S. Xu, MD
Resident Physician
Division of Neurological Surgery
Barrow Neurological Institute
St. Joseph's Hospital and Medical Center
Phoenix, AZ, USA
Case 78: Normal Pressure
Hydrocephalus

Derek Yecies, MD
Resident
Department of Neurosurgery
Stanford Hospitals and Clinics
Stanford, CA, USA
Case 29: Radiation Necrosis versus
Tumor Recurrence

Nathan T. Zwagerman, MD
Department of Neurological Surgery
University of Pittsburgh Medical Center
Pittsburgh, PA, USA
Case 50: Cervical Spondylotic
Myelopathy

Acknowledgements

For those that have not had the opportunity to assemble a text, the immense collaborative effort can be lost behind the bold, large font names on the cover. Yes, the editors are key to the process. Equally important is the publishing team. Alexandra Mortimer, Louisa Talbott and Andrew Riley have been thoughtful and attentive companions in making this book. The book would be porous and flawed without them. Most importantly Charlotta Kryhl has helped shepherd us through the original idea, its need in the neurosurgical community and ultimately the spirit of this textbook. Thank you for your support and leadership.

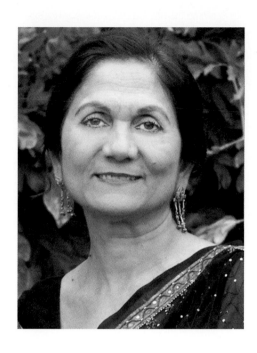

For boundless love
For unwavering support
For my mother, Sushma Jandial
Rahul Jandial

Chen, Ph.D, for gifting me his disdain of the conventional-and to my mother, Professor S.J. Chen, for my brutal endurance and voice of reason.

Mike Y. Chen

I am grateful to all of my colleagues for their collaboration, expertise, and friendship. I am appreciative of our residents who motivate us to be even better. Also, my patients, who inspire me to persevere.

I dedicate this book to family: My mother, Lenore, for her endless commitment to our happiness. My father, Stephen, who is missed beyond words. My in-laws, Shari and Ali, for their undying love and support. My husband, Shervin, for his sacrifices for my dedication to my profession. My children, Ava and Cyrus, who have enriched my life in ways I never thought possible, making me a better person and surgeon.

Michele R. Aizenberg

Section I Vascular Neurosurgery

Case 1

Cerebral Arteriovenous Malformation

Jason W. Signorelli ● J. Scott Pannell, MD ●
Alexander A. Khalessi, MD

Presentation

An 18-year-old female presents to the ED with severe headaches, nausea, vomiting, and complex partial seizure beginning on the right side of the body. She has no history of prior seizures. She has had headaches in the past, but this headache is worse than usual.

- PMH: otherwise unremarkable; no recent trauma
- Exam: mild left-sided weakness

Differential Diagnosis

- Vascular
  - Ischemic/embolic stroke
  - Arteriovenous malformation (AVM)
  - Cavernous hemangioma
  - Aneurysm rupture
  - Moyamoya disease
- Infectious
  - CNS infection (herpes simplex encephalitis)
- Neoplastic
  - Primary cerebral tumor
  - Metastasis (most commonly lung, renal cell carcinoma, melanoma, breast)
- Metabolic/toxic/nutritional
  - Alcohol withdrawal
  - Drug intoxication
  - Electrolyte abnormalities
  - Hypoglycemia
- Congenital/developmental
  - Osler-Weber-Rendu disease
  - Sturge-Weber syndrome
  - Wyburn-Mason syndrome ("Bonnet–Dechaume–Blanc syndrome")

Initial Imaging

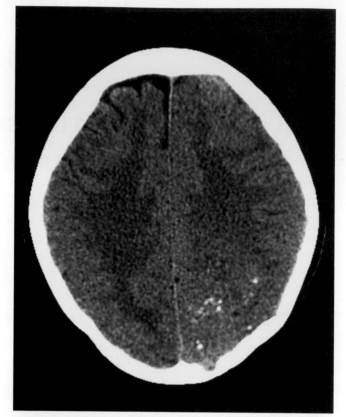

FIGURE 1-1

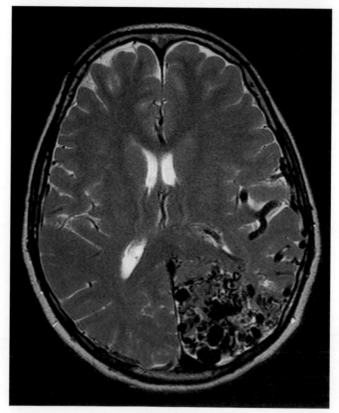

FIGURE 1-2

Imaging Description and Differential

- Axial noncontrast head CT demonstrates serpiginous calcified structures in the left parieto-occipital region, concerning for vascular malformation.
- Axial T2-weighted MRI demonstrates cortical AVM and numerous flow voids in the left parieto-occipital region.

Further Imaging

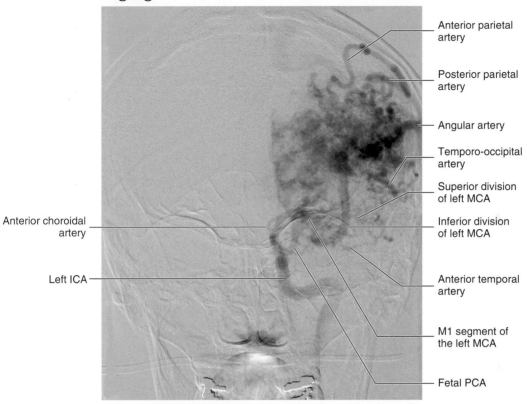

FIGURE 1-3 PA and lateral left anterior circulation digital subtraction angiogram.

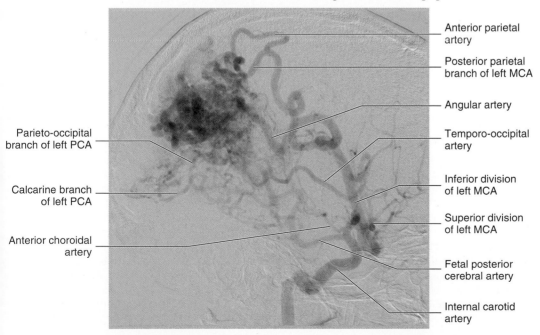

FIGURE 1-4 PA and lateral left anterior circulation digital subtraction angiogram.

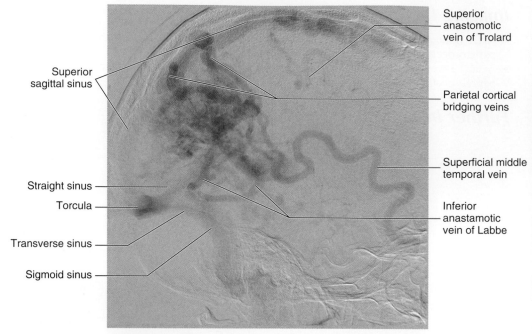

Superior anastomotic vein of Trolard

Superior sagittal sinus

Parietal cortical bridging veins

Superficial middle temporal vein

Straight sinus

Torcula

Inferior anastamotic vein of Labbe

Transverse sinus

Sigmoid sinus

FIGURE 1-5   Lateral venous phase digital subtraction angiogram.

- Figures 1-3 and 1-4 are digital subtraction angiograms of PA and lateral left anterior circulation performed by left ICA injection. They depict a large 6 cm AVM nidus supplied by multiple MCA and foetal variant PCA pedicles.
- Figure 1-5 is a lateral venous phase digital subtraction angiogram performed by left ICA injection and demonstrates superficial and deep venous drainage from the AVM.
- Findings are consistent with Spetzler-Martin (SM) scale grade 5 AVM.

Further Workup

- Imaging
  - ECG
- Grading
  - SM or supplemented SM grading (SM-supp)
- Laboratory
  - CMP, CBC, ESR, and CRP
- Consultants
  - Cardiology (ECHO)

Pathophysiology

Cerebral AVM is a rare disorder with an estimated prevalence of 0.01% to 0.5% that commonly presents with intracranial hemorrhage or seizures. It is the most common cause of spontaneous intraparenchymal hemorrhage in adults <40 years old. The majority of lesions (~88%) are superficially located, with approximately 20% having associated aneurysms. The natural history is heterogeneous, with an approximate 2.2% annual risk of rupture for previously unruptured AVMs and 4.5% for ruptured. This risk is significantly altered by several factors including prior hemorrhage, venous drainage, and associated aneurysms; increasing the annual risk of hemorrhage to as high as 34% in patients having all three risk factors. Furthermore, the cumulative risk of rupture increases with age. Ruptured AVMs result in major mortality and morbidity; the associated death rate is as high as 29% and only 55% of survivors are capable of independent living (mRS ≤2). A majority of patients will be diagnosed with an AVM before the age of 40, and there is substantial risk of at least one hemorrhage during their lifetime; therefore these lesions should be treated.

Of note, the recently published ARUBA trial argued for the superiority of medical management versus interventional therapy for unruptured AVMs; however, methodological flaws within the trial and other more recent studies cast significant doubt on those findings.

Treatment Options

Treatment of AVMs is often multimodal, tailored to the specifics of the lesion, and commonly assessed by the SM grading scale.

- Surgery
  - Resection is the most definitive treatment, resulting in complete obliteration of the AVM in nearly all patients
  - Appropriate for lesions with SM grade ≤5 or SM-supp grade ≤6
  - May be combined with embolization for larger AVMs
- Stereotactic radiosurgery
  - Appropriate for lesions ≤3cm in diameter with a compact nidus or location in an eloquent area where resection would result in significant neurologic deficits
  - Long latency to lesion obliteration period (1–3 years) and does not completely eliminate the risk of hemorrhage
  - May be combined with embolization
- Embolization
  - Facilitates both surgery and stereotactic radiosurgery
  - May be appropriate for complete AVM obliteration in select cases

Surgical Technique

The approach must be tailored to the AVM location and key associated vascular structures, including arterial feeders, draining veins, and boundaries of the nidus. Extranidal aneurysms should also be accounted for when planning an approach. Intraoperative monitoring is important when the AVM is located in or near an eloquent cortex; electrophysiological monitoring with continuous bilateral upper and lower somatosensory and motor evoked potentials may aid in the resection. Preoperative staging for embolizations may be performed if deemed appropriate. The significant majority of AVMs are located in the cerebral convexity, and this surgical approach is outlined next.

Surgical Resection: Cerebral Convexity (85% of AVMs)

The head is placed in rigid fixation with the cortical surface of the AVM parallel to the floor. The skin is incised in standard fashion and a wide craniotomy/durotomy is performed to ensure adequate access and visualization of all key vascular structures.

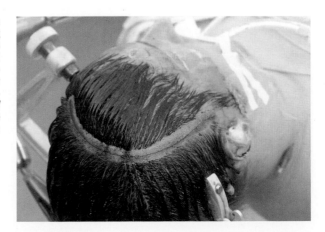

FIGURE 1-6 Skin is incised in standard fashion. Extra precaution should be taken if arterial feeders emanating from the external carotid arteries feed the AVM nidus since this can lead to significant bleeding. When the skull is exposed, the AVM is mapped out using a neuronavigation system for bone flap planning. To avoid unnecessary bleeding, care should be exercised when crossing locations of draining veins with a craniotomy. *(Reprinted with permission. Jandial R, McCormick P, Black PM. Core Techniques in Operative Neurosurgery. Philadelphia: Philadelphia: Elsevier/Saunders; 2011, ©2011.)*

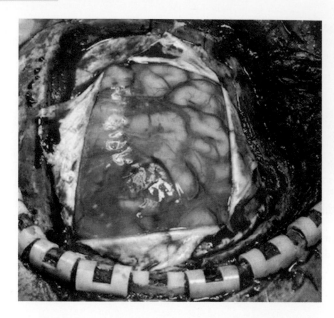

FIGURE 1-7   When the bone flap has been removed, the dura should be tacked up to the surrounding bone taking care not to penetrate vessels underlying the dura. The dural opening should adequately expose the entire AVM nidus, feeding arteries, and draining veins of the cortical surface. The dura should be reflected very gently because vessels associated with the AVM can be adherent to the dura, and tearing could result in AVM bleeding. *(Reprinted with permission. Jandial R, McCormick P, Black PM. Core Techniques in Operative Neurosurgery. Philadelphia: Philadelphia: Elsevier/Saunders; 2011, ©2011.)*

Next, surface feeding arteries are identified and occluded. The dissection of the nidus may then begin in a circumferential pattern. Deep feeding arteries should be coagulated and cut or clipped as needed. Upon completion of the nidus dissection, the deep arterial pedicles must be identified and dissected.

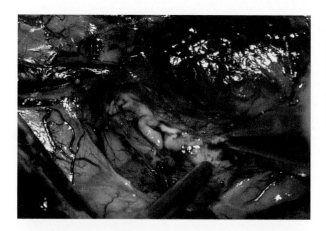

FIGURE 1-8   When all components of the AVM are identified on the cortical surface, the parenchymal phase of the dissection can begin, dissecting around the AVM in a spiral fashion. A gliotic tissue plane frequently exists because of chronic ischemic changes that facilitate identification of such a plane. Retraction during dissection should always be on the AVM nidus and not on the surrounding brain parenchyma. *(Reprinted with permission. Jandial R, McCormick P, Black PM. Core Techniques in Operative Neurosurgery. Philadelphia: Philadelphia: Elsevier/Saunders; 2011, ©2011.)*

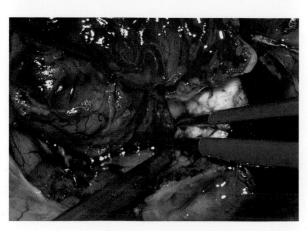

FIGURE 1-9   When the dissection plane has led to the apex of the nidus, special attention must be paid to the deep arterial supply. Often these arterial feeders are small and high flow, making their control difficult with electrocautery. Small AVM clips are useful. If the bleeding cannot be controlled, it may be necessary to remove the bulk of the AVM nidus so that the remaining AVM deep in the resection bed can be better controlled. *(Reprinted with permission. Jandial R, McCormick P, Black PM. Core Techniques in Operative Neurosurgery. Philadelphia: Philadelphia: Elsevier/Saunders; 2011, ©2011.)*

Deep venous drainage is approached last. Major draining veins must first be occluded with a temporary aneurysm clip and the AVM observed to identify indications of intact arterial pedicles, such as increased distension of the AVM. Following control of these veins, the AVM is removed en bloc and blood pressure may be transiently elevated to confirm adequate hemostasis.

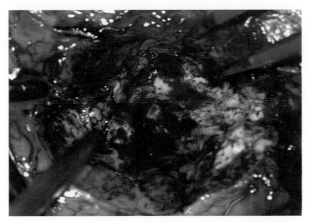

FIGURE 1-10 After the AVM nidus has been removed, the resection bed must be examined for residual nidi and areas of bleeding. Continuous bleeding often means residual nidi and should be examined closely. Intraoperative imaging may consist of digital subtraction angiography, with or without supplementary indocyanine green dye video angiography. The resection bed must be completely dry because increases in systolic blood pressure can easily lead to re-bleeds, necessitating evacuation. Systolic blood pressure can be increased temporarily to high-normal levels to check for areas of potential bleeding. *(Reprinted with permission. Jandial R, McCormick P, Black PM.* Core Techniques in Operative Neurosurgery. *Philadelphia: Philadelphia: Elsevier/Saunders; 2011, ©2011.)*

Once confirmed, an EVD or ICP monitor is placed if deemed appropriate. The dura is then closed, bone flap replaced, and skin closed.

Surgical Resection: Deep Brain

For AVMs with a nidus in the deep brain, preoperative staged embolizations should be incorporated and an anatomically suitable approach used including options such as:

- Interhemispheric transcallosal (frontal, parietal, or occipital)
- Transsylvian
- Occipital transtentorial infrasplenial
- Infratentorial supracerebellar

Complication Avoidance and Management

- Craniotomy must be wide enough to visualize all surface vascular structures and minimize brain retraction.
- The AVM must be resected as a whole; partial resection is likely to lead to severe hemorrhage.
- Venous drainage should always be addressed last. Early elimination of venous drainage increases the risk of rupture and bleeding into the parenchyma or ventricles.
- A noncontrast head CT should be obtained postoperatively to monitor for hematoma formation.
- Normotensive or hypotensive blood pressure should be targeted postoperatively to reduce the risk of hematoma formation in the residual cavity.

KEY PAPERS

Al-Shahi R, Bhattacharya JJ, Currie DG, et al. Prospective, population-based detection of intracranial vascular malformations in adults the Scottish intracranial vascular malformation study (SIVMS). *Stroke.* 2003;34(5):1163-1169.

Brown RD, Wiebers DO, Forbes G, et al. The natural history of unruptured intracranial arteriovenous malformations. *J Neurosurg.* 1988;68(3):352-357.

Friedlander RM. Arteriovenous malformations of the brain. *N Engl J Med.* 2007;356(26):2704-2712.

Gross BA, Du R. Natural history of cerebral arteriovenous malformations: a meta-analysis. *J Neurosurg.* 2013;118(2):437-443.

Kim H, Abla AA, Nelson J, et al. Validation of the supplemented Spetzler-Martin grading system for brain arteriovenous malformations in a multicenter cohort of 1009 surgical patients. *Neurosurgery.* 2015;25-31.

Korja M, Bervini D, Assaad N, et al. Role of surgery in the management of brain arteriovenous malformations prospective cohort study. *Stroke.* 2014;45(12):3549-3555.

Mohr JP, Parides MK, Stapf C, et al. Medical management with or without interventional therapy for unruptured brain arteriovenous malformations (ARUBA): a multicentre, non-blinded, randomised trial. *Lancet.* 2014;383(9917):614-621.

Potts MB, Zumofen DW, Raz E, et al. Curing arteriovenous malformations using embolization. *Neurosurg Focus.* 2014;37(3):E19.

Stapf C, Mast H, Sciacca RR, et al. Predictors of hemorrhage in patients with untreated brain arteriovenous malformation. *Neurology.* 2006;66(9):1350-1355.

van Beijnum J, van der Worp H, Buis DR, et al. Treatment of brain arteriovenous malformations: a systematic review and meta-analysis. *JAMA.* 2011;306(18):2011-2019.

Case 2

Cavernous Malformation

Jeffrey A. Steinberg, MD ● J. Scott Pannell, MD ●
Alexander A. Khalessi, MD

Presentation

A healthy 45-year-old female presents to the emergency room with seizure.

- PMH: otherwise unremarkable
- Exam: mildly slowed cognition
  - Pupils equal and reactive
  - Moves all extremities with full strength
  - Face/smile symmetric
  - No drift

Differential Diagnosis

- Vascular
  - Stroke/TIA
  - Hemorrhage of vascular malformation
- Neurologic
  - Seizure
- Neoplastic
  - Brain tumor
- Infectious
  - Meningitis, abscess
- Other
  - MS
  - Systemic/metabolic

Initial Imaging

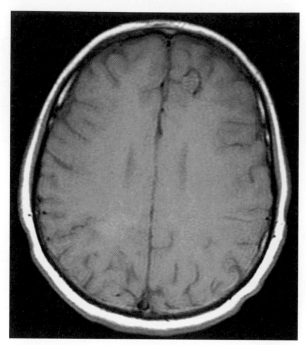

FIGURE 2-1

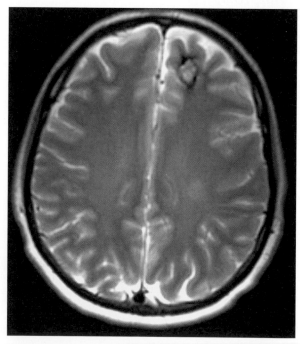

FIGURE 2-2

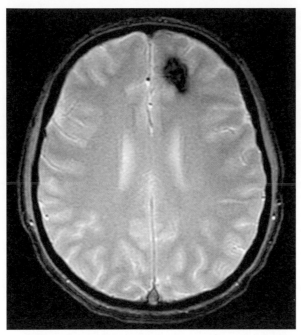

FIGURE 2-3

Imaging Description and Differential

- MRI of the brain depicts typical representation of cavernous malformation, evident by the popcorn/mulberry shape and surrounding rim of signal loss, secondary to hemosiderin deposit, with increased signal on T2 compared with T1. Gradient echo sequences are most sensitive in picking up these lesions because of the increased susceptibility effect.

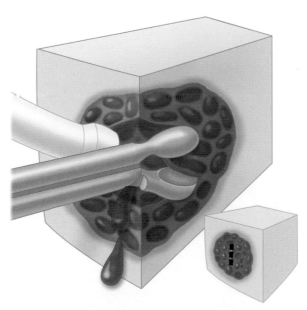

FIGURE 2-4   Brainstem cavernous malformations are often removed through a parenchymal incision much smaller than the malformation itself. In contrast to many supratentorial cavernous malformations, the principles of piecemeal resection are applied here. After incision the lesion is emptied, internally targeting cavities with liquefied old blood. *(Reprinted with permission. Jandial R, McCormick P, Black PM. Core Techniques in Operative Neurosurgery. Philadelphia: Elsevier/Saunders, ©2011.)*

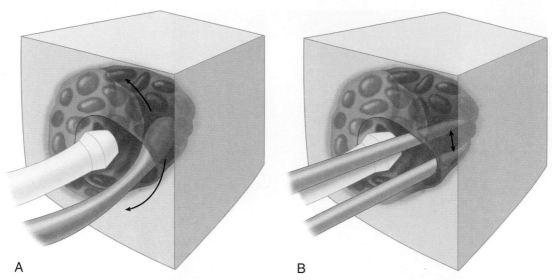

A   B

FIGURE 2-5   When the malformation has been partially internally decompressed, a cleavage plane between the lesion and the surrounding gliotic hemosiderin-stained parenchyma is developed beginning in the portion of the capsule and surface of the malformation closest to the entry point. Specifically designed round dissectors (A) or gentle spread of the bipolar forceps (B) can be used for this maneuver. During this maneuver, gentle traction is applied to the cavernous malformation with the suction in the surgeon's left hand, minimizing the mechanical trauma to the surrounding parenchyma. *(Reprinted with permission. Jandial R, McCormick P, Black PM.* Core Techniques in Operative Neurosurgery. *Philadelphia: Elsevier/Saunders, ©2011.)*

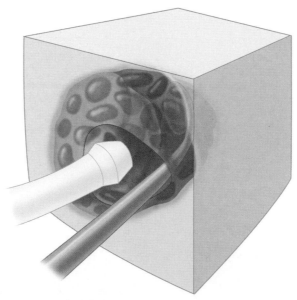

FIGURE 2-6   After further internal emptying of the malformation, the cleavage plane is dissected further with a round dissector. Because of the depth of the field and the limited size of the entry incision, this portion of the operation is done more by "feel" than by direct vision. Extreme caution and gentle touch must be exercised to avoid any damage to portions of parenchyma not in direct vision. *(Reprinted with permission. Jandial R, McCormick P, Black PM.* Core Techniques in Operative Neurosurgery. *Philadelphia: Elsevier/Saunders, ©2011.)*

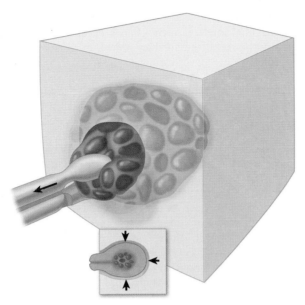

FIGURE 2-7   After the bulk of the cavernous malformation has been released from the surrounding paren-chyma, gentle traction with pituitary forceps is applied to the edges of the most superficial portion of the lesion. If the cavernous malformation has been properly separated, very gentle but steady traction at this point often leads to the malformation eventually "giving in." *(Reprinted with permission. Jandial R, McCor-mick P, Black PM. Core Techniques in Operative Neurosurgery. Philadelphia: Elsevier/Saunders, ©2011.)*

- Differential: cerebral amyloid angiography, diffuse axonal injury, hemorrhagic metasta-ses, capillary telangiectasia, or arteriovenous malformation

Further Workup

- Laboratory
  - Routine labs
- Imaging
  - MRI brain including gradient echo sequences
  - Cerebral angiography generally not necessary for classically appearing lesions, but may be useful in atypical lesions to rule out other vascular anomalies

Pathophysiology

Cavernoma is defined as a vascular malformation composed of dilated capillary-like vessels without intervening neuronal parenchyma. Cavernomas may occur in the brain or spinal cord; they can range in size from a few millimeters to several centimeters, are often associ-ated with venous lesions, and may be congenital or acquired. Grossly they appear as purple-blue multilobulated "mulberry" lesions, often with gliotic, yellow-stained sur-rounding tissue from repeated small hemorrhages. Microscopically cavernomas are thin-walled vessels that lack smooth muscle and elastin and are composed of a single cell layer of endothelial cells that can contain areas of thrombosis.

Treatment Options

- Observation
  - Serial imaging in patients with asymptomatic lesions, lesions in deep locations, or eloquent regions
  - Monitor for hemorrhage or secondary growth/changes in recurrent hemorrhage.
- Medical management
  - Focus on symptom management of headaches and seizures.

- Surgery
  - Surgical resection is the only treatment that is curative for cavernomas. Complete resection eliminates the risk of hemorrhage and improves seizures and headaches.
- Stereotactic radiosurgery
  - Controversial in the treatment of cavernomas, generally only considered for inoperable lesions with progressive symptoms. Results and evidence vary.

Surgical Technique

The goal of surgery is complete removal of the cavernoma. As with many other neurosurgical pathologies, the approach is critical in facilitating resection without injury to normal parenchyma. Intraoperative navigation and ultrasound may be beneficial for localization. Because these lesions are not highly vascularized, piecemeal removal is possible (Figure 2-4, cavernoma dissection). Dissection between the lesion and the surrounding gliotic hemosiderin-stained parenchyma is achieved. Decompression of the cavernoma may facilitate dissection by allowing folding in of the lesion from the normal tissue (Figures 2-4, 2-5, 2-6, Cavernoma dissection). Once the lesion is completely removed, hemostasis of the cavity should be achieved with irrigation and a hemostatic agent, as opposed to bipolar cautery, to decrease risk of injury to parenchymal tissue.

Complication Avoidance and Management

- Cavernoma Resection
  - Resection 2 to 4 weeks after hemorrhage allows for liquefaction of the hematoma, aiding in decompression and delivery of the lesion. Monitoring of tissue color changes from shades of brown to yellow typically demarcates the plane between cavernoma and normal tissue. Deep-seated lesions should be approached with minimal disruption of parenchymal tissue, specifically avoiding eloquent brain regions, and targeting the most superficial aspect of the cavernoma. Dissection through tissue should occur parallel to neuronal tracts to better preserve these structures. Co-occurring venous malformations should be preserved. Hemostasis should be achieved with irrigation and hemostatic agents, as opposed to bipolar cautery, to decrease the risk of injuring normal tissue.

KEY PAPERS

Brown RD Jr, Flemming KD, Meyer FB, et al. Natural history, evaluation, and management of intracranial vascular malformations. *Mayo Clin Proc.* 2005;80:269-281.

Lanzino G, Spetzler RF. *Cavernous Malformations of the Brain and Spinal Cord.* New York: Thieme; 2008.

Porter RW, Detwiler PW, Spetzler RF, et al. Cavernous malformations of the brainstem: experience with 100 patients. *J Neurosurg.* 1999;90:50-58.

Case 3

Ruptured Middle Cerebral Artery Aneurysm

Vincent J. Cheung, MD ● Jayson A. Sack, MD ●
J. Scott Pannell, MD ● Alexander A. Khalessi, MD

Presentation

A 47-year-old woman with no significant past medical history presents to the emergency department with acute onset headache, nausea, and vomiting. Upon presentation, she is lethargic but able to answer orientation questions and briskly follow commands in all extremities. Cranial nerves and motor strength are all grossly intact.

Differential Diagnosis

- Vascular
  - Ruptured aneurysm
  - Ruptured dural arteriovenous fistula
  - Ruptured arteriovenous malformation
  - Hypertensive hemorrhage
- Infectious
  - Rupture of mycotic cerebral aneurysm (in setting of IV drug use)
  - Meningitis
- Other
  - Traumatic hemorrhage
  - Cocaine-induced intracerebral hemorrhage
  - Migraine

Initial Imaging

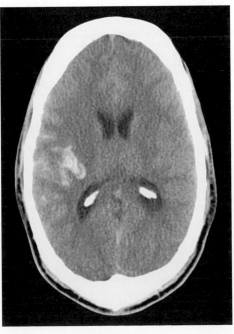

FIGURE 3-1

15

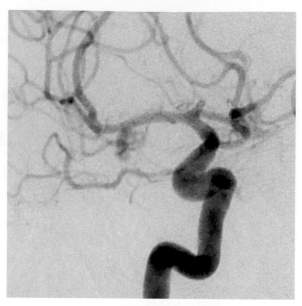

FIGURE 3-2

Imaging Description

- Figure 3-1: Noncontrast CT scan of the head. Dense subarachnoid hemorrhage is present in the right sylvian fissure.
- Figure 3-2: AP projection digital subtraction angiography, right internal carotid injection. An elongated M1 segment MCA aneurysm is shown.

Further Workup

Following a subarachnoid hemorrhage, the first priority should be given to "ABCs" (airway, breathing, circulation). If there is significant intraventricular hemorrhage, or the patient must be intubated and sedated for airway protection or poor neurologic status, an external ventricular drain should be placed. Strict blood pressure control is critical.

Following subarachnoid hemorrhage, patients are at risk for vasospasm. Vasospasm is a pathologic constriction of blood vessels that can result in ischemic stroke and is a major cause of morbidity and mortality after aneurysmal rupture. After securing a ruptured aneurysm through endovascular embolization or craniotomy for clip ligation, patients are typically observed for at least 2 weeks. Vasospasm risk peaks from 3 to 14 days after rupture. During this time, efforts are made to monitor for and mitigate the effects of vasospasm.

Pathophysiology

Aneurysms are pathologic dilatations in the wall of a blood vessel. When the aneurysm weakens to the point of rupture, blood extravasates into the subarachnoid space. The development of a cerebral aneurysm is multifactorial and includes focal structural defects in the vessel wall, hemodynamic stress from turbulent blood flow or branch point, and familial factors. Hereditary syndromes associated with cerebral aneurysms include Ehlers-Danlos syndrome, fibromuscular dysplasia, Osler-Weber-Rendu syndrome, and polycystic kidney disease. Aneurysms may also form from trauma or infection. Traumatic aneurysms differ from true aneurysms in that they typically result from dissection between layers of a vessel wall. In contrast, saccular aneurysms involve all layers of the vessel wall. Infectious aneurysms (also known as mycotic aneurysms) typically occur in distal cortical branches and can form in response to focal weakening of the vessel wall due to septic emboli from bacterial endocarditis, meningitis, or fungal infection.

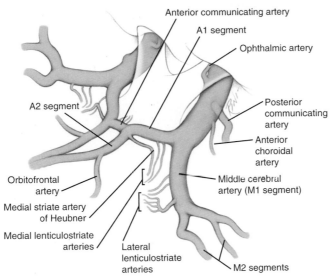

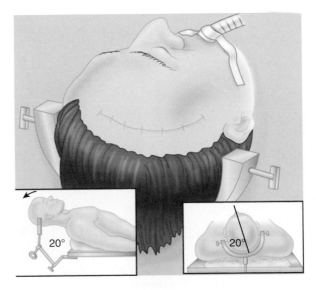

Anterior communicating artery

A1 segment

Ophthalmic artery

A2 segment

Posterior communicating artery

Anterior choroidal artery

Orbitofrontal artery

Middle cerebral artery (M1 segment)

Medial striate artery of Heubner

Medial lenticulostriate arteries

Lateral lenticulostriate arteries

M2 segments

FIGURE 3-3   Anatomy of anterior circulation with the major branches and perforators of the internal carotid artery, of the M1 segment of the middle cerebral artery, of the A1 and A2 segments of the anterior cerebral artery, and of the anterior communicating artery. *(Reprinted with permission. Winn HR. Youmans Neurological Surgery. 6th ed. Elsevier; 2011.)*

Treatment Options

- Craniotomy for clip ligation
- Endovascular embolization

Surgical Technique

The patient is positioned supine in a head holder, and the head is maintained in a 15- to 20 degree rotation away from the side of the aneurysm. Additionally, the head is extended roughly 20 degree to allow gravity to retract the frontal lobe from the anterior cranial fossa. A curvilinear skin incision is performed inferiorly from the zygomatic arch (<1 cm from tragus) and superiorly to the midline, staying just behind the hairline. The skin and temporalis muscle are elevated together and retracted forward with skin hooks. A standard frontotemporal craniotomy is performed. Additional bone of the pterion and lesser wing of the sphenoid are drilled down and/or rongeured until the lateral edge of the superior orbital fissure is reached. The dura is then opened with a semicircular incision.

FIGURE 3-4   Positioning of the patient for the right-sided lateral supraorbital approach. *(Reprinted with permission. Quiñones-Hinojosa A. Schmidek and Sweet Operative Neurosurgical Techniques. 6th ed. Elsevier; 2012.)*

20°

20°

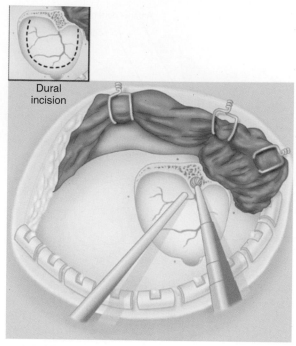

FIGURE 3-5   Removal of the sphenoid wing with high-speed drill and dural incision. *(Reprinted with permission. Quiñones-Hinojosa A. Schmidek and Sweet Operative Neurosurgical Techniques. 6th ed. Elsevier; 2012.)*

Next, opening of the arachnoid of the sylvian fissure is undertaken. Proximal-to-distal dissection of the arachnoid and underlying vasculature may be preferred in the setting of ruptured aneurysms, as this allows for early proximal control of the M1 segment. The arachnoid overlying the carotid cistern is identified and incised. At this point, frontal and temporal retractors may be placed to assist with stretching of the arachnoid overlying the sylvian fissure so that the arachnoid can be sharply cut and the fissure opened. Next, the supraclinoid ICA is dissected to its bifurcation. The A1 of the Anterior cerebral artery (ACA) and the M1 segment of the MCA are then identified and the proximal M1 segment

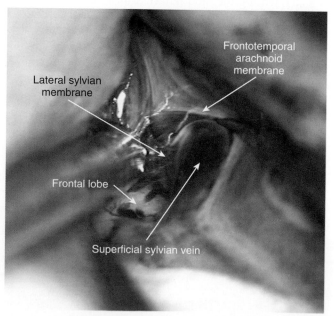

FIGURE 3-6   Intraoperative photograph showing the course of the superficial sylvian vein between the two arachnoid membranes. *(Reprinted with permission. Quiñones-Hinojosa A. Schmidek and Sweet Operative Neurosurgical Techniques. 6th ed. Elsevier; 2012.)*

is cleared for placement of the temporary clip. Once the proximal sylvian dissection is complete, attention is turned toward distal dissection, whereby the superior M1 trunk is followed retrograde to the frontal side of the aneurysm neck and the inferior M1 trunk is followed retrograde to the temporal side of the aneurysm neck. Once the aneurysm neck has been dissected adequately for clip placement, a temporary clip is placed on the proximal M1 segment, followed by permanent clipping of the MCA aneurysm.

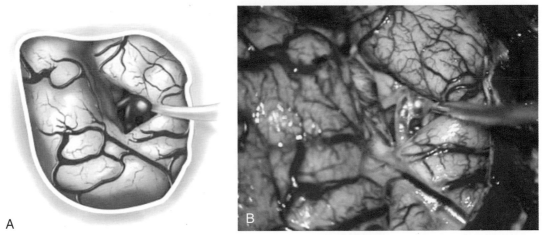

FIGURE 3-7   Once proximal control has been established at the proximal M1, further dissection of the aneurysm and associated branches can proceed. Sharp dissection around the aneurysm itself limits inadvertent tearing or rupture of the aneurysm complex. Establishing the local vascular anatomy and correlating this with the known angiographic anatomy is important at this stage. (A) and (B), Final dissection of a small right MCA aneurysm is demonstrated, with the dome adjacent to the suction device. *(Reprinted with permission. Winn HR. Youmans Neurological Surgery. 6th ed. Elsevier; 2011.)*

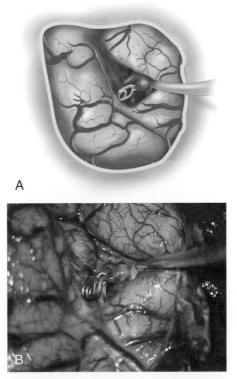

FIGURE 3-8   (A) and (B) A small straight clip has been applied across the neck of the aneurysm. This ideally should be placed parallel to the bifurcation to avoid residual "dog ears" that can result from other configurations. Clip selection varies, but should be kept as straightforward as possible. Intraoperative Doppler should be employed before and after clipping to establish baselines and to immediately detect any sonographic changes. We also use intraoperative indocyanine green angiography and digital subtraction. *(Reprinted with permission. Winn HR. Youmans Neurological Surgery. 6th ed. Elsevier; 2011.)*

Complication Avoidance and Management

- As with clipping of any ruptured aneurysm, intraoperative rupture is a major risk that should be anticipated and efficiently managed. Therefore establishing proximal control before dissection of the aneurysm neck is critical. The approach to intraoperative rupture depends upon the timing of rupture during the procedure. If the rupture occurs before aneurysm exposure, first proximal control must be established by placement of temporary clips on the proximal control vessel and the distal vessel if accessible. Next, place two large suctions and patties to clear the field of blood. Then, dissect out the neck of the aneurysm and clip the aneurysm under local flow arrest. If the rupture occurs after aneurysm exposure, place clip with suction without local flow arrest if possible. During evaluation of clipped aneurysm if bleeding persists then its not adequately clipped. Advancing blades blindly should be avoided due to the risk of perforation of the aneurysm or entry of the parent vessel with the clip blade. Reapplication of temporary clips and repeat application of permanent clips is preferred. Alternatively, a second clip could be placed. Patency of the vessel should be assessed by doppler or fluorescein angiography. Meticulous exposure of the aneurysm neck and avoiding unintended clip occlusion of any adjacent perforating vessels or trapping of the superior/inferior trunk can prevent iatrogenic morbidity. Though there is much debate regarding the optimal timing of intervention, it is our practice to perform early intervention (within 24 hours) due to risk of rerupture. Attentive postoperative care, with special emphasis on vasospasm management, is important to prevent secondary injury from delayed stroke.

KEY PAPERS

Molyneux A, Kerr R, Stratton I, et al. International Subarachnoid Aneurysm Trial (ISAT) Collaborative Group. International Subarachnoid Aneurysm Trial (ISAT) of neurosurgical clipping versus endovascular coiling in 2143 patients with ruptured intracranial aneurysms: a randomized trial. *Lancet.* 2002;360:1267-1274.

Rinne J, Hernesniemi J, Niskanen M, et al. Analysis of 561 patients with 690 middle cerebral artery aneurysms: anatomic and clinic features as correlated to management outcome. *Neurosurgery.* 1996;38:2-11.

Case 4

Unruptured Anterior Communicating Artery Aneurysm

Vincent J. Cheung, MD ● Jayson A. Sack, MD ●
J. Scott Pannell, MD ● Alexander A. Khalessi, MD

Presentation

A 55-year-old man with a history of poorly controlled hypertension presents to the emergency department after an acute episode of dizziness and confusion. Upon initial evaluation, the patient has returned to his neurologic baseline and is without focal deficit. Imaging workup reveals an unruptured anterior communicating artery aneurysm.

Differential Diagnosis

With the wide availability of CT and MR angiography at many centers, there is often little doubt regarding radiologic diagnoses of incidental, unruptured aneurysms. However, it may be difficult to distinguish smaller aneurysms from infundibular dilations without a formal cerebral angiogram. When a patient exhibits acute symptoms, it is critical to confirm whether the aneurysm is ruptured or unruptured. Patients should also be asked about symptoms of meningismus and any other neurologic complaints that may suggest subarachnoid hemorrhage. A lumbar puncture for the evaluation of xanthochromia is the gold standard in ruling out subarachnoid hemorrhage.

Initial Imaging

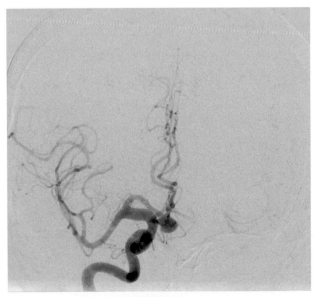

FIGURE 4-1

Imaging Description

Figure 4-1: AP projection digital subtraction angiography by right internal carotid injection. 9 mm diameter broad-based aneurysm encompassing origins of both A2 segments.

Further Workup

Basic laboratory evaluation. Evaluation of renal function is a prerequisite for endovascular intervention due to the increased risk of contrast-induced nephropathy in patients with renal insufficiency.

Pathophysiology

Please see Case 3 for a discussion of cerebral aneurysm pathophysiology.

Treatment Options

- Craniotomy for clip ligation
- Endovascular embolization
- Observation

Surgical Technique

A standard pterional (see prior chapters) or frontal craniotomy with orbital osteotomy is sufficient for most anterior communicating aneurysms; however, a greater orbitozygomatic approach may be advantageous for large and complex aneurysms. A right side approach is used in patients with symmetric A1 segments, whereas the dominant side is chosen in patients with asymmetric A1 segments. Additionally, a lumbar drain may be placed before surgery to assist with brain relaxation and to minimize retraction.

Once the craniotomy and dural opening are completed, the carotid cistern and proximal sylvian cistern are opened to expose the distal ICA and proximal A1. The ipsilateral recurrent artery of Huebner is often visualized before the A1 segment, and can serve as a landmark to the Acomm artery. A retractor tip can be placed on the posterior portion of the medial gyrus rectus to increase visualization of the A1 segment and the proximal Acomm artery. Next, the ipsilateral A2 segment is found by opening the interhemispheric fissure. The Acomm artery is then followed to the contralateral side, whereby proximal control is completed by identifying the opposite A1 segment. Finally, the contralateral A2 segment is located by entering the interhemispheric fissure distal to the aneurysm dome. The Acomm artery perforators are then dissected from the neck and the aneurysm is prepared for clip placement.

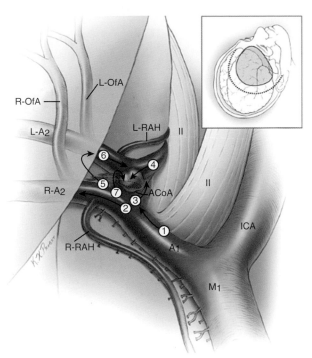

FIGURE 4-2   ACoA aneurysm dissection steps: (1) Follow the A1 segment and recurrent artery of Heubner, (2) identify A2 segment, (3) cross the midline via the ACoA, (4) control the contralateral A1 segment, (5) enter the distal interhemispheric fissure, (6) trace the contralateral A2 segment proximally, and (7) separate the perforator from the aneurysm neck. *(Reprinted with permission. Lawton MT. Seven Aneurysms: Tenets and Techniques for Clipping. New York: Thieme; 2010.)*

Complication Avoidance and Management

- Avoiding injury or inadvertent clipping of the medial lenticulostriate arteries, the recurrent artery of Huebner, and the anterior choroidal artery is of utmost importance. A stroke related to the injury of the medial lenticulostriate arteries and recurrent artery of Huebner can result in contralateral face and arm weakness as well as anesthesia and expressive aphasia in the dominant hemisphere (i.e., from involvement of the head of the caudate, the putamen, the outer segment of the globus pallidus, and the anterior limb of the internal capsule). Anterior choroidal distribution strokes typically result in contralateral hemiplegia, hemianesthesia and hemianopia from involvement of the posterior limb of the internal capsule, thalamus, and optic radiations. Additionally, careful dissection of perforating arteries originating from the surface of the anterior communicating artery is of equal importance, as injury to the hypothalamus, fornix, corpus callosum and optic chiasm may result from a compromised blood supply. As with the clipping of any aneurysm, intraoperative rupture is a major risk that should be anticipated and efficiently managed. Therefore establishing proximal control before dissection of the aneurysm neck is critical.

KEY PAPERS

International Study of Unruptured Intracranial Aneurysms Investigators. Unruptured intracranial aneurysms: natural history, clinical outcome, and risks of surgical and endovascular treatment. *Lancet.* 2003;362: 103-110.

Perlmutter D, Rhoton AL Jr. Microsurgical anatomy of the anterior cerebral-anterior communicating-recurrent artery complex. *J Neurosurg.* 1976;45(3):259-272.

Case 5

Intradural Internal Carotid Artery Fusiform Aneurysm

Gunjan Goel, MD ● J. Scott Pannell, MD ●
Alexander A. Khalessi, MD

Presentation

A 69-year-old female with progressively worsening headaches and visual loss.

- PSH: previous cigarette smoker
- Exam
  - AO × 3
  - Speech and language intact
  - Pupils equal, round, and reactive
  - Left lower quadrant visual field deficit
  - Rest of cranial nerves intact
  - Normal strength in bilateral extremities

Differential Diagnosis

- Neoplastic
  - Metastases (e.g., ocular melanoma)
  - Meningioma/hemangiopericytoma/optic nerve sheath tumor
- Vascular
  - Dural AVM/AVF
  - Aneurysm
- Inflammatory
  - Temporal arteritis
  - Takayasu arteritis
- Traumatic
  - Dissecting aneurysm
- Other
  - Ocular migraine

Initial Imaging

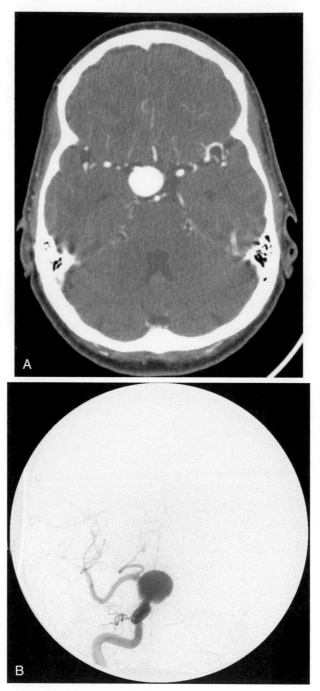

FIGURE 5-1

Imaging Description and Differential

CT angiogram in Figure 5-1A shows a large 1.8 cm supraclinoid right internal carotid artery with a wide neck projecting posteriorly and medially.

PA angiogram of anterior circulation in Figure 5-1B, performed by injection of the right internal carotid, demonstrates a large 1.8 cm supraclinoid right internal carotid artery with a wide neck projecting posteriorly and medially.

Differential: fusiform giant aneurysm, less likely dissecting aneurysm.

Further Workup

- Laboratory
  - Routine labs
  - Lipid profile
- Imaging
  - Magnetic resonance angiography (MRA)
  - Cerebral angiography

Pathophysiology

Fusiform cerebral aneurysms are nonsaccular dilations involving the entire vessel wall of a segment of a cerebral artery. They can progress from a small focal dilation or vessel narrowing, to a relatively thick-walled, tortuous dilation and elongated artery. Symptoms may include nonspecific headaches without hemorrhage, ischemia, transient ischemic attack, stroke, a mass effect with or without seizure, or hemorrhage. This type of aneurysm may be caused by vessel dissection or atherosclerosis; by disorders of collagen and elastin metabolism such as neurofibromatosis 1, fibromuscular dysplasia, or systemic lupus erythematosus; by infections; and very rarely, by neoplastic invasion of the arterial wall.

Treatment Options

- Conservative medical management
  - Some large asymptomatic aneurysms may be treated conservatively with risk factor modification. This may include prescribing a statin and/or antiplatelet drug, systemic hypertension control, and cessation of smoking to decrease risk of subarachnoid hemorrhage. This aneurysm has an annual rupture rate of 2.9% as per the ISUIA study, and the mortality of a ruptured large/giant aneurysm is known to be higher.
- Endovascular
  - Flow diversion stent: pipeline embolization device
  - Stent with coiling
  - Coiling with balloon assistance: This may be done in poor surgical candidates having large aneurysms (>4 mm) and a dome/neck ratio >1.5.
  - Proximal occlusion: Balloon occlusion test is performed to ascertain that good collateral blood flow is present; then ICA proximal to the ophthalmic segment can be sacrificed with detachable coils or microvascular plugs.
- Microsurgical
  - Clip reconstruction: This can be attempted when there is a neck present, minimal atherosclerosis, and there are two or fewer branches arising from the neck. However, in this case no neck was present.
  - Bypass with ICA occlusion: When ICA occlusion is planned, a selective approach to revascularization may be employed in patients with inadequate collateral circulation who require bypass in conjunction, or a universal approach. This involves angiographic evaluation of the competence of the circle of Willis and balloon text occlusion. Type 1: interposition vein graft (Figure 5-2) and type 2: extracranial to intracranial bypass with a saphenous vein or radial artery graft (Figure 5-3) (described in the Surgical Technique section).

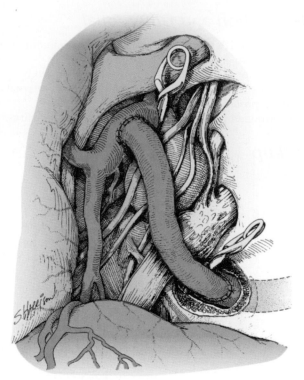

FIGURE 5-2 A petrous-to-supraclinoid carotid skull base bypass showing a saphenous interposition graft from the petrous segment of the carotid artery (exposed by drilling the middle cranial fossa floor) to the supraclinoid carotid artery (for the treatment of an intracavernous aneurysm in this case). *(Reprinted with permission. Spetzler RF, Fukushima T, Martin NA, et al. Petrous carotid–to–intradural carotid saphenous vein graft for intracavernous giant aneurysm, tumor, and occlusive disease.* J Neurosurg. *1990;73:496-501.)*

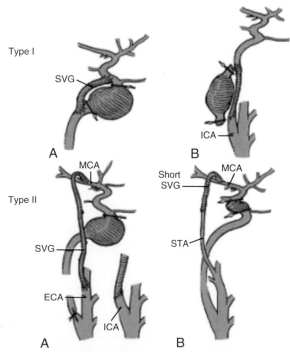

FIGURE 5-3 Arterial bypass types. Type I: saphenous vein interposition graft for carotid artery replacement. Type II: saphenous vein bypass graft from the extracranial carotid artery to the middle (A) and (B). *(Reprinted with permission. Martin NA. Arterial bypass for the treatment of giant and fusiform intracranial aneurysms.* Tech Neurosurg. *1998;4:153-178.)*

- Combined surgical/endovascular approach
  - Proximal occlusion with coils with extracranial-intracranial bypass

Surgical Technique

Extracranial carotid to middle cerebral artery (MCA) bypass with saphenous vein interposition graft (Figure 5-4)

After the carotid bifurcation is exposed and a pterional craniotomy performed, the sylvian fissure is opened widely. The ideal M2 arterial recipient site is then exposed. Next the saphenous vein is exposed but left in situ for continuity. Using a clamp, blunt dissection creates a subcutaneous tunnel from the cranial incision, behind the root of the zygomatic arch, to the cervical incision. The vein graft is gently drawn through a large chest tube, which is then pulled from the cervical to cranial incision with a clamp. The tube is removed, leaving the vein in place. The graft is filled with cool, heparinized saline and occluded proximally and distally with temporary clips. Intracranial anastomosis is then

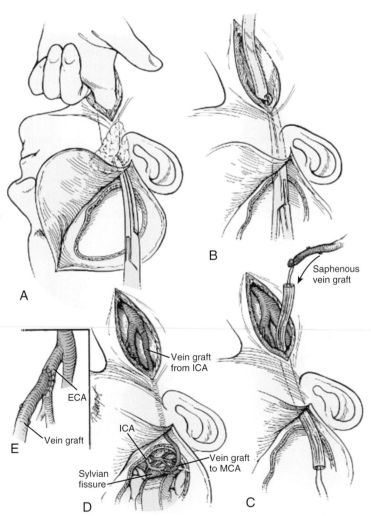

FIGURE 5-4 ECA–to–MCA saphenous vein bypass graft. (A) A clamp is passed from the cranial incision behind the root of the zygomatic arch to the cervical incision. (B) A chest tube is pulled from the cervical incision to the cranial incision. (C) The harvested saphenous vein graft is passed through the chest tube, which is removed, leaving the graft in its subcutaneous tunnel. (D) Completed bypass after end-to-end anastomosis to the ICA and end-to-side anastomosis to the MCA. (E) Alternative technique showing end-to-side anastomosis to the ECA. *(Reprinted with permission. Martin NA. Arterial bypass for the treatment of giant and fusiform intracranial aneurysms. Tech Neurosurg. 1998;4:153-178.)*

performed. The terminal 5 to 6 mm portion of the vein graft is trimmed of loose adventitia, and the end is beveled to create an orifice that is 5 to 6 mm in diameter.

After barbiturates are administered and blood pressure is stabilized at 20% higher than the patient's baseline, a 10 to 15 mm length of the MCA is occluded between temporary clips. A linear MCA arteriotomy is matched to the diameter of the vein graft orifice. The vein graft is fixed to the MCA branch with 8-0 monofilament nylon sutures, which are then used to complete a running closure. After the anastomosis is completed, blood flow is restored. The vein graft is pulled gently into the cervical incision to remove slack and redundancy. The proximal anastomosis can be constructed end to end to the ICA. The vein-carotid anastomosis is completed with 6-0 Prolene sutures. After removal of the temporary occluding clips, if the proximal and distal anastomoses are widely patent, a bounding pulse should be visible and palpable in the vein graft. A normal flow signal should be confirmed with intraoperative Doppler assessment. The craniotomy is closed and a notch for the graft is cut in the bone flap. The cervical incision is closed in routine fashion

Complication Avoidance and Management

- Early graft occlusion: Patency grafts can be ensured through a gentle and meticulous surgical technique. Careful avoidance of twisting, kinking, stretching, or any tension in the graft is imperative. Graft spasm should be avoided by adventitial papaverine irrigation. And finally, conclude with administration of perioperative antiplatelet therapy. If the graft is found to be severely stenotic or occluded, the bypass vessel or anastomosis should be revised. Sometimes simply repositioning the bypass vessel is adequate. Other cases require undoing at least one of the anastomoses, removing the thrombus, and then resuturing.
- Aneurysmal rupture: May be caused by hemodynamic stress associated with the presence of the distal high-flow bypass. These complications emphasize the need to isolate the aneurysm completely from circulation by trapping it whenever possible.
- Ischemic neurologic deficits: May be from a prolonged period of temporary arterial occlusion during bypass anastomosis construction. Cerebral protection with moderate hypothermia, induced arterial hypertension, and barbiturate administration may minimize this risk.
- Hematoma: To avoid this complication, it is wise not to use systemic heparinization for bypass procedures. Instead, local anticoagulation by filling the saphenous vein with heparinized saline should be performed.

KEY PAPERS

Day AL, Gaposchkin CG, Yu CJ, et al. Spontaneous fusiform middle cerebral artery aneurysms: characteristics and a proposed mechanism of formation. *J Neurosurg.* 2003;99:228-240.

Findlay JM, Hao C, Emery D. Non-atherosclerotic fusiform cerebral aneurysms. *Can J Neurol Sci.* 2002;29:41-48.

Park SH, Yim MB, Lee CY, et al. Intracranial fusiform aneurysms: its pathogenesis, clinical characteristics and managements. *J Korean Neurosurg Soc.* 2008;44(3):116-123.

Youman's Neurological Surgery Sixth edition. Chapter 380: Revascularization techniques for complex aneurysm and skull base tumors.

Case 6

Spinal Arteriovenous Malformations

J. Scott Pannell, MD ● Alexander A. Khalessi, MD

Presentation

An 8-year-old male has a 6-month history of back pain and lower extremity paresthesia and numbness. He denies any weakness, incontinence, or urinary hesitancy. No history of trauma.

- PMH: otherwise unremarkable
- Exam:
  - Normal UE examination
  - Slightly increased DTR in the bilateral lower extremities
  - Decreased sensation to pin prick from T6 and below
  - No visible sacral dimple, lipoma, hair patch, or dermal sinus tract

Differential Diagnosis

- Congenital
  - Tethered cord/filum terminale lipoma
  - Spinal dysraphism (diastomyelia given lack of cutaneous findings)
  - Congenital stenosis and/or scoliosis
- Neoplastic
  - Teratoma
  - Spinal cord glioma
  - Neurenteric cyst
  - Osseous spinal tumors
  - Metastatic disease
- Vascular
  - Arteriovenous malformation (AVM)
  - Invasive hemangioma
- Inflammatory
  - Neuromyelitis optica (Devic's disease)
- Metabolic
  - B_{12} deficiency (vegan)
  - Leukodystrophy
  - Copper deficiency
- Traumatic
  - Child abuse
  - Other unreported trauma

Initial Imaging

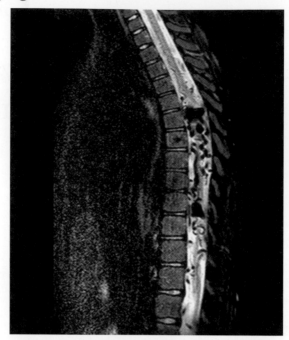

FIGURE 6-1

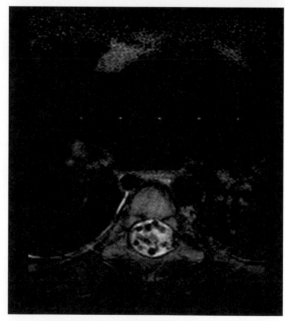

FIGURE 6-2

Imaging Description and Differential

- Thoracic T2-weighted sagittal and axial images MRI, respectively. Thoracic MRI of the spine demonstrates a serpiginous pattern of intradural, extraaxial, and intraaxial flow voids from T4 to T12 with large venous pouches occupying a large portion of the central canal at T4 and T8.
- Differential:
  - Type III or juvenile spinal AVM
  - Type IV-3 spinal AVF (giant perimedullary fistula)

Further Workup

- Imaging
  - Spinal angiogram (gold standard for suspected vascular lesions)

Further Imaging

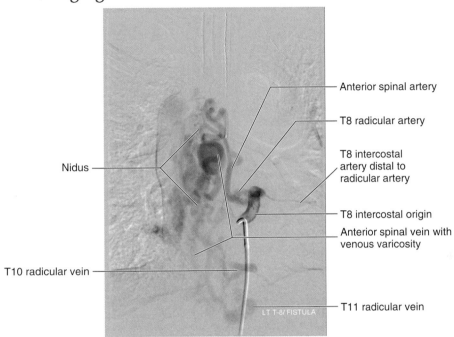

FIGURE 6-3   Diagnostic left T8 intercostal injection performed in the PA plane demonstrates an extensive spinal vascular malformation with complex nidal vasculature near the cephalad most portion of the malformation at T3, a fistulous venous pouch at T4, and numerous engorged draining veins.

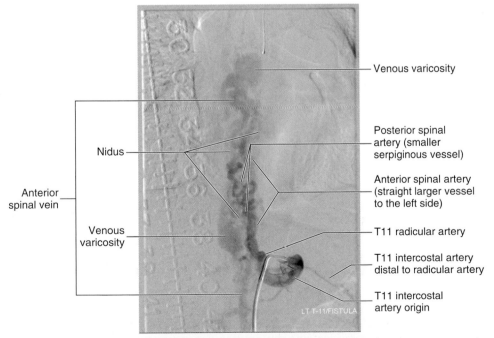

FIGURE 6-4   Diagnostic left T11 intercostal injection performed in the PA plane demonstrates an extensive spinal vascular malformation with complex nidal vasculature extending from T4 to T10, a fistulous venous pouch at T4 and T8, and numerous engorged draining veins.

Pathophysiology

A clear understanding of normal vascular supply to the spinal cord is imperative. Spinal dural AVMs are categorized into two separate categories: glomus (type II) and juvenile (type III).

Glomus AVMs are exclusively intraaxial lesions and are the second most common type of spinal vascular malformation, accounting for 19% to 45% of cases. Glomus AVMs usually present between the third and fifth decade of life.

Juvenile AVMs are the least common type of spinal vascular malformation and often have extensive involvement in the surrounding subdural and epidural space. In some cases, juvenile AVMs may involve adjacent bones or soft tissues. Juvenile AVMs typically present in the first two decades of life.

Both types of AVMs are congenital. Symptoms may arise as a result of intramedullary hemorrhage, subarachnoid hemorrhage, arterial steal, venous hypertension, or compression by distended vessels.

Treatment Options

The definitive treatment for type II or glomus AVMs is complete surgical resection. Endovascular treatment can be a useful adjunct in high-flow glomus AVMs to reduce bleeding risk, and may temporize symptomatic patients by reducing venous hypertension. However, similar to cerebral AVMs, endovascular techniques rarely result in complete obliteration.

The treatment for type III or juvenile AVMs is largely palliative and consists of surgical or endovascular ligation of the arterial supply.

Endovascular Technique

We recommend the use of general endotracheal anaesthesia and neurophysiologic monitoring for embolization procedures. Once access to the common femoral artery is obtained, a 5 Fr short sheath is introduced into the external iliac artery.

Using a 5 Fr HS1/2, C2, or reverse curve catheter, a complete spinal and cerebral angiogram is performed to evaluate the presence of nidal vasculature and early draining veins. The artery of Adamkiewicz is also identified. After identifying a supplying pedicle (under overlay guidance), microcatheter exploration with supraselective angiography is performed to confirm the architecture of the potential embolization targets. Provocative testing may also be performed with sodium amytal and/or lidocaine.

A liquid embolic is then chosen. We typically use onyx for AVMs that require the catheter to be flushed with DMSO. The onyx is then infused into the fistula, under fluoroscopic guidance, making sure the liquid embolic remains cohesive, opacifies only abnormal nidal vasculature, and does not reflux into normal arterial structures nor occlude draining veins. Diagnostic angiography is repeated to evaluate for residual nidi.

Surgical Technique

The goal of surgery for glomus (type II) AVM is complete resection of the nidus.

The goal of surgery for type III or juvenile AVMs is palliative and may be accomplished by relief of compressive symptoms by partial resection and/or reduction of venous hypertension via progressive arterial ligation.

Complication Avoidance and Management

- Endovascular
  - The radicular arteries can variably anastomose with the anterior and posterior spinal arteries. An improper liquid embolization technique and an incomplete understanding of the angiographic anatomy can result in devastating infarcts of the spinal cord. These procedures are best performed at centers with high volume and experience.

Meticulous catheter hygiene and adequate heparinization are essential in avoidance of embolic complications.
- Surgical
  - The complete resection of juvenile AVMs carries a significant risk of neurologic deterioration and is rarely attempted. Early sacrifice of venous structures in glomus type II AVM resection may result in devastating intramedullary hemorrhage.

KEY PAPERS

Aminoff MJ, Logue V. The prognosis of patients with spinal vascular malformations. *Brain*. 1974;97:211-218.

Kim LJ, Spetzler RF. Classification and surgical management of spinal arteriovenous lesions: arteriovenous fistulae and arteriovenous malformations. *Neurosurgery*. 2006;59:S3-195–S3-201.

Velat GJ, Chang SW, Abla AA, et al. Microsurgical management of glomus spinal arteriovenous malformations: pial resection technique. *J Neurosurg Spine*. 2012;16:523-531.

Wilson DA, Abla AA, Uschold TD, et al. Multimodality treatment of conus medullaris arteriovenous malformations: 2 decades of experience with combined endovascular and microsurgical treatments. *Neurosurgery*. 2012;71:100-108.

Case 7

Cranial Dural Arteriovenous Fistula

Reid Hoside, MD ● J. Scott Pannell, MD ●
Alexander A. Khalessi, MD

Presentation

A 19-year-old male was seen by his primary care physician for left-sided pulsatile tinnitus that began after a skateboarding accident. He denies other symptoms.

- PMH: unremarkable
- Neurologic examination: unremarkable

Differential Diagnosis

- Vascular (arterial)
  - Arteriovenous malformation (AVM)
  - Dural arteriovenous fistula (dAVF)
  - Carotid cavernous fistula
  - Internal carotid artery dissection
  - Internal carotid artery aneurysm
- Vascular (venous)
  - Jugular vein diverticulum and/or dehiscence
  - Dominant transverse sinus
  - Abnormal condylar or emissary vein
- Neoplastic
  - Glomus jugulare tumors
  - Facial nerve hemangioma
  - Cavernous hemangioma

Initial Imaging

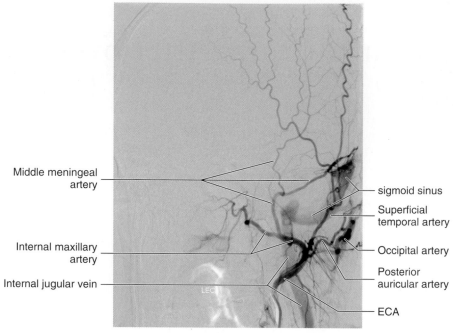

Middle meningeal artery

sigmoid sinus

Superficial temporal artery

Internal maxillary artery

Occipital artery

Internal jugular vein

Posterior auricular artery

ECA

FIGURE 7-1

Imaging Description and Differential

Figure 7-1 shows a left external carotid artery angiogram performed in the PA plane, revealing middle meningeal and occipital artery supply to a dural arteriovenous fistula.

Further Workup

- Laboratory
  - Routine analysis
- Imaging
  - MRI and A/V of the brain
  - Six vessel digital subtraction angiogram of the brain

Pathophysiology

Much debate has contributed to whether dAVFs are congenital or acquired. The etiology of acquired dAVFs includes posttraumatic, infection, or sinus thrombosis. Engorgement of the dural sinus from thromboses, or thrombophlebitis, can lead to venous hypertension and subsequent engorgement of the normal arteriovenous shunts that exist in the sinus, thereby creating a dAVF. Recanalization events and angiogenic factors from phlebitis can also contribute to these fistulae formations. The majority of dAVFs exists at the transverse-sigmoid sinus junction, followed by the cavernous sinus. In a patient with transverse-sigmoid sinus dAVFs, the most commonly occurring symptom is pulsatile tinnitus. This occurs as a result of arterial systolic-diastolic rhythm in the venous system, which can be audible, especially when in the vicinity of the acoustic structures. Likewise, carotid-cavernous dAVFs result in situations of pulsatile exophthalmos; the cavernous sinus takes on arterial pressure, leading to poor venous outflow of the orbit, causing swelling and pain. Headaches can occur in dAVFs as a result of intracranial hypertension, related to venous hypertension, causing cerebral edema and poor resorption of cerebrospinal fluid through the arachnoid villi. Moreover, engorgement of the sinuses can cause mass effect. Cranial nerve dysfunction may also be seen as a result of vascular steal phenomena. Vascular supply to the cranial nerves takes place via the dural arteries, which can be compromised when the arterial supply is shunted to the venous system. Most dAVFs carry a benign natural history; however, some aspects of previous or active hemorrhage, retrograde cortical venous drainage, or venous aneurysmal dilatation make the natural history of these fistulae more dangerous and provide an argument for treatment rather than observation.

Treatment Options

- Medical
  - Observation and anticoagulation of a transverse sinus thrombosis, if present
- Surgical
  - Ligation of arterial feeders and venous outflow of the dAVF, with or without excision of the intervening dura
- Endovascular
  - Transarterial, transvenous, or a combined access to the embolization of the fistulous tract
- Radiation
  - Stereotactic ablation using 16–20 Gy, but no more than 32 Gy
  - A latency period exists with radiosurgery, from the time of treatment to the time of cure. Radiosurgery is usually reserved for inaccessible lesions, or when other management strategies have failed.

Surgical Technique

The operative approach for dAVF cases is selected depending on the region of the lesion. Surgical management is started by coagulation and ligation of the fistula's arterial feeders. Next, the sinus and venous involvement can be ligated. Excision of the fistula is then performed, which includes the intervening dura. Intraoperative angiography can be employed to confirm successful obliteration. That excision of the fistulous dura is unnecessary, and that adequate disconnection of the fistula is sufficient, has been suggested.

Endovascular

Transarterial obliteration of the fistula involves the following steps: a sheath is placed in the femoral artery, and a guide catheter is employed to advance into the arterial circulation of the brain. A six-vessel angiogram is then performed to identify the vascular suppliers of the fistula. Microcatheterization of the arterial feeder to the fistula is accessed and embolysate is then introduced as close to the fistula as possible. This process is repeated for each arterial feeder. See Figures 7-2 to 7-4 demonstrating post-transarterial embolization angiographic and fluoroscopic images of above-depicted dAVF.

Transvenous obliteration of the fistula is favored over transarterial access, because of fewer complications associated with distal emboli formation. The following steps are involved: access via the femoral vein is achieved and microcatheterization of the venous structures to the fistula is performed. Embolysate is then introduced in a similar fashion to that of the transarterial obliteration procedure. This process is repeated for each arteriovenous anastomoses. Coursing through the valves of the venous system may be cumbersome, but is achievable with the Valsalva maneuver.

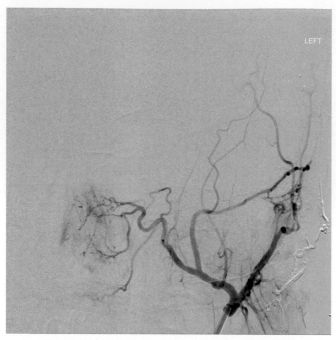

FIGURE 7-2 A left-sided angiogram taken after external carotid embolization of the dAVF depicted above.

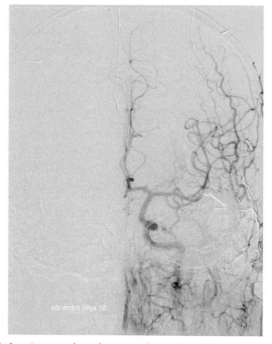

FIGURE 7-3 A left-sided angiogram taken after internal carotid embolization of the dAVF depicted above.

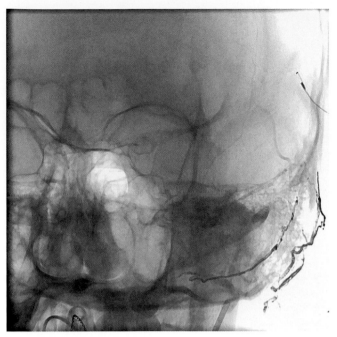

FIGURE 7-4   An unsubtracted angiogram demonstrating the embolysate cast of the dAVF depicted above.

Complication Avoidance and Management

- Endovascular Complication Avoidance
  - Embolysate migration is worrisome, especially in high-flow fistulae, and can be avoided by selecting the proper embolysate. The typical complications of endovascular procedures may occur and include stroke, vascular injury, and groin hematoma. Postembolization pain is common and occurs as a result of the inflammatory response to the presence of the embolysate, especially against the dura. A short course of steroidal, or nonsteroidal, anti-inflammatory drugs may be used to alleviate post-embolization pain. Hemodynamics and hypertension should be closely managed to prevent venous stroke and hypertensive hemorrhage.
- Surgical Complication Avoidance
  - The use of a lumbar drain may be considered to minimize brain retraction. Surgical after endovascular treatment of the dAVF may also be considered, and could alleviate blood loss during surgery. Intraoperative angiography can be used to determine success. Positioning of the patient with the head below the heart can prevent air emboli, a high-risk complication in these procedures.

KEY PAPERS

Kim M, Han D, Kwon O, et al. Clinical characteristics of dural arteriovenous fistula. *J Clin Neurosci.* 2002;9(2):147-155.

Kopitnik T, Samson D. Management of dural arteriovenous malformation. *Contemp Neurosurg.* 1995;9:1-7.

Case 8

Spinal Dural Arteriovenous Fistulas

David R. Santiago-Dieppa, MD ● J. Scott Pannell, MD ●
Scott E. Olson, MD ● Alexander A. Khalessi, MD

Presentation

A 55-year-old male presented with a 3-year history of progressive left lower extremity weakness. The patient also endorsed back pain that radiated to the bilateral lower extremities. The pain was described as "shock like" and was exacerbated by strenuous exercise and activity.

- PMH: otherwise unremarkable
- Exam:
  - Normal UE examination
  - LLE strength 4/5
  - Decreased DTR in the LLE
  - Decreased sensation to pin prick from T7 and below

Differential Diagnosis

- Degenerative
  - Spinal stenosis resulting in neurogenic claudication
- Neoplastic
  - Metastasis
  - Primary spinal cord tumor
- Vascular
  - dAVF (favored given slow progressive onset of symptoms in an older patient)
  - AVM (usually acute presentation in younger patient)
- Infectious
  - Spinal abscess

Initial Imaging

Thoracic T2-weighted MRI sequences. Sagittal (left) and axial (right) projections.

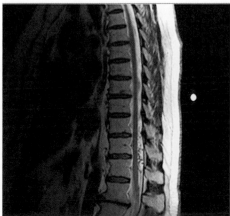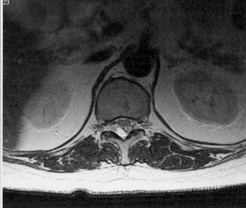

FIGURE 8-1

Imaging Description and Differential

- Thoracic T2-weighted MRI of the spine. Sagittal and axial projections demonstrate a serpentine pattern of intradural flow voids from T10-T12, and overlying the dorsal surface of the spinal cord.
- Differential
  - Vascular lesion (spinal AVM, spinal dAVF, and radicular varicosity)
  - Collateral venous flow from IVC occlusion
  - Spinal cord tumor
  - Normal CSF pulsations

Further Workup

- Imaging
  - Spinal angiogram: gold standard for suspected vascular lesions

Further Imaging

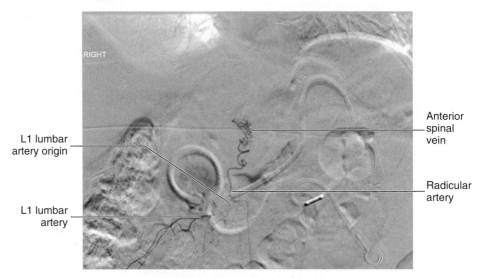

FIGURE 8-2   Diagnostic spinal angiogram.

Diagnostic spinal angiogram. AP projection. Right L1 lumbar injection demonstrates a spinal dural arteriovenous fistula arising from the right L1 lumbar artery with a serpiginous early draining vein overlying the dorsal surface of the spinal cord.

Pathophysiology

SDAVF is the most common form of spinal vascular malformation. The exact etiology of SDAVF is not known; however, they are thought to be acquired. SDAVFs are more common in men and tend to present later in life, more specifically the 51- to 60-year-old age group. These lesions are composed of dural branch of the dorsal ramus intercostal artery that drains into an engorged spinal vein. The nidus by definition is located within the dura, often near the nerve root sleeve. This pathologic arteriovenous shunt leads to venous congestion and hypertension, and as a result of the reduced arterial perfusion pressure the cord experiences ischemia.

Treatment Options

- Endovascular
  - Pros: liquid embolization is highly effective and less invasive than traditional open microsurgical techniques
  - Cons: associated with a variable recurrence rate

- Surgical
  - Historically considered the more definitive treatment
  - Cons: more invasive than endovascular techniques

Endovascular Technique

We recommend the use of general endotracheal anesthesia and neurophysiologic monitoring for embolization procedures. Access to the common femoral artery is obtained and a sheath is introduced into the external iliac artery.

Using a diagnostic catheter, the bilateral superior thoracic arteries, bilateral intercostal arteries (from T4 to T12), and bilateral lumbar arteries at each level are catheterized. Arterial pedicles with filling patterns suspicious of SDAVF are then catheterized with a micro wire and catheter. A microcatheter angiogram is then performed to confirm the architecture of the embolization target.

A liquid embolic is then chosen. We typically use onyx which requires the catheter to be flushed with DMSO. The onyx is then infused into the fistula under fluoroscopic guidance, making sure the liquid embolic remains cohesive and does not reflux in normal arterial structures. Diagnostic angiography is repeated to ensure no fistula remains.

Surgical Technique

The goal of surgery is obliteration of the draining arterialized vein. Laminectomies should be performed at least one level above and below the involved level(s). Adequate exposure is imperative and may require facetectomy in order to expose the proximal vein near the fistula in the nerve root sleeve. Once the arterialized vein of the SDAVF is identified, it is traced in a retrograde fashion until the point of dural entry is located. The vein is then coagulated and cut; this results in the restoration of physiologic cord perfusion in the majority of cases.

Complication Avoidance and Management

- Endovascular
  - The radicular arteries can variably anastomose with the anterior and posterior spinal arteries. An improper liquid embolization technique and an incomplete understanding of the angiographic anatomy can result in devastating infarcts of the spinal cord. These procedures are best performed at centers with a high volume and experience.
- Surgical
  - The fistula may be difficult to localize intraoperatively. We recommend placement of a femoral artery sheath before initiating surgery so that intraoperative angiography can be performed.

KEY PAPERS

Aminoff MJ, Barnard RO, Logue V. The pathophysiology of spinal vascular malformations. *J Neurol Sci.* 1974;23(2):255-263.

Oldfield EH. Surgical treatment of spinal dural arteriovenous fistulas. *Semin Cerebrovasc Dis Stroke.* 2002;2:209-226.

Rosenblum B, Oldfield EH, Doppman JL, et al. Spinal arteriovenous malformations: a comparison of dural arteriovenous fistulas and intradural AVM's in 81 patients. *J Neurosurg.* 1987;67(6):795-802.

Strugar J, Chyatte D. In situ photocoagulation of spinal dural arteriovenous malformations using the Nd:YAG laser. *J Neurosurg.* 1992;77(4):571-574.

Case 9

Vertebral Artery Dissection

Robert C. Rennert, MD ● Jayson A. Sack, MD ●
J. Scott Pannell ● Alexander A. Khalessi, MD

Presentation

A 42-year-old female with a history of migraines and oral contraceptive use has subacute complaints of neck pain, headaches, acute onset of vertigo, dysphagia, and right-sided facial and left-sided body numbness 3 months after a minor automobile accident.

- PMH: otherwise unremarkable
- Exam: mild tenderness to palpation over occiput and upper cervical spine
  - Decreased pain and temperature sensation over left hemibody and extremities
  - Decreased sensation on right face
  - Diminished gag reflex
  - Normal motor exam

Differential Diagnosis

- Neoplastic
  - Medullary or cervical spine metastasis (h/o cancer)
  - Primary medullary or cervical spine tumor
- Vascular
  - Spontaneous vertebral artery dissection with lateral medullary syndrome
  - Vertebral artery dissecting aneurysm (altered consciousness if ruptured)
  - Isolated lateral medullary syndrome
  - Bow hunter's stroke syndrome (i.e., rotational vertebrobasilar insufficiency)
- Infectious
  - Medullary abscess (h/o IV drug abuse, manifestations of infection)
- Traumatic
  - Traumatic vertebral artery dissection (h/o recent C-spine injury)
- Other
  - Fibromuscular dysplasia (FMD) underlying vertebral artery dissection

Initial Imaging

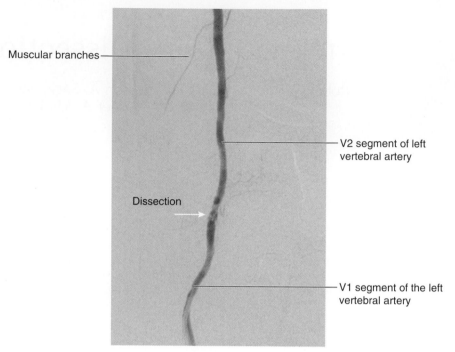

FIGURE 9-1

Muscular branches

V2 segment of left vertebral artery

Dissection

V1 segment of the left vertebral artery

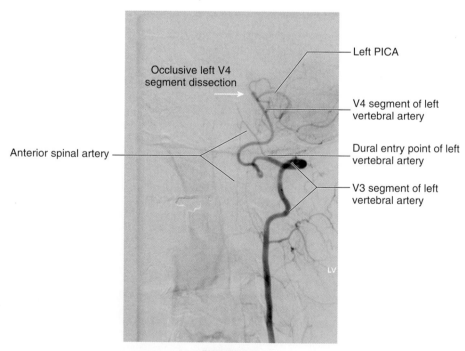

FIGURE 9-2

Occlusive left V4 segment dissection

Left PICA

V4 segment of left vertebral artery

Anterior spinal artery

Dural entry point of left vertebral artery

V3 segment of left vertebral artery

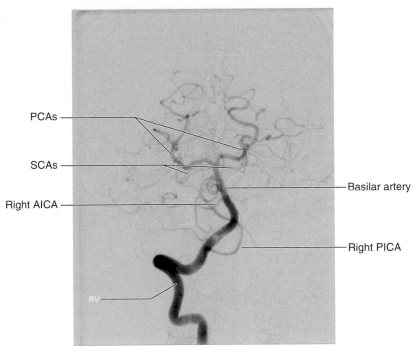

PCAs

SCAs

Right AICA

Basilar artery

Right PICA

RV

FIGURE 9-3

Imaging Description

- Figure 9-1: digital subtraction angiography (DSA) demonstrating an irregular, flow-limiting dissection of the right V2 segment as a result of a C5-C6 facet fracture.
- Figure 9-2: DSA demonstrating a near occlusive dissection of the left V4 segment beyond the origin of the anterior spinal artery in a patient with exertional headaches and left vertebral intracranial narrowing noted on an MRA.
- Figure 9-3: DSA of the posterior circulation performed by injection of the right vertebral artery.

Further Workup

- Laboratory
  - Routine labs
  - Coagulation panel
- Imaging
  - CT of the C-spine to assess for bony injury
  - CT of the head for assessment of hemorrhagic stroke or late ischemic stroke
  - MRI of the head to assess for early ischemic stroke
  - CT or MRA for initial cerebral vessel imaging (although limited sensitivity)
  - Angiography: definitive diagnostic study; "string of pearls" commonly seen with dissection and a "stack of coins" with FMD
- Consultants
  - Stroke neurology, if associated with lateral medullary syndrome

Pathophysiology

Vertebral artery dissections can be spontaneous or secondary to blunt trauma. Spontaneous dissections are most common in middle-aged adults in their 30s to 50s, are associated with FMD and oral contraceptive use, and may be preceded by minor or forgotten traumas. Similar to spontaneous tears in the carotid artery, they are secondary to intimal tears that allow blood to enter the arterial wall. Luminal narrowing is seen if the resulting hematoma dissects the vessel intima from the internal elastic lamina. Pseudoaneurysm formation is seen if the hematoma enters the subadventitial plane. Traumatic vertebral artery dissections are more commonly seen after brunt traumas, such as a motor vehicle accident, and are associated with acute cervical spine injuries. The risk of TIA or stroke, commonly manifested as lateral medullary syndrome or cerebellar infarct, from vertebral artery dissection is highest with V3 or V4 segment involvement.

Treatment Options

- Medical
  - Antithrombotic therapy with either antiplatelet agents or anticoagulation, consisting of therapeutic heparin bridged to warfarin for 6 months (in the absence of hemorrhagic or large ischemic stroke)
- Interventional
  - Endovascular intervention is reserved for symptomatic or progressive lesions, despite antithrombotic therapy, or for lesions presenting with subarachnoid hemorrhage (SAH)
    - Typically consists of vessel embolization and occlusion and is done after balloon test occlusion to confirm adequate posterior circulation filling via the contralateral vertebral artery. Stenting or angioplasty is also possible.
- Surgical
  - Vertebral artery occlusive clipping (intradural lesions when endovascular therapy is not an option), with or without bypass (if unilateral vertebral artery occlusion not tolerated)
  - Nonocclusive clipping (i.e., fusiform aneurysms), or vessel wrapping (limited benefit)
  - Approaches include lateral suboccipital and the more complex far lateral suboccipital and far lateral retrosigmoid craniotomies
- Other
  - For FMD, antiplatelet therapy combined with angioplasty with or without stenting is the preferred treatment approach.

Endovascular Technique

For endovascular interventions, position the patient on the angiography table, asleep or awake, depending on the operator's comfort. Access the femoral artery and perform a four vessel diagnostic angiogram to ensure adequate understanding of the distal vertebrobasilar and posterior circulation anatomy.

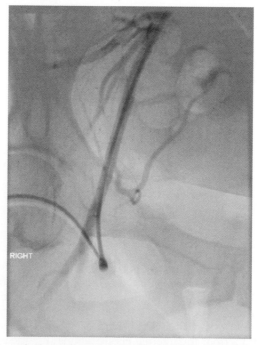

FIGURE 9-4 DSA of the right femoral artery demonstrating entry point of the sheath in the common femoral over the mid-femoral head above the bifurcation and below the inferior epigastric.

Following a balloon test occlusion to ensure vertebral takedown will be tolerated, the guide catheter is positioned proximal to the dissection in the affected vertebral artery so both can be visualized on the same screen. A microwire is used to advance a microcatheter just proximal to the dissection and coils are deployed to create an occlusive coil mesh. PA and lateral high magnification runs should be performed to ensure adequate proximal occlusion. The contralateral vertebral artery is then selected and an angiogram from this position is used to assess dissection filling via retrograde flow. If needed, the distal affected vertebral artery is accessed using the microcatheter from the contralateral vertebral artery and a second coil mass is deposited. Final angiogram runs are obtained before and after microcatheter removal to ensure complete vascular integrity.

For endovascular stenting, the microcatheter is advanced past the level of the dissection under microwire guidance. The microcatheter is then removed and the stent delivery system is raised to the dissection location over the microwire. The stent is deployed and the stent delivery system is removed with the microwire in place. If stenosis remains, a low compliance balloon (sized smaller than the stent length and normal vessel diameter) can be positioned and inflated. Final angiogram runs are obtained before and after microwire removal to ensure complete vascular integrity.

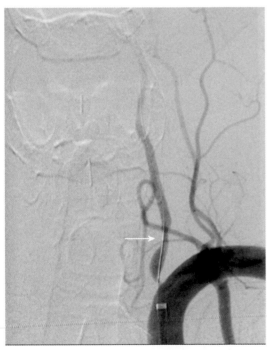

FIGURE 9-5 DSA of the left subclavian artery demonstrating the guide catheter in the subclavian artery immediately below the left vertebral origin and a microwire beyond dissection.

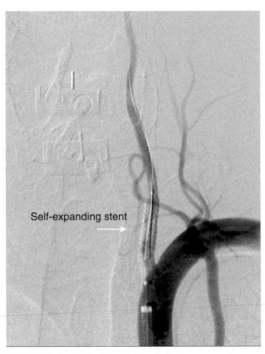

FIGURE 9-6 DSA of the right subclavian artery demonstrating complete luminal restoration after stent deployment. The microwire access is maintained until luminal restoration is confirmed.

Surgical Technique

For occlusion via surgical clipping, balloon testing is similarly used to first assess tolerance of vertebral takedown. For lateral suboccipital craniotomies, the patient is positioned in the lateral position, with the head flexed and rotated 30 degrees toward the contralateral side. Upon completion of the craniotomy, the dura is opened and the CSF is drained from the cisterna magna to assist with cerebellar relaxation. The cerebellum is gently retracted, allowing direct visualization of the vertebral artery, which is followed medially until the PICA is identified. The vertebral segment to be clipped is dissected from the surrounding arachnoid and placement of an occlusive clip is performed.

Arterial bypass is reserved for patients intolerant of vertebral occlusion. Options include PICA-PICA anastomosis, PICA origin transplantation, and extracranial to intracranial bypass via an occipital artery to PICA anastomosis.

Complication Avoidance and Management

- Endovascular
  - If distal coils are needed as a result of retrograde dissection filling after proximal embolization, it is critical to ensure the PICA is not included in the vertebral segment sacrificed. If stents are used, self-expanding stents are preferred over balloon expanding stents in particularly mobile areas of the neck (i.e., at the level of C2), as they are less prone to kinking.
- Surgical
  - Clip placement in surgical vessel occlusion is determined by the PICA's relation to the dissection. If the PICA is involved in the dissection, the clip should be placed proximal to allow reversal of blood flow to the PICA, thereby promoting tamponade of the dissection flap. If the dissection does not involve the PICA, it can be clipped proximally and/or distally.

KEY PAPERS

Halbach VV, Higashida RT, Dowd CF, et al. Endovascular treatment of vertebral artery dissections and pseudo-aneurysms. *J Neurosurg.* 1993;79:183-191.

Iihara K, Sakai N, Murao K, et al. Dissecting aneurysms of the vertebral artery: a management strategy. *J Neurosurg.* 2002;97:259-267.

Case 10

Basilar Tip Aneurysm

Robert C. Rennert, MD ● Jayson A. Sack, MD ●
J. Scott Pannell, MD ● Alexander A. Khalessi, MD

Presentation

A 55-year-old male with a history of hypertension and tobacco and alcohol use with sudden onset of severe headache, nausea, vomiting, double vision, and neck pain that started while playing golf.

- PMH: hypertension, tobacco and alcohol use
- Exam: Lethargic, mild confusion, oriented to person and place, not date
  - Bilateral cranial nerve III palsy
  - Pain with neck flexion
  - Pain with leg extension b/l with thigh flexed
  - Follows commands in all four extremities with 5/5 strength
  - Sensation to light touch intact

Differential Diagnosis

- Neoplastic
  - Hemorrhage from primary (rare) or metastatic tumor (h/o cancer)
- Vascular
  - Aneurysmal subarachnoid hemorrhage
  - Vascular malformation rupture (AVM, cavernous hemangioma, more common in young patients)
  - Hemorrhagic stroke (more common in older patients)
    - Hypertensive (basal ganglia most common)
    - Vasculitis (amyloid angiopathy)
  - Reversible cerebral vasoconstrictive syndrome ("string of beads" on angiography)
  - Perimesencephalic nonaneurysmal subarachnoid hemorrhage
- Infectious
  - Rupture of mycotic cerebral aneurysm (in setting of IV drug use)
- Other
  - Benign thunderclap headache, differentiated by negative head imaging

Initial Imaging

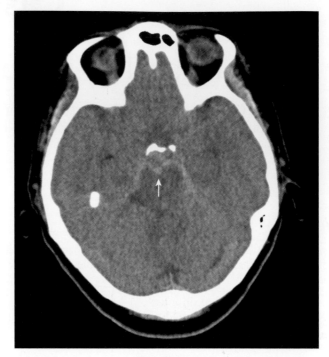

FIGURE 10-1

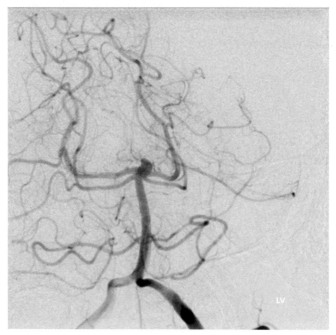

FIGURE 10-2

Imaging Description

- Figure 10-1: Noncontrast head CT showing an acute subarachnoid hemorrhage within the interpeduncular and ambient cisterns (white arrow). Blood pattern is consistent with the posterior circulation aneurysm rupture, or perimesencephalic nonaneurysmal SAH.
- Figure 10-2: Digital subtraction angiography demonstrating a 4 mm irregular aneurysm projecting superiorly from the basilar tip.

Further Workup

- Laboratory
  - ABG, CBC, coags, electrolytes
  - LP if imaging negative and high suspicion for subarachnoid hemorrhage (SAH)
- Imaging
  - Non contrast head CT
  - CT angiogram, MRA, or digital subtraction angiography (the gold standard) for vessel imaging
    - Patency and size of Pcomms important for surgical and interventional planning

Pathophysiology

Propensity for aneurysm formation in intracranial vessels is thought to result from decreased thickness of vessel wall media and adventitia, combined with vessel location in the subarachnoid space with relatively little supporting connective tissue. Noninfectious intracranial aneurysms typically occur near the circle of Willis, form at vessel curves or branch points, and point in the direction of proximally flowing blood. Risk factors include hypertension, smoking, alcohol and cocaine abuse, pregnancy, autosomal dominant polycystic kidney disease, and connective tissue disorders. Risk factors for basilar apex aneurysms include conditions with increased blood flow through the vertebrobasilar system (i.e., posterior circulation AVMs and subclavian steal syndrome). Approximately 5% of intracranial and 50% of posterior circulation aneurysms occur at the basilar apex and, if large enough, can compress the third nerve and/or brainstem. Posterior circulation aneurysms have a relatively high risk of rupture even when small (0.5% annual risk for aneurysms <7 mm). Basilar apex aneurysmal rupture has an increased theoretical risk of brainstem dysfunction (i.e., apnea and neurogenic pulmonary edema) and perimesencephalic blood patterning, but is often clinically and radiographically indistinguishable from anterior circulation lesions.

Treatment Options

- Medical
  - Sodium for hyponatremia, prophylactic anticonvulsants, sedation, analgesia, nimodipine for vasospasm prevention, and blood pressure control
- Interventional
  - Aneurysm coiling is the preferred treatment modality for basilar apex aneurysms because of difficult surgical access. Relatively high rate of recurrence after coiling as a result of end arterial location.
- Surgical
  - Surgical clipping is the standard of care before endovascular techniques. Challenging access and anatomy has increasingly limited surgical treatment of basilar apex aneurysms.
    - Approaches include subtemporal (posterior or posteroinferiorly directed aneurysms) and most commonly, pterional craniotomies. Nondominant (right side) craniotomies are typically preferred if the aneurysm anatomy is amenable.

Interventional Technique

For endovascular interventions, position the patient on the angiography table, asleep or awake, depending on the operator's comfort and the patient's mental status. Access the femoral artery and perform a four vessel diagnostic angiogram to ensure adequate understanding of the distal vertebrobasilar and posterior circulation anatomy, as well as aneurysm morphology. If ruptured, heparin is routinely held until the aneurysm is secured.

A guide catheter is positioned so it can be simultaneously visualized onscreen with the aneurysm and parent artery. The aneurysm is accessed with a microcatheter via microwire guidance. Coils are deployed and detached to a goal of approximately 30% packing density. PA and lateral high magnification runs should be performed to ensure adequate coiling before microcatheter removal. Final angiogram runs are obtained after microcatheter removal to ensure complete vascular integrity.

Surgical Technique

For a subtemporal approach, supine positioning with the head rotated 80 degrees to 100 degrees from the midline is used (zygomatic arch horizontal) (Figures 10-3 and 10-4). Following the craniotomy, the dura is opened and CSF is drained to allow for the temporal lobe to fall away from the middle cranial fossa floor (Figure 10-5). Additionally, a lumbar drain is often used to assist with brain relaxation. The temporal lobe is then gently elevated and the underlying tentorium is visualized. The uncus and third nerve are gently elevated to visualize the interpeduncular cistern. The membrane of Liliequist is sharply divided and the superior cerebellar artery is identified and followed back to the basilar artery (Figure 10-6).

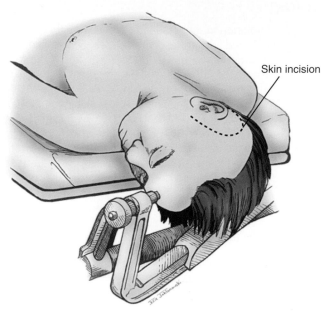

FIGURE 10-3   Patient positioning for a subtemporal approach. *(Reprinted with permission from Quiñones-Hinojosa A. Schmidek and Sweet Operative Neurosurgical Techniques. 6th ed. Elsevier; 2012.)*

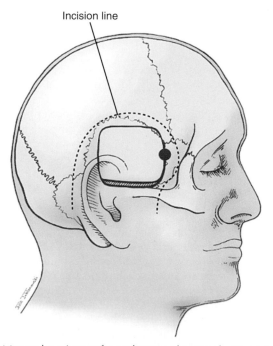

FIGURE 10-4   Skin incision and craniotomy for a subtemporal approach. *(Reprinted with permission from Quiñones-Hinojosa A. Schmidek and Sweet Operative Neurosurgical Techniques. 6th ed. Elsevier; 2012.)*

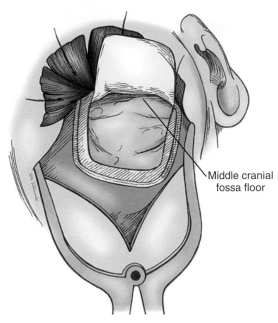

Middle cranial
fossa floor

FIGURE 10-5   Subtemporal approach: dural opening and tack up, allowing for retraction of the temporal lobe. *(Reprinted with permission from Quiñones-Hinojosa A. Schmidek and Sweet Operative Neurosurgical Techniques. 6th ed. Elsevier; 2012.)*

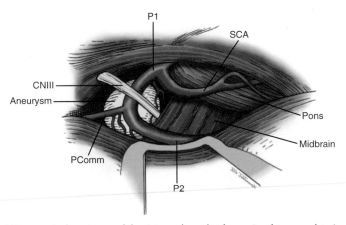

P1

SCA

CNIII

Aneurysm

Pons

Midbrain

PComm

P2

FIGURE 10-6   Microsurgical anatomy of the interpeduncular fossa. A subtemporal trajectory allows for visualization of the posterior perforating arteries. *(Reprinted with permission from Quiñones-Hinojosa A. Schmidek and Sweet Operative Neurosurgical Techniques. 6th ed. Elsevier; 2012.)*

For a pterional approach, supine positioning with head rotated 30 degrees from the midline is used (malar eminence upward) (Figure 10-7). After the craniotomy, the sphenoid wing, orbital roof, and posterior clinoid can be drilled down to improve exposure (Figures 10-8 and 10-9). The sylvian fissure is split, and the M1 takeoff, third nerve, Pcomm, and anterior choroidal arteries are identified. The Pcomm is followed to the PCA (at the P1/P2 junction), and P1 is followed back retrograde to the basilar bifurcation. The proximal basilar is then exposed for arterial control in case of rupture.

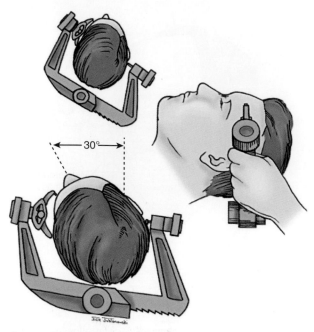

FIGURE 10-7   Head positioning for a half-and-half approach for BA aneurysms with the head slightly extended and turned 30 degrees to the left, placing the malar eminence at the highest point of the operating field. *(Reprinted with permission from Quiñones-Hinojosa A. Schmidek and Sweet Operative Neurosurgical Techniques. 6th ed. Elsevier; 2012.)*

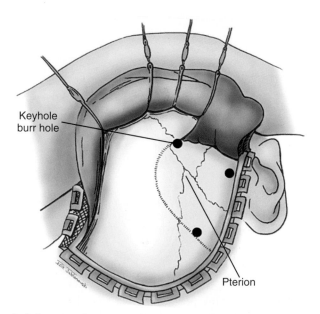

FIGURE 10-8   Burr hole locations for a half-and-half craniotomy. A burr hole is placed at the keyhole, a second hole is placed at the root of the zygoma, and a third is placed at the posterior extent of the superior temporal line. *(Reprinted with permission from Quiñones-Hinojosa A. Schmidek and Sweet Operative Neurosurgical Techniques. 6th ed. Elsevier; 2012.)*

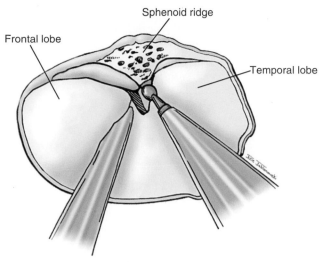

FIGURE 10-9 A high-speed drill is used to extensively drill the lateral sphenoid wing, extending to the base of the anterior clinoid process and the squamosal portion of the temporal bone to the floor of the middle cranial fossa. *(Reprinted with permission from Quiñones-Hinojosa A. Schmidek and Sweet Operative Neurosurgical Techniques. 6th ed. Elsevier; 2012.)*

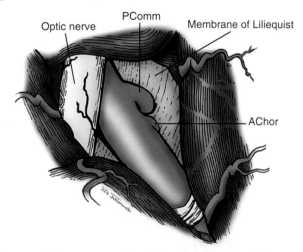

FIGURE 10-10 Microsurgical anatomy once the sylvian fissure is dissected, freeing the frontal and temporal lobes. The ICA is identified, along with the Pcomm and anterior choroidal artery. The membrane of Liliequist is identified lateral to the ICA. *(Reprinted with permission from Quiñones-Hinojosa A. Schmidek and Sweet Operative Neurosurgical Techniques. 6th ed. Elsevier; 2012.)*

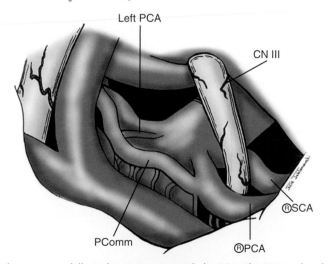

FIGURE 10-11 The Pcomm is followed to its junction with the PCA. The SCA is identified inferior to CN III. The basilar trunk is followed superiorly to the aneurysm neck. *(Reprinted with permission from Quiño-nes-Hinojosa A. Schmidek and Sweet Operative Neurosurgical Techniques. 6th ed. Elsevier; 2012.)*

With either approach, the aneurysm is then carefully dissected from surrounding arachnoid and perforators. A temporary then permanent clip is placed across the aneurysm neck, minimizing neck residual (Figures 10-10 to 10-12).

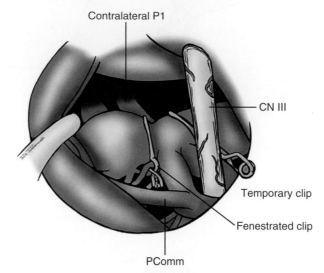

FIGURE 10-12   Temporary clip placement as more aggressive dissection of the aneurysm is performed. Using a retractor or the side of a suction tip, the Pcomm and overlying vessels can be retracted to allow better visualization of the aneurysm neck. Several techniques can be utilized to clip BA aneurysms. In this instance, a fenestrated clip is utilized to avoid compromising perforators adjacent to the neck of the aneurysm. *(Reprinted with permission from Quiñones-Hinojosa A.* Schmidek and Sweet Operative Neurosurgical Techniques. *6th ed. Elsevier; 2012.)*

Complication Avoidance and Management

With either endovascular or surgical approaches, care must be taken to avoid disruption of the perforating brainstem vessels. Early intervention is now generally preferred should there be a rupture, and standard secondary treatment for SAH is critical to prevent vasospasm and secondary stroke.

- Endovascular coiling
  - Stent-assisted coiling can be used for wide-necked aneurysms to hold coils inside the aneurysm. A "Y" or P1-to-P1 stent configuration may be needed for very wide-necked basilar apex aneurysms to ensure adequate coil containment.
- Microsurgical clipping
  - Systemic hypotension or basilar occlusion is used during temporary and permanent clip placement to reduce rupture risk. In low-lying basilar apex aneurysms, a subtemporal approach with division of the tentorium is necessary. Operative planning for a more posterior approach and a larger bone flap are needed. With any surgical approach, preservation of the perforating arteries of the posterior basilar, proximal P1, and distal PCA is critical to avoid lacunar, thalamic, and midbrain stroke.

KEY PAPERS

Sekhar LN, Tariq F, Morton RP, et al. Basilar tip aneurysms: a microsurgical and endovascular contemporary series of 100 patients. *Neurosurgery.* 2013;72:284-298, discussion 298-299.
Wiebers DO, Whisnant JP, Huston J 3rd, et al. Unruptured intracranial aneurysms: natural history, clinical outcome, and risks of surgical and endovascular treatment. *Lancet.* 2003;362:103-110.

Case 11

Endovascular Treatment of Unruptured Aneurysms

J. Scott Pannell, MD ● Alexander A. Khalessi, MD

Presentation

A 40-year-old female with 2-week history of left-sided ptosis and intermittent diplopia.

- PMH: otherwise unremarkable
- Exam
  - Left medial gauze CN III palsy
  - Mild left-sided ptosis

Differential Diagnosis

- Neoplastic
  - Nasopharyngeal carcinoma
  - Sphenoid meningioma
  - Metastasis
- Vascular
  - Hypertension
  - Posterior communicating (PCOM) aneurysm
  - Cavernous sinus thrombosis
- Inflammatory
  - Multiple sclerosis
  - Sarcoidosis
- Metabolic
  - Diabetes
- Trauma (typical or iatrogenic)

Initial Imaging

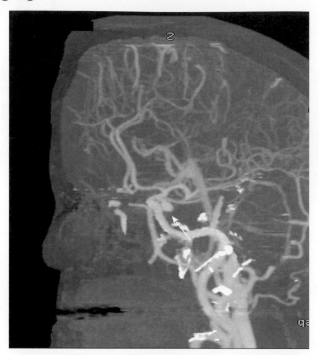

FIGURE 11-1

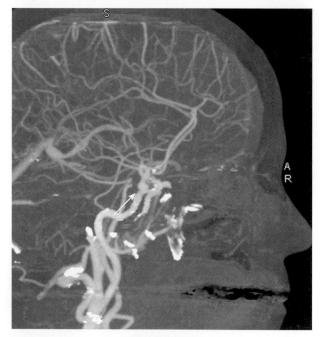

FIGURE 11-2

Imaging Description and Differential

- Figures 11-1 and 11-2 PA and lateral oriented CTA – 3D MIP demonstrates a 5 × 7 × 10 mm left PCOM aneurysm. The neck of the aneurysm appears narrow.
- Differential:
  - PCOM artery aneurysm

Further Workup

- Imaging:
  - Diagnostic cerebral angiography, the gold standard

Further Imaging

Figures 11-3 and 11-4 left anterior circulation angiogram, performed in the PA and lateral plane by left internal carotid artery (ICA) injection, and demonstrates the same $5 \times 7 \times 10$ mm left PCOM aneurysm. The neck of the aneurysm is narrow, measuring 3 mm in diameter. The aneurysm appears irregular, particularly at the neck.

Pathophysiology

Aneurysms are pathologic dilations of the blood vessel wall. The development of a cerebral aneurysm is multifactorial and includes focal structural defects in the vessel wall, hemodynamic stress as a result of turbulent blood flow or a branch point, and familial factors. Hereditary syndromes associated with cerebral aneurysms include Ehlers-Danlos syndrome, fibromuscular dysplasia, Osler-Weber-Rendu syndrome, and polycystic kidney disease. Unruptured aneurysms may present with symptoms related to mass effect on adjacent structures, or may be discovered incidentally during the workup of unrelated symptoms. The case presented demonstrates a large PCOM aneurysm; however, attention to the morphology is necessary to distinguish smaller blister aneurysms from infundibula. Infundibula are typically smaller than 3 mm, triangular shaped, and give rise to a vessel at the apex of the triangle.

Treatment Options

Endovascular coil embolization has demonstrated a survival advantage over neurosurgical clipping in the immediate perioperative period. However, the survival advantage erodes over time because of recurrence in the endovascular group. Rates of long term morbidity are similar between the two groups when the anterior circulation is considered in isolation.

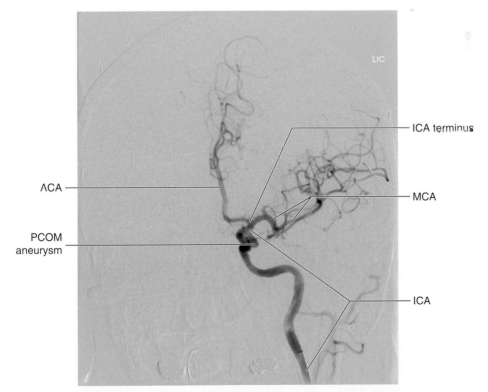

FIGURE 11-3 Left anterior circulation angiogram showing the narrow neck of the aneurysm measuring at 3 mm in diameter.

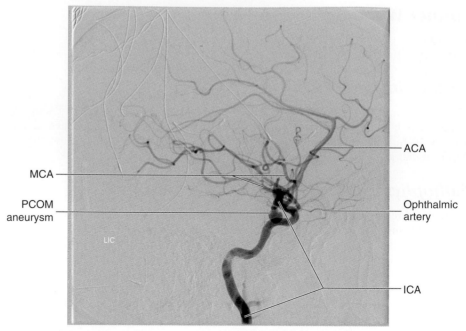

MCA

PCOM
aneurysm

LIC

ACA

Ophthalmic
artery

ICA

FIGURE 11-4 Left anterior circulation angiogram showing the irregular appearance of the aneurysm, particularly at the neck.

However, long term morbidity rates are higher in the surgical group for posterior circulation aneurysms. The cost is lower in the endovascular group, despite the need for potential retreatments.

The choice of endovascular repair verses surgical repair should take into consideration the age of the patient, patient preference, appearance of the aneurysm, and its location. Microneurosurgical clipping should be considered in younger patients <50 years of age with anterior circulation aneurysms. Endovascular repair should be considered in patients >50 years of age, or patients with posterior circulation aneurysms. However, endovascular repair may not be feasible in all circumstances, particularly in but not limited to large fusiform MCA aneurysms which often necessitate clip remodeling or clip sacrifice with ECA-MCA bypass.

Endovascular Technique

We recommend the use of general endotracheal anesthesia and neurophysiologic monitoring for embolization procedures. Access to the common femoral artery is obtained, and a 6 Fr long sheath is introduced into the distal aorta over a 0.35 inch wire.

Using a 4 Fr diagnostic catheter, the bilateral vertebral and ICAs are selected. Diagnostic angiography is performed of the bilateral anterior and posterior circulation. If performing a combined diagnostic angiogram and embolization, the angiogram is generally concluded in the artery of interest. A 3D rotational angiogram is then obtained. Working projections are then acquired from the 3D rotational angiogram. Next, the 4 Fr diagnostic is exchanged for a 6 Fr guide catheter. We recommend exchanging the catheter with the exchange wire in the external carotid. Alternatively, a tri-axial approach may be employed with the diagnostic catheter placed through the guide catheter for access. After the guide is introduced, the patient is heparinized.

Next, using the previously obtained working projections, the aneurysm is catheterized with a microcatheter and a 0.14 inch wire. The aneurysm is embolized with a framing coil, and filling coils, based upon the size of the aneurysm and/or residual. Many aneurysms can be primarily coiled. The patient in this case was primarily coiled with complete obliteration. See Figures 11-5 to 11-8.

Figures 11-5 and 11-6 are PA and lateral spot fluoroscopic images of the coil construct used in the embolization.

Figures 11-7 and 11-8 are PA and lateral left anterior circulation angiograms demonstrating complete obliteration of the aneurysm.

However, wider necked aneurysms may require balloon assistance with a compliant balloon or stent assistance. The stent may be deployed before catheterizing the aneurysm, or after catheterization, which results in jailing of the microcatheter in the aneurysm.

Repair of aneurysms at the basilar tip or MCA bifurcation may necessitate a Y-stent construct to protect the parent vessels. Most operators deploy an open cell stent, followed by a close cell stent, in Y-stent reconstruction to facilitate better vessel apposition and parent artery protection.

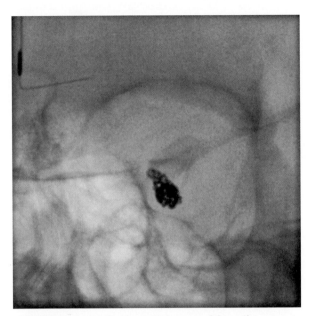

FIGURE 11-5 PA fluoroscopic images of the coil construct.

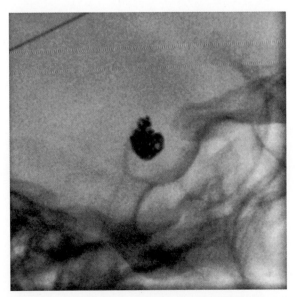

FIGURE 11-6 Lateral spot fluoroscopic images of the coil construct.

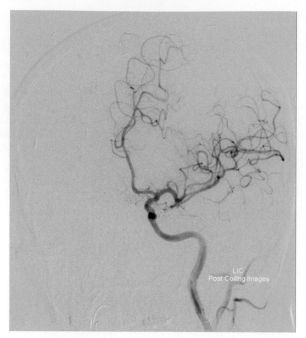

FIGURE 11-7   PA circulation angiogram.

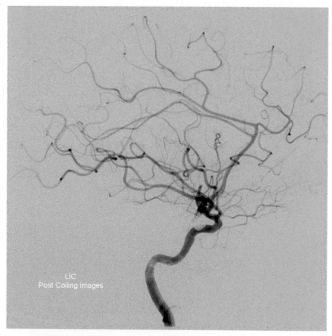

FIGURE 11-8   Lateral left anterior circulation angiogram.

Surgical Technique

Please see Chapter 3 and Chapter 4 for surgical techniques.

Complication Avoidance and Management

- Complications in the endovascular technique are often ischemic or embolic. Meticulous catheter hygiene, adequate heparinization, and exquisite parent artery preservation are all key in avoiding embolic complications. Ischemic complications can be avoided by minimizing the use of occlusive catheter systems and avoiding dissections, often a function of vessel size and catheter mismatch or step-offs.

KEY PAPERS

Alshekhlee A, Mehta S, Edgell RC, et al. Hospital mortality and complications of electively clipped or coiled unruptured intracranial aneurysm. *Stroke.* 2010;41:1471-1476.

Gonda D, Khalessi A, McCutcheon B, et al. Long-term follow-up of unruptured intracranial aneurysms repaired in California. *J Neurosurg.* 2014;120:1349-1357.

Molyneux A, Kerr R, Stratton I, et al. International Subarachnoid Aneurysm Trial (ISAT) Collaborative Group. International Subarachnoid Aneurysm Trial (ISAT) of neurosurgical clipping versus endovascular coiling in 2143 patients with ruptured intracranial aneurysms: a randomized trial. *Lancet.* 2002;360:1267-1274.

Rinne J, Hernesniemi J, Niskanen M, et al. Analysis of 561 patients with 690 middle cerebral artery aneurysms: anatomic and clinic features as correlated to management outcome. *Neurosurgery.* 1996;38:2-11.

Case 12

Dominant Hemisphere Hemorrhagic Stroke

J. Scott Pannell, MD ● Robert C. Rennert, MD ●
Scott E. Olson, MD ● Alexander A. Khalessi, MD

Presentation

A 63-year-old female with a history of left MCA occlusion with persistent right hemiparesis, following TICI 3 reperfusion after mechanical thrombectomy.

- PMH: Graves' disease
- Exam: lethargic, moderate confusion, and oriented to person only
  - Cranial nerves intact
  - Sensation intact
  - Right 1/5 strength in upper and lower extremity

Differential Diagnosis

- Vascular
  - Progression of ischemic stroke
  - Hemorrhagic transformation of ischemic stroke (h/o ischemic stroke)

Initial Imaging

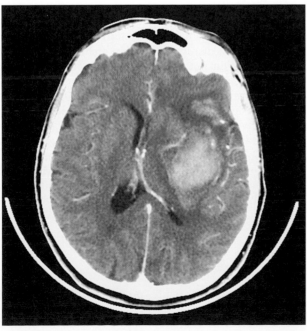

FIGURE 12-1

Imaging Description

- Figure 12-1 is an axial CTA centered at the level of the basal ganglia, demonstrating a 50cc hematoma in the left basal ganglia with an 11 mm midline shift and perihematomal edema.

Imaging Differential

- Neoplastic
  - Hemorrhage from a primary or metastatic tumor
- Vascular
  - Progression of ischemic stroke
  - Vascular malformation (AVM) rupture and cavernous hemangioma (more common in younger patients)
  - Hemorrhagic stroke (more common in older patients)
    - Hypertensive (basal ganglia most common)
    - Vasculitis (amyloid angiopathy is most common in the elderly)
  - Traumatic intraparenchymal hemorrhage (h/o trauma)
  - Hemorrhagic transformation of ischemic stroke (h/o ischemic stroke)
  - Rupture of arterial aneurysm (h/o perianeurysmal fibrosis from previous rupture)
- Infectious
  - Rupture of mycotic cerebral aneurysm (in a setting of IV drug use)

Further Workup

- Laboratory
  - ABG, CBC, coagulation panel, and electrolytes
- Imaging
  - Noncontrast CT most important
  - MRI secondary choice, because of changes in blood patterning that occur over time
  - Cerebral imaging via CT angiogram, MRA, or digital subtraction angiography (the gold standard) for assessment of underlying vascular abnormalities

Pathophysiology

Hemorrhagic strokes are the result of hemorrhage into the brain parenchyma. These hemorrhages cause local mass effect, disrupting cerebral architecture, and causing perihematomal ischemia. Secondary brain injury from blood product breakdown, and resulting edema, can also occur. Hemorrhagic strokes can result from a variety of underlying pathologies, including hypertension, vasculopathy, trauma, tumors, or vascular malformations. Hemorrhage location and patient age can help predict the underlying cause. Elderly patients (≥70 years of age) with lobar hemorrhages are often as a result of cerebral amyloid angiopathy, where the incidence of this disease is highest. Conversely, patients aged 45 to 70 years with basal ganglia hemorrhages are likely to be hypertensive in nature. In patients younger than 45 years, underlying vascular lesions such as AVMs, cavernomas, or aneurysms must be highly considered. Trauma, hemorrhagic transformation of an ischemic stroke, cirrhosis, and anticoagulant use are other causes of hemorrhagic stroke that occur across age groups.

Treatment Options

- Medical
  - BP control, target of 140/90, seizure prophylaxis, correct coagulopathies, ICP management
  - BP control, with a target of 140/90, prophylactic anticonvulsants, sedation, analgesia, and nimodipine for vasospasm prevention if SAH is a component

- Surgical (controversial)
  - Standard craniotomy and microsurgical evacuation is considered in patients with lobar clots >30 mL and within 1 cm of the cortical surface.
  - Decompressive craniectomy without clot evacuation
  - Minimally invasive evacuation plus thrombolysis (trials ongoing)
  - Endoscopic hematoma evacuation (trials ongoing)

Surgical Technique

For microsurgical evacuation, positioning and craniotomy are dependent upon hemorrhage location. After craniotomy, the dura is opened and any overlying parenchyma is carefully dissected to expose the clot. A combination of microaspiration and forceps evacuation is used depending on the clot consistency. The resection cavity is thoroughly flushed and hemostasis is ensured prior to closure.

For minimally invasive hematoma evacuation, positioning is based on hematoma location and a cannula is stereotactically placed into the center of the clot. Hand aspiration, using a 10 mL syringe, is performed until resistance is noted. A soft ventriculostomy catheter is placed through the rigid cannula, a thrombolytic agent is injected, and closed for 1 hour prior to being opened for gravity drainage.

For endoscopic hematoma evacuation, positioning is based on hematoma location and access is planned using neuronavigation software. A Burr hole is created at the access site and the endoscopic sheath is inserted to the distal aspect of the hematoma. Evacuation typically proceeds distal to proximal, with slow withdrawal of the sheath.

Complication Avoidance and Management

While clot evacuation is theoretically advantageous for avoidance of secondary injury following hemorrhagic stroke, clinical data have inconsistently demonstrated a significant benefit of surgery. Careful patient selection and surgical planning are needed to avoid complications.

- Surgical evacuation
  - Manipulation of penumbral ischemic tissue is thought to contribute to secondary injury and should be minimized.
- Endoscopic evacuation
  - The limited field of view and potentially distorted anatomy requires an operator with a baseline technical skill set to practice endoscopic neurosurgery. Current guidelines for endoscopic evacuation are for supratentorial clots >30 mL.

KEY PAPERS

Hemphill JC 3rd, Farrant M, Neill TA Jr. Prospective validation of the ICH score for 12-month functional outcome. *Neurology*. 2009;73:1088-1094.

Mendelow AD, Gregson BA, Fernandes HM, et al. Early surgery versus initial conservative treatment in patients with spontaneous supratentorial intracerebral haematomas in the International Surgical Trial in Intracerebral Hemorrhage (STICH): a randomised trial. *Lancet*. 2005;365:387-397.

Morgenstern LB, Hemphill JC 3rd, Anderson C, et al. Guidelines for the management of spontaneous intracerebral hemorrhage: a guideline for healthcare professionals from the American Heart Association/American Stroke Association. *Stroke*. 2010;41:2108-2129.

Case 13

Hypertensive Thalamic Hemorrhage

Jason W. Signorelli ● J. Scott Pannell, MD ●
Alexander A. Khalessi, MD

Presentation

A 53-year-old male with a history of uncontrolled hypertension presents to the ED with left hemiparesis of 2 hours duration and decreased level of consciousness. There is no history of trauma.

- PMH: otherwise unremarkable
- Exam
  - Complete left hemisensory loss
  - Left hemiparesis
  - Miotic pupils

Differential Diagnosis

- Vascular
  - Hypertensive hemorrhage
  - Aneurysm
  - Moyamoya disease
  - Arteriovenous or dural vascular malformations
  - Venous thrombosis
  - Vasculitis
- Infectious
  - Septic embolism
  - Mycotic aneurysm
  - CNS infection (herpes simplex encephalitis)
- Neoplastic
  - Primary cerebral tumor
  - Metastasis (most commonly lung, renal cell carcinoma, melanoma, or breast)
- Other
  - Cerebral amyloid angiopathy
  - Drugs – cocaine, amphetamine

Initial Imaging

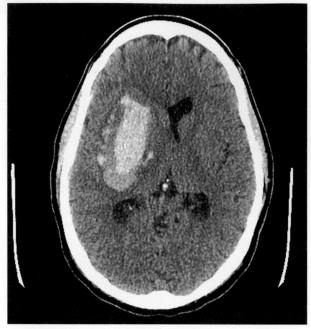

FIGURE 13-1

Imaging Description and Differential

- CT head without contrast demonstrating acute thalamic hematoma

Further Imaging

- Laboratory
  - CBC, CMP, PT, PTT, INR, toxicology screen, urinalysis, urine culture, pregnancy test in women of childbearing age
- Imaging
  - CXR, ECG
- Prognostic indicators
  - Intracerebral hemorrhage (ICH) score – predicts 30-day mortality based on GCS at presentation
  - Patient's age, supra versus infratentorial location, ICH volume, intraventricular blood
- Consultants
  - Neurocritical care

Pathophysiology

Thalamic hemorrhage is the second most common cause of ICH, occurring in approximately 6% to 25% of all cases. The most common etiology of thalamic hemorrhage is hypertension, which is believed to induce pathologic changes in the vascular wall, leading to rupture. It can be categorized by anatomic location: dorsal, medial, anterior-lateral, and posterior-lateral, with the latter being both the most common and most likely to hemorrhage into the ventricle. Hematoma growth is common, with lesions demonstrating up to 37% expansion within 3 hours of onset. Perihematomal edema and neurotoxic products of blood degradation may also play a significant role in pathological progression. Patients classically present with a predominance of sensory over motor deficits, but usually have both, oculomotor abnormalities, language disturbances if the dominant hemisphere is affected, and neglect syndrome if in the nondominant hemisphere. Decreased mental status, headaches, nausea, and vomiting are also seen in 20% to 30% of patients. The overall mortality rate ranges from 13%, for restricted intrathalamic lesions, to >50% in patients with concomitant intraventricular hemorrhage (IVH).

Treatment Options

Current treatment recommendations for thalamic hemorrhages are primarily medical. Large-scale randomized trials, such as STITCH, have not demonstrated a benefit to deep hematoma evacuation unless it is complicated by IVH resulting in acute hydrocephalus or mass effect. However, novel and minimally invasive techniques continue to be investigated and may alter these recommendations in the near future.

- Medical
  - ICU monitoring
  - ICP monitoring in patients with GCS ≤8, and evidence of IVH, herniation, or hydrocephalus
  - Rapid correction of coagulopathies and reversal of warfarin as required
  - BP control, target of 140/90, in patients with systolic blood pressure <220; otherwise permissive hypertension to maintain a target cerebral perfusion pressure of 50–70 mmHg
  - Antiepileptic drugs (AEDs) in patients with clinical or EEG proven seizures. Prophylactic AEDs are not recommended.
- Surgical
  - EVD placement: standard care for increased ICP
  - Neuroendoscopy with EVD placement, with or without intraventricular fibrinolysis
  - Stereotactic aspiration with thrombolysis
  - Decompressive craniectomy

Surgical Technique

EVD Placement

The nondominant side is used when possible. The skin is clipped and prepped in standard fashion. Using a twist drill, a burr hole is drilled 1 to 2 cm anterior to the coronal suture in the midpupillary line and 2 to 3 cm lateral to the midline. The meninges may be opened using the drill. The catheter should be inserted perpendicular to the cortical surface and aimed toward the ipsilateral medial canthus and the ipsilateral tragus in the mediolateral and anteroposterior planes, respectively. Do not insert the catheter more than 5 to 7 cm deep. If no CSF is encountered by the third attempt, a CT scan should be obtained to check the position.

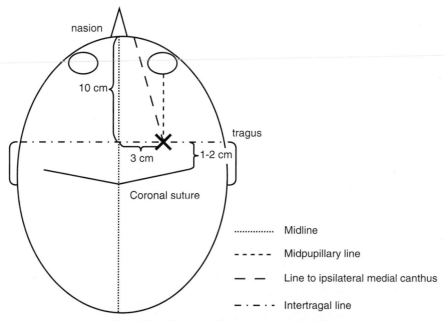

FIGURE 13-2   Reproduced from Schmidek HH and Roberts DW. *Schmidek and Sweet Operative Neurosurgical Techniques: Indications, Methods, and Results.* 5th ed. Elsevier; 2006.

Neuroendoscopic Approach

Keen's point (2.5 to 3 cm posterior and superior to the pinna) is commonly used for the endoscopic approach. The patient is placed in supine position with the head turned approximately 60 degrees away. A 3- to 4-cm incision is made in the scalp ipsilateral to the hemorrhage and a 1-cm burr hole placed at Keen's point. An endoscopic sheath is used to perform a transcortical, transventricular perforation and the endoscope/suction tube is then inserted through the sheath to allow for evacuation of hematomas from both intraventricular and intrathalamic locations. An EVD is placed and the dura and skin are closed.

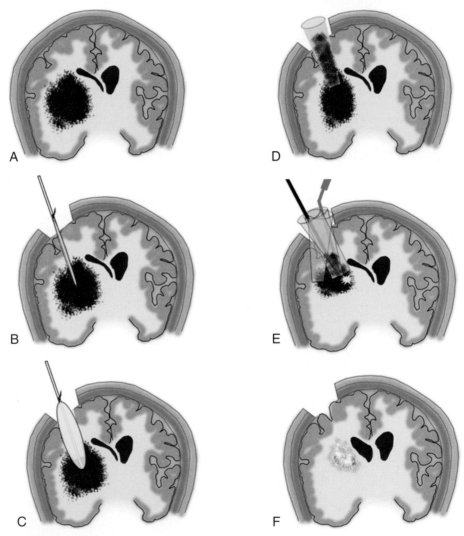

FIGURE 13-3 Cartoon picture diagram of the strategy for endoscopic hematoma evacuation. **(A)** Intracerebral hematoma usually has a mass effect and causes midline shift. **(B)** Incise the cortex and insert the ventricular catheter with a sutured glove. **(C)** Dilate the working channel by ballooning the glove. **(D)** Introduce the transparent sheath and begin central decompression. Hematoma will gush out under high intracranial pressure. **(E)** Change the angle of the transparent sheath and use different angles of endoscope and angles of suction tips to remove residual hematoma. As the sheath is withdrawn, the cavity created by the hematoma will collapse. The resting hematoma will be pushed within view of the sheath. **(F)** A layer of hemostatic agents is paved for hemostasis. *(Reproduced from Wang W-H, Hung Y-C, Hsu SPC, et al. Endoscopic hematoma evacuation in patients with spontaneous supratentorial intracerebral hemorrhage.* J Chin Med Assoc [Internet]. *2014 Nov [cited 02.02.15].)*

Decompressive Craniectomy

The decompressive craniectomy, via trauma flap, is a more commonly used approach. The patient is placed in supine position with the head rotated to the contralateral side. The skin is opened with a large reverse question mark incision beginning at the zygoma, extending posteriorly to the ear (approximately 4 to 6 cm), and then curving upward, remaining 1 to 2 cm lateral of the sagittal suture. The underlying temporalis muscle and subcutaneous tissue are reflected anteriorly and secured with scalp hooks. Raney clips should be used to assist with scalp hemostasis.

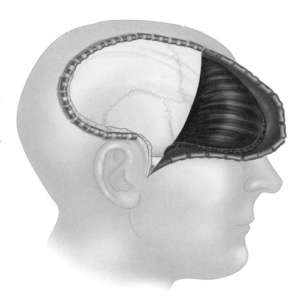

FIGURE 13-4   Muscle and soft tissue dissection. The incision is carried through the subcutaneous tissue, including the temporalis muscle, down to the cranium. The musculocutaneus flap is reflected anteriorly and fixed with scalp hooks. Ideally, this muscle dissection extends down to the root of the zygoma and as far beneath the keyhole as possible, to maximize the temporal decompression. *(Reprinted with permission from Jandial R, McCormick, P and Black PM.* Core Techniques in Operative Neurosurgery. *Elsevier; 2011.)*

Three or more burr holes should be placed to create a bone flap of no less than 10 × 15 cm in size. The burr holes are connected and particular attention should be paid to avoiding the transverse and superior sagittal sinuses.

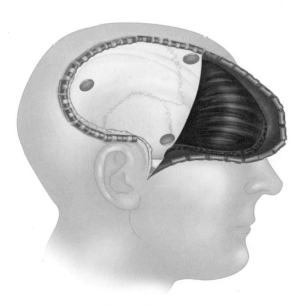

FIGURE 13-5   Burr holes and bone flap. Several burr holes (at least three) are made to create a bone flap that is at least 10 × 15 cm. Bone flaps smaller than this would not sufficiently decompress the brain and would reduce the ICP. When possible, a small ruler can be used to measure back from the keyhole to ensure that the anteroposterior extent of the bone flap is 15 cm. *(Reprinted with permission from Jandial R, McCormick P, and Black PM.* Core Techniques in Operative Neurosurgery. *Elsevier; 2011.)*

The bone flap is then removed, the requisite temporal craniectomy completed, and the durotomy performed.

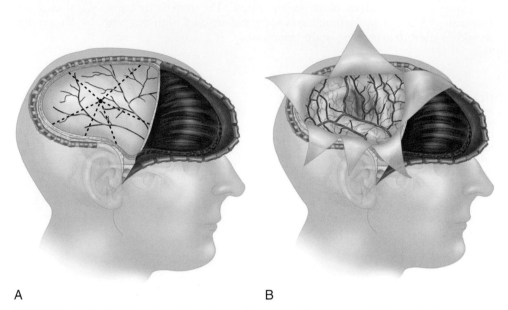

A   B

FIGURE 13-6   The dural opening. After achieving hemostasis, there are several choices for the durotomy. Our preferred method is to open the dura slowly with multiple radial incisions (in a stellate fashion) to provide maximal cerebral decompression **(A)** Associated hematomas can be removed, and hemostasis can be achieved **(B)** When the dural opening is complete, closure can be undertaken. Although some surgeons perform a duraplasty, we prefer to leave the durotomy open and simply cover the brain with a dural substitute or similar material to protect the brain surface and reduce adhesions. The leaves of the dura are folded over the dural substitute. Unless there is an urgent need to leave the operating room, drains are placed over the surface of the dural substitute and tunneled externally. The galea should be closed with numerous and closely spaced interrupted 2-0 absorbable braided sutures. The skin is closed with a running 4-0 absorbable monofilament suture. To ensure a watertight closure, the sutures are placed very close together. *(Reprinted with permission from Jandial R, McCormick P, and Black PM.* Core Techniques in Operative Neurosurgery. *Elsevier; 2011.)*

A duraplasty may be completed, or the durotomy left open, at the discretion of the surgeon. If open, the brain is covered with a dural substitute, the previously incised portions of dura situated over the dural substitute, drains placed, galea and skin then closed.

Stereotactic Aspiration with Thrombolysis

A CT scan without contrast should be obtained. The CT slice with the largest area of thalamic hemorrhage is first identified and the center of the hematoma on this image marked. Vertical and horizontal lines are drawn, crossing through the center of the hematoma. The entrance point on the scalp is marked as the intersection between the horizontal line and the neurocranium.

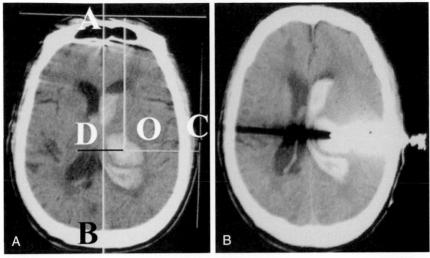

FIGURE 13-7   (A) The stereotactic methods before puncture of the thalamic hematoma: point "O" is the target of puncture and the central point of the hematoma in the CT slice, in which the hematoma is the largest. A median sagittal line "AB" is drawn, intersecting the frontal bone at "A," and intersecting the occipital bone at "B." The line "CD" is perpendicular to the median sagittal line "AB" through "O." Point "C," at which "CD" intersects the surface of the skull, is chosen as the puncture point, and the length of "CO" is the depth of the puncture. **(B)** CT scan performed immediately after operation showing the puncture needle on the right side of the brain and the black shadow on the left is an image artifact from the needle. *(Reproduced from Chen M, Wang Q, Zhu W, et al. Stereotactic aspiration plus subsequent thrombolysis for moderate thalamic hemorrhage.* World Neurosurg. *2012;77(1):122-129.)*

A burr hole is then made and the meninges opened via incision. A cannula is inserted to the level of the hematoma, which is aspirated until resistance is felt and the residual cavity flushed with saline.

FIGURE 13-8   The inner portion of the cannula is carefully removed, allowing the cannula to remain in the clot. Using a 10-mL syringe, manual aspiration is performed until resistance is met. *(Reprinted with permission from Jandial R, McCormick P, and Black PM.* Core Techniques in Operative Neurosurgery. *Elsevier; 2011.)*

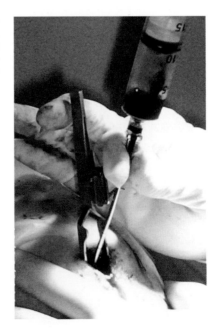

A flexible catheter may be placed via the cannula into the residual cavity and the cannula removed. The catheter is tunneled through and secured to the skin. Recombinant tPA is injected, allowed to stand for 1 hour with the system closed, and then aspirated through the tube. This process is repeated three times a day until a reduction in the hematoma volume, by at least 80%, is achieved. The catheter remains connected to a closed bag drainage system between treatments and is placed at head level.

Complication Avoidance and Management

It is important to approach via the nondominant hemisphere when possible. Aberrant placement too lateral or medial may result in damage to key structures such as the basal ganglia or internal capsule.

- Decompressive craniectomy
  - Several complications are common to all craniectomies. Laceration of a herniating brain on the bone edges is best avoided with a wide craniectomy. Extraaxial fluid collections are seen in approximately 20% of craniectomies and best treated with drainage. Infection should be controlled with meticulous closure and prolonged drain use, including two or more JP drains. Other infrequent complications include syndrome of the trephined (treated with cranioplasty), seizures, and cranioplasty failure.
- Neuroendoscopic approach and stereotactic aspiration with thrombolysis
  - Both procedures present a risk of new onset neurologic deficits and hemorrhage, which may be minimized with careful trajectory selection and postoperative CT scanning. Postprocedural infections are best avoided with perioperative antibiotics.

KEY PAPERS

Arboix A, Rodríguez-Aguilar R, Oliveres M, et al. Thalamic haemorrhage vs internal capsule-basal ganglia haemorrhage: clinical profile and predictors of in-hospital mortality. *BMC Neurol.* 2007;7(1):32.

Chen C-C, Liu C-L, Tung Y-N, et al. Endoscopic surgery for intraventricular hemorrhage (IVH) caused by thalamic hemorrhage: comparisons of endoscopic surgery and external ventricular drainage (EVD) Surgery. *World Neurosurg.* 2011;75(2):264-268.

Chen M, Wang Q, Zhu W, et al. Stereotactic aspiration plus subsequent thrombolysis for moderate thalamic hemorrhage. *World Neurosurg.* 2012;77(1):122-129.

Fung C, Murek M, Z'Graggen WJ, et al. Decompressive hemicraniectomy in patients with supratentorial intracerebral hemorrhage. *Stroke.* 2012;43(12):3207-3211.

Kumral E, Kocaer T, Ertübey NÖ, et al. Thalamic hemorrhage: a prospective study of 100 patients. *Stroke.* 1995;26(6):964-970.

Mendelow AD, Gregson BA, Fernandes HM, et al. Early surgery versus initial conservative treatment in patients with spontaneous supratentorial intracerebral haematomas in the International Surgical Trial in Intracerebral Haemorrhage (STICH): a randomised trial. *The Lancet.* 2005;365(9457):387-397.

Morgenstern LB, Hemphill JC, Anderson C, et al. Guidelines for the management of spontaneous intracerebral hemorrhage: a guideline for healthcare professionals from the American Heart Association/American Stroke Association. *Stroke.* 2010;41(9):2108-2129.

Steinke W, Sacco RL, Mohr JP, et al. Thalamic stroke: presentation and prognosis of infarcts and hemorrhages. *Arch Neurol.* 1992;49(7):703-710.

Tokgoz S, Demirkaya S, Bek S, et al. Clinical properties of regional thalamic hemorrhages. *J Stroke Cerebrovasc Dis.* 2013;22(7):1006-1012.

Van Asch CJ, Luitse MJ, Rinkel GJ, et al. Incidence, case fatality, and functional outcome of intracerebral haemorrhage over time, according to age, sex, and ethnic origin: a systematic review and meta-analysis. *Lancet Neurol.* 2010;9(2):167-176.

Case 14

Cerebellar Hemorrhage

Reid Hoside, MD ● J. Scott Pannell, MD ●
Alexander A. Khalessi, MD

Presentation

A 38-year-old male presents to the emergency room with a sudden onset of headache, dizziness, and ataxia since this morning. According to his wife, he became more somnolent as the day progressed.

- PMH: poorly controlled hypertension and chronic methamphetamine use.
- Neurologic exam
  - Somnolent and falls asleep frequently during exam
  - Cranial nerves intact
  - Pupils are 4 mm and briskly responsive to light
  - Markedly diminished right-sided capabilities in coordination, which include finger-to-nose, heel-to-shin, and rapid alternation by foot tap and hand clap
  - Left side is normal
  - Blood pressure is 197/115

Differential Diagnosis

- Vascular
  - Rupture of arteriovenous malformation
  - Aneurysmal rupture
  - Embolic ischemia, with or without hemorrhagic conversion
  - Hypertensive intracerebral hemorrhage
  - Cavernous malformation rupture
  - Venous sinus thrombosis
- Neoplastic
  - Hemorrhagic tumor (hemangioblastoma, primary brain tumor, or metastatic lesion)
- Other
  - Spontaneous intracerebral hemorrhage in a setting of a hypocoagulable state (medication effects or inherited blood dyscrasias)
  - Spontaneous intracerebral hemorrhage in a setting of drug use (cocaine or amphetamines)

Initial Imaging

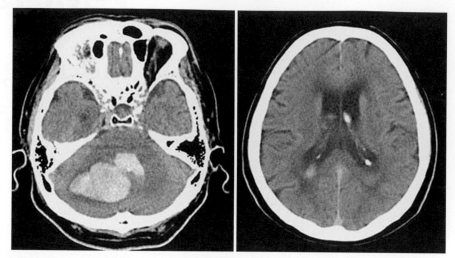

FIGURE 14-1

Imaging Description and Differential

Figure 14-1: CT imaging of the head showing significant right-sided parenchymal hemorrhage of the cerebellum, with fourth ventricular extension and slightly dilated lateral ventricles.

Further Workup

- Laboratory
  - Routine labs (CBC, CMP, PT, PTT)
- Imaging
  - Vascular imaging (CTA, MRA, DSA) can be considered if initial imaging is suspicious for an underlying lesion, or if the clinical picture does not suggest a hypertensive etiology. Yield may be compromised due to the presence of a clot, which can mask vascular or neoplastic lesions.

Pathophysiology

Spontaneous hypertensive intracerebral hemorrhage (ICH) is easily the most common cause of cerebellar hemorrhage. These hemorrhages are usually centered in the watershed areas between the superior cerebellar artery (SCA) and anterior inferior cerebellar artery (AICA), routinely at the region of the dentate nucleus. The nature of ICH alone is morbid; however, more worrisome are the mass effects created by the hematoma in the enclosed and limited space of the posterior fossa. Closer inspection of overall mass effect is imperative, which includes the patency of the fourth ventricle, posterior elements of the basal cisterns, and the third ventricle. Clinically, these manifestations are translated into the patient becoming more somnolent, nonresponsive, and can quickly progress to death if not managed quickly. Neurosurgeons should maintain a low threshold to surgically manage patients of posterior fossa ICHs. Even without surgical management, the placement of an external ventricular drain should be considered to alleviate any presence of, or impending of, hydrocephalus from the hematoma's mass effect.

Treatment Options

- Medical: airway management, reversal of anticoagulation, blood pressure management (SBP <140), and placement of external ventricular drain to ensure that aggressive drainage is avoided to upward herniation

Case 15

Moyamoya Disease

Brandon C. Gabel, MD ● J. Scott Pannell, MD ●
Alexander A. Khalessi, MD

Presentation

The patient, a 38-year-old Japanese male, presents after several transient episodes of right arm weakness. These episodes resolve, but have become more frequent. They typically occur after periods of strenuous exercise.

- Exam
  - Alert and oriented to person, place, and time
  - Extraocular movements intact
  - Slight flattening of the left nasolabial fold and tongue midline
  - Moves all four extremities with full strength and no focal weakness is apparent

Differential Diagnosis

- Vascular
  - Cerebrovascular ischemia
    - Thromboembolic stroke
    - Intracranial atherosclerotic disease
    - Moyamoya disease
    - Carotid dissection
  - Transient ischemic attack
- Other
  - Partial complex seizure
  - Hypoglycemia or hyperglycemia can often mimic ischemic stroke
    - Migraine aura

Initial Imaging

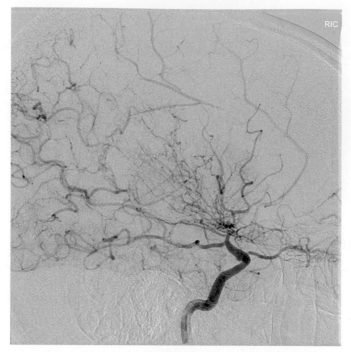

FIGURE 15-1

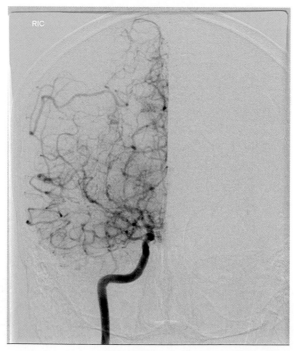

FIGURE 15-2

Imaging Description

Figure 15-1 shows a right lateral internal carotid artery angiogram. Figure 15-2 shows a right anteroposterior internal carotid artery angiogram. The imaging reveals the classic "puff of smoke" consistent with recruitment of moya moya vessels near the carotid terminus. These findings were present bilaterally in this patient.

Further Workup

- Routine laboratory analysis including CBC, CMP, PT, PTT, and INR
- ECG and echocardiogram
- Carotid duplex
- Lipid panel
- Workup for hypercoagulopathy
- Imaging
  - MRI and MR angiogram
  - MR or CT perfusion studies
  - CT angiogram
  - Formal catheter angiogram

Pathophysiology

The pathophysiology of MMD remains elusive. For unknown reasons, MMD has a much higher incidence and prevalence among the Japanese and Asian populations. Genetic links have been found, but the inheritance pattern is complicated. MMD is associated with many other diseases. Connective tissue and autoimmune diseases, such as Marfan's disease or systemic lupus erythematosus, have been associated with MMD. Patients with chromosomal disorders, such as Down's syndrome, are also at higher risk.

Regardless of the cause, the ultimate outcome is abnormal stenosis and occlusion of the supraclinoid intracranial carotid arteries. On pathological analysis, the vessel walls show intimal thickening and disruption of the internal elastic lamina. This process is generally considered slowly progressive. In order to cope with hypoperfusion, the brain is believed to release angiogenetic factors that recruit collateral flow from tortuous moya moya vessels at the base of the brain. These vessels give angiograms the classic "puff of smoke" appearance.

Treatment Options

Surgical treatment of MMD involves bypass procedures. Both direct and indirect bypass procedures have been used with success. Direct bypass grafting is usually done by suturing a branch of the superior temporal artery directly to a cortical branch of the middle cerebral artery, and less commonly the anterior cerebral or posterior cerebral artery. Direct bypass procedures have an increased risk of hyperperfusion syndrome.

Indirect bypass procedures are technically easier to perform and have outcomes comparable to direct procedures. One of the most common types of indirect bypass is encephalomyosynangiosis (EMS) in which the temporalis muscle is laid over the chronically ischemic brain. Vessels from the muscle are then slowly recruited by the adjacent brain. A similar procedure known as encephaloduroarteriosynangiosis involves laying a branch of the superficial temporal artery directly over exposed cortex. Indirect bypass procedures avoid hyperperfusion syndrome, but results take longer because collateralization of the ischemic brain takes time.

Antiplatelet agents, such as acetylsalicylic acid or clopidogrel, are also commonly prescribed to prevent thrombus formation in the diseased vessels. Some authors advocate using calcium channel antagonists and steroids if transient ischemic attacks are frequent.

Surgical Technique

In direct bypass procedures a branch of the superficial temporal artery is located using Doppler ultrasonography before making a skin incision. Great care is taken to avoid sacrificing the vessel during initial dissection. Once the vessel is adequately exposed and skeletonized, a craniotomy is performed. A donor MCA (or ACA/PCA) cortical vessel is then located. The skeletonized vessel is then directly approximated to the receiving vessel using microsutures. When repeating the craniotomy, it is important to not trap the anastomosed vessel.

In indirect bypass procedures, the temporalis muscle is dissected free from the underlying cranium. A frontotemporal craniotomy is performed and the dura is opened. The muscle is then flapped over the exposed brain tissue and tacked to the dural edges. In an indirect bypass, the craniotomy should be of sufficient size to allow as much collateralization as possible.

Complication Avoidance and Management

- MR or CT perfusion can help locate areas of the brain at most risk for infarct, and patients should be counseled about the importance of hydration. Neuromonitoring potentials may be used intraoperatively to help rule out ischemic complications during bypass grafting.

KEY PAPERS

Fukui M. Members of Research Committee on Spontaneous Occlusion of the Circle of Willis (Moyamoya Disease) of the Ministry of Health and Welfare, Japan. Guidelines for the diagnosis and treatment of spontaneous occlusion of the circle of Willis ("moyamoya" disease). *Clin Neurol Neurosurg.* 1997;99:S238-S240.

Khan N, Schuknecht B, Boltshauser E, et al. Moyamoya disease and moyamoya syndrome: Experience in Europe: choice of revascularisation procedures. *Acta Neurochir (Wien).* 2003;145:1061-1071.

Scott RM, Smith ER. Moyamoya disease and moyamoya syndrome. *N Eng J Med.* 2009;360:1226-1237.

Case 16

Venous Sinus Thrombosis

Brandon C. Gabel, MD ● J. Scott Pannell, MD ●
Alexander A. Khalessi, MD

Presentation

A 28-year-old female on birth control presented to an emergency room with a headache. This was managed conservatively and the patient was discharged. The patient returned 1 day later with a worsening headache, confusion, vomiting, and lethargy.

- Exam
  - Lethargic
  - Alert and oriented to person, but not place or time
  - Extraocular movements are intact, pupils are equal, round, and reactive to light.
  - Formal strength examination shows no focal weakness.

Differential Diagnosis

The differential diagnosis of lethargy, headache, and confusion in a young, otherwise healthy female is large. Neurologic diagnoses that should be considered include migraine, aneurysmal subarachnoid hemorrhage, meningitis, ischemic stroke, and arteriovenous malformations.

Initial Imaging

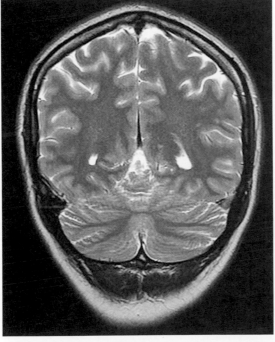

FIGURE 16-1

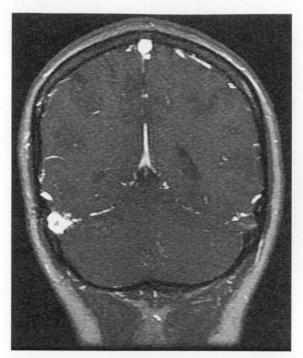

FIGURE 16-2

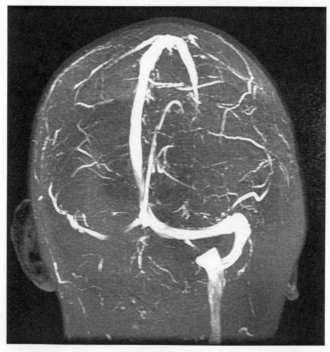

FIGURE 16-3

Imaging Description and Differential

Figure 16-1 shows a T2 weighted MRI, Figure 16-2 shows a T1 weighted MRI with contrast, and Figure 16-3 shows an MR venogram. This imaging reveals a left-sided transverse sinus thrombosis. The MRI and MRV imaging reveals opacification of the left transverse sinus by thrombus. The main differential diagnosis is an atretic or congenitally absent sinus.

Further Workup

- Routine labs (CBC, CMP, PT, INR, D-dimer)
- ECG and echocardiogram
- Continuous EEG
- Workup for hypercoagulopathy
  - Antithrombin, protein C, protein S, factor V Leiden, prothrombin mutations, lupus anticoagulant, anticardiolipin, etc.
- Imaging
  - MRI, MRA/MRV to aid in assessment of vascular anatomy
  - Noncontrast head CT
  - CT venogram (in lieu of MRV)
  - Formal catheter venography

Pathophysiology

Patients who develop sinus thrombosis often have predisposing risks. Those at risk of hypercoagulability have a higher incidence of sinus thrombosis. This includes young women who are pregnant or on birth control, patients with underlying hypercoagulopathies, and patients with a history of malignancy. Infection of the mastoid can cause thrombophlebitis, which can result in sinus thrombosis. Additionally, traumatic head injuries can also cause sinus thrombosis.

Regardless of the etiology, the end result is obliteration or severe stenosis of the affected thrombosis sinus. Venous pooling behind the thrombus causes engorgement of cortical veins and capillaries. The resulting increase in intravascular pressure leads to blood-brain-barrier disruption and cerebral edema. If severe, cortical veins may rupture and cause venous hemorrhage. Thrombosis of the transverse sinus can be difficult to recognize both on imaging and clinically. Patients with unilateral thrombosis of the transverse sinus not involving the torcula may be asymptomatic. However, some patients will present with ipsilateral hemorrhage or edema in the posterior temporal vein of Labbe distribution. Other subtle findings such as ipsilateral mastoid air cell opacification may be present.

Treatment Options

The mainstay of treatment for cerebral sinus thrombosis remains as systemic anticoagulation. Most physicians use intravenous heparin with a goal of 2.0 to 2.5 times the normal PTT. Once therapeutic, the patient is commonly started on long-term systemic anticoagulation medication (i.e., warfarin). If no hypercoagulopathy is identified, anticoagulation is usually continued for 3 to 6 months; if an underlying hypercoagulopathy is identified, then anticoagulation is usually lifelong. Endovascular transvenous treatment with tPA or urokinase has also been shown to be effective, but many of these studies used small cohorts of patients.

In addition to systemic anticoagulation, supportive care should be provided. This includes airway management, seizure precautions, hypertonic fluids (i.e., mannitol and/ or hypertonic saline), or external ventricular drainage to aid in intracranial pressure management. A craniotomy, to evacuate any intraparenchymal hematomas, may be necessary in some cases. It is also important to treat the underlying etiology of the thrombosis. Infection may necessitate IV antibiotics and surgical debridement. A workup for underlying hypercoagulopathy is also essential and frequently dictates the length of anticoagulant therapy. Workup for systemic malignancy may also be warranted in certain patients.

Complication Avoidance and Management

- Cerebral sinus thrombosis can be insidious with no specific symptoms; therefore, a high index of suspicion is often necessary to make the diagnosis.
- False positive MR or CT venograms may occur, especially in patients with a congenitally atretic or absent sinus.
- The underlying etiology for thrombosis should be thoroughly evaluated because it can dictate treatment regimens and durations.

KEY PAPERS

Barnwell SL, Higashida RT, Halbach VV, et al. Direct endovascular thrombolytic therapy for dural sinus thrombosis. *Neurosurgery*. 1991;28(1):135-142.

Ferro JM, Canhao P, Stam J, et al. Prognosis of cerebral vein and dural sinus thrombosis: results of the International Study on Cerebral Vein and Dural Sinus Thrombosis (ISCVT). *Stroke*. 2004;35:664-670.

Soleau SW, Schmidt R, Stevens S, et al. Extensive experience with dural sinus thrombosis. *Neurosurgery*. 2003;52:534-544.

Case 17

Carotid Stenosis

Jeffrey A. Steinberg, MD ● J. Scott Pannell, MD ●
Alexander A. Khalessi, MD

Presentation

An obese 65-year-old male with a history of smoking and hypertension presents with an acute 10-minute episode of aphasia and left-sided facial droop. The patient returned to baseline after the event.

- PMH: hypertension, 40 pack year smoking hx, obesity
- Exam: obese male in no acute distress
  - AAO × 3
  - PERRL, EOMI
  - Smile and forehead wrinkle symmetric
  - Tongue midline
  - Full strength in all extremities
  - Carotid bruit auscultated over left carotid artery

Differential Diagnosis

The differential diagnosis for symptomatic carotid stenosis involves pathologies that can mimic a transient ischemic attack or stroke.

- Neurologic
  - Seizure
  - Vertigo
  - Migraine
- Neoplastic
  - Brain tumor
- Cardiovascular
  - Aneurysm, AVM, or cavernoma
  - Cardioembolic disease
  - Spontaneous intracerebral hemorrhage
- Infectious
  - Meningitis
- Other
  - MS
  - Toxic metabolic disorders
  - Hypercoagulable state

Initial Imaging

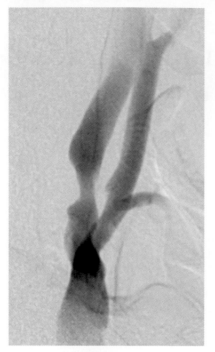

FIGURE 17-1

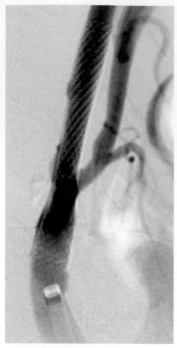

FIGURE 17-2

Imaging Description and Differential

- Diagnostic cerebral angiogram demonstrates a 70% stenosis of the left ICA in a patient who presented with recurrent TIAs as evidenced by right arm weakness/numbness and word finding difficulties (Figure 17-1). A diagnostic cerebral angiogram performed after stent placement and angioplasty demonstrates resolution of stenosis (Figure 17-2).
- Differential: ulcerated versus stable ICA plaque

Further Workup

- Laboratory
  - Serum chemistry
  - CBC, coagulation panel
  - Cardiac enzymes
  - Lipid profile
- Imaging
  - Ultrasound carotids
  - MRI brain including DWI/ADC
  - CTA neck, MRA neck, and/or diagnostic cerebral angiogram
  - ECG and ECHO
- Consultants
  - Stroke neurology

Pathophysiology

Atherosclerosis results from genetic predispositions and lifestyle choices. It is defined as arterial buildup of cholesterol, fat, and other substances that commonly occur at arterial bifurcations. Symptoms typically result from thromboembolia to the distal branches, including the retinal or cerebral arteries, but can also exist as hemodynamic instabilities,

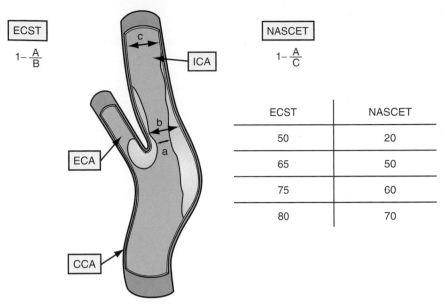

FIGURE 17-3 Methods of assessing carotid stenosis severity. **(A)** Residual lumen diameter at most stenotic portion of the vessel. **(B)** Estimated diameter of carotid wall at the level of the lesion. **(C)** Diameter of normal carotid artery just distal to stenosis. *(Reprinted with permission from Ellenbogen RG, Abdulrauf SI, Sekhar LN. Principles of Neurological Surgery. 3rd ed. Elsevier; 2012.)*

secondary to gross reduction in cerebral perfusion. Elevated levels of LDL correlate with increased plaque formation and this is further exacerbated by oxidative processes. Disruption of a plaque results in platelet activation, which can potentiate embolic events. The degree of stenosis, and symptomatic versus asymptomatic lesions, have been shown to correlate with the risk of TIA/stroke. Percent stenosis can be measured with different methods, but the NASCET and ECST methods are most common (Figure 17-3). As outlined in numerous landmark papers, the degree of stenosis and symptomatology dictate management. More specifically, carotid revascularization confers greater benefit in symptomatic patients with greater than 50% stenosis and in asymptomatic patients with greater than 60% stenosis. However, treatment in asymptomatic stenosis is more controversial. See Table 17-1 for a summary of the major trial results.

Treatment Options

- Lifestyle risk reduction
  - Smoking cessation, diet, exercise, and blood pressure reduction
- Medical management
  - Blood pressure medications, ensuring that no episodes of hypotension occur, which can result in hypoperfusion of cerebral tissue
  - Statin drugs for stabilization of intimal plaques and treatment of hyperlipidemia
  - Antiplatelet agents to reduce embolic events secondary to platelet activation at plaque sites
- Surgery
  - Carotid endarterectomy
- Interventional
  - Carotid angioplasty and stenting

Surgical Technique

Supine position with head extended and slightly turned to contralateral side with small bump placed between shoulder blades. Electroencephalogram (EEG) and somatosensory evoked potentials (SSEP) are monitored. A curvilinear incision is made along the anterior

TABLE 17-1

Trial	Summary of Results
The North American Symptomatic Carotid Endarterectomy Trial (NASCET) • Surgical endarterectomy trial • Enrolled patients with TIAs or non-disabling stroke • Primary endpoints: death or disabling stroke defined as mRS ≥3 at 2 years • Required surgeons to have less than 6% stroke or death rate in 50 consecutive cases over 2 years	Critical, 90–99% stenosis: 26% ARR Severe, >70% stenosis: 17% ARR Moderate, 50–69% stenosis: 7% ARR No statistically significant benefit for < 50% stenosis Perioperative stroke risk: 6%; death: 7% Results were durable to 8 years post procedure
European Carotid Surgery Trial (ECST) • Surgical endarterectomy trial • Enrolled patients with TIAs or non-disabling stroke • Primary endpoints: any ipsilateral stroke or death at 3 years	Severe, >70% stenosis: 21% ARR Moderate, 50–69%: 6% ARR Perioperative stroke and death risk: 7.5% Results durable to 10 years No clear benefit in near-occlusion group
Stenting versus Endarterectomy for Treatment of Carotid-Artery Stenosis (CREST) • Stenting vs CEA • Enrolled asymptomatic patients and patients with TIAs or non-disabling stroke • Primary endpoints: any stroke, myocardial infarction (MI), or death within 4 years	No statistically significant difference in primary endpoints between the two groups More perioperative strokes in the stenting group (4.1 vs 2.3%)* MIs in the CEA group (2.3 vs 1.1)
Asymptomatic Carotid Atherosclerosis Study (ACAS) • Surgical CEA trial • Enrolled asymptomatic patients • Primary endpoints: stroke or death at 3 years	>60% stenosis: 6% ARR Perioperative stroke and death risk 3% 70% relative risk reduction in men 16% relative risk reduction in women

*Rate of use of embolic protection devices not reported.
ARR, absolute risk reduction.

border of the sternocleidomastoid, beginning 1 cm beneath the mastoid, and down to the sternoclavicular joint. Dissection is carried out through the skin and platysma until the sternocleidomastoid muscle is visualized. Dissection is then carried out down anterior and deep to the sternocleidomastoid, freeing it from underlying fascia, until the carotid sheath is encountered. The jugular vein typically lies parallel and anterolateral within the carotid sheath, and is dissected from the carotid artery (Figure 17-4). Division of the common facial vein allows for enhanced visualization of the carotid artery and dissection of each of its branches. Then 3000 to 5000 units of heparinized saline are given before dissection of the carotid branches. Once each branch is dissected, umbilical tape is wrapped around the CCA, ICA, and ECA. Bradycardia can be treated with lidocaine injection into the carotid bulb. The ICA should be clamped distal to the plaque to prevent dislodging of emboli.

Clamping of the ICA first, followed by the CCA and ECA, reduces the risk of plaque embolization into the cerebral circulation. EEG and SSEP changes should be monitored closely at this point, and any changes treated with induced hypertension or the use of a shunt.

An arteriotomy is made with a number 11 blade and opening is done with Potts scissors from the CCA into the ICA (Figures 17-5 and 17-6). The plaque is dissected from the arterial wall, ensuring all intimal flaps are removed (Figure 17-7). At this point, tacking sutures may be placed. Attention is then turned toward closure of the arteriotomy with or without a patch graft and 6-0 proline sutures are employed for closure (Figure 17-8). Opening of the ECA, CCA, followed by the ICA, allows for any remaining debris to flow out of the ECA before declamping of the ICA. The incision is then closed (Figure 17-9).

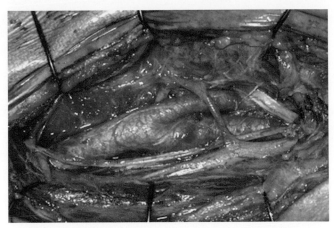

FIGURE 17-4   The common internal and external carotid vessels are dissected free. The facial vein can be seen crossing the carotid bifurcation and should be doubly ligated and divided. The hypoglossal nerve and descendens hypoglossi are easily visible and carefully protected during the operation. The superior thyroid artery is also identified and controlled. The internal jugular vein is well exposed in this dissection, but does not need to be seen extensively. *(Reprinted with permission from Winn HR. Youmans Neurological Surgery. Elsevier ©2011.)*

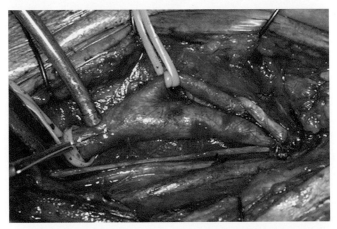

FIGURE 17-5   An arteriotomy is made in the common carotid artery with a number 11 knife blade. *(Reprinted with permission from Winn HR. Youmans Neurological Surgery. Elsevier ©2011.)*

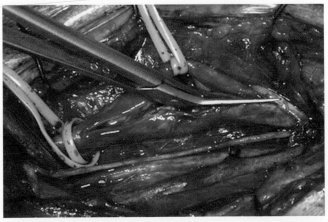

FIGURE 17-6   The arteriotomy is extended up the internal carotid artery with Pott's scissors. *(Reprinted with permission from Winn HR. Youmans Neurological Surgery. Elsevier ©2011.)*

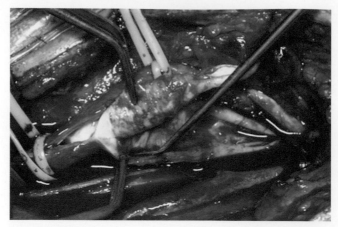

FIGURE 17-7   After an appropriate break point is established in the distal internal carotid artery, the plaque is dissected proximally into the common carotid artery. *(Reprinted with permission from Winn HR.* Youmans Neurological Surgery. *Elsevier ©2011.)*

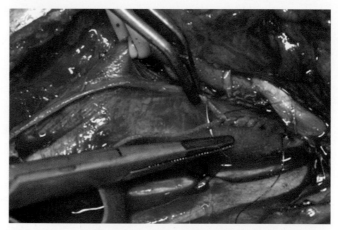

FIGURE 17-8   The forehand side of the graft is sewn in place with a running Prolene suture first. It is very important to keep the sutures uniform in their depth and distance from one another. *(Reprinted with permission from Winn HR.* Youmans Neurological Surgery. *Elsevier ©2011.)*

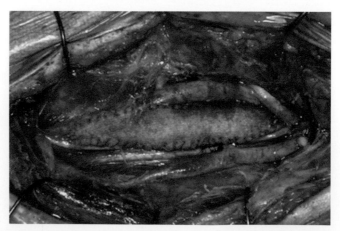

FIGURE 17-9   The final result after an endarterectomy, patch closure angioplasty, and restoration of flow. *(Reprinted with permission from Winn HR.* Youmans Neurological Surgery. *Elsevier ©2011.)*

Carotid Artery Stenting

Patients should be taking aspirin and a thienopyridine antiplatelet agent before stenting and angioplasty of carotid stenosis lesions. Access and angiography are performed, taking measurements of the carotid lesion's length, the tapering portions, and the vessel caliber proximal and distal to the stenosis. An appropriately sized distal protection device is then deployed. The stent and balloon delivery system are then crossed across the stenosis. The stent is deployed, ensuring an appropriate vessel landing length. Angioplasty before placing the stent may be utilized if the stent cannot be passed through the stenosis. Once the stent system is removed, post stent angioplasty is performed, and finally, the protection device is removed.

Complication Avoidance and Management

- Carotid endarterectomy
  - Hypoperfusion syndrome: intraoperative monitoring should be employed to identify patients who develop hypoperfusion syndrome intraoperatively. The risk of intraprocedural hypoperfusion during the period of cross-clamping of the ICA should be assessed by imaging the circle of Willis prior to the procedure. A dual balloon shunt (CCA to ICA) should be available and utilized for all cases if a hypoperfusion event occurs.
  - Embolic complications: heparinization during the procedure reduces the risk of embolic complications intraprocedurally. Use of antiplatelet agents varies; however, most surgeons will maintain a patient on at least one agent after the procedure.
  - Bleeding: Lining the arteriotomy site with absorbable hemostatic gauze such as Surgicel after closure of the arteriotomy and monitoring for 5 minutes prior to closure of the overlying soft tissues will help to ensure no bleeding occurs. If a large hematoma occurs which compromises the airway, intubate the patient and open and evacuate the hematoma (this can be opened at the bedside in emergent situations). CTA or ultrasound should be performed to evaluate for pseudoaneurysm or lumenal compromise in smaller hematomas that do not compromise the airway. Ultrasound may be nondiagnostic in the immediate postoperative period due to air in the operative site.
  - Cranial nerve injury
    - Facial nerve: occurs more frequently in high-riding bifurcation. Consider stenting if significantly high-riding bifurcation. Injury can be avoided by careful extension of the incision to the mastoid and avoidance of retraction against the mandibular ramus and avoidance of opening the parotid fascia.
    - Hypoglossal nerve: occurs more frequently with medialized internal carotid. If the ICA stenosis is significantly medialized, consider stenting. Injury can be avoided by carefully splitting the digastric and avoiding aggressive retraction against the body of the mandible.
    - Recurrent laryngeal nerve: the recurrent laryngeal nerve is a branch of the vagus nerve near the bifurcation. Dissection lateral to the carotid bulb should be minimized. Avoid lateral deep soft tissue retraction against the jugular or SCM and deep medial soft tissue retraction against the trachea.
  - Carotid occlusion: may result from intimal dissection flap, intramural hematoma at the clamp site, or thrombus formation in the lumen. If evident during the procedure due to lack of back bleeding, extend the arteriotomy incision and explore. If the occlusion is not identified, consider intraoperative angiography and endovascular intervention.
  - New postoperative deficit: CT head and CTA head and neck should be performed. If not large vessel occlusion, observe and consider MRI. If occlusion is at the level of the endarterectomy, consider re-exploration. However, if the occlusion is intracranial or at the skull base, angiogram and endovascular intervention should be considered.
  - Intraoperative bradycardia and hypotension: typically due to stimulation of the carotid body and occurs more frequently with left-sided CEA. Lidocaine can be

administered locally above the carotid bulb to block the carotid body. If not effective, glycopyrrolate, pressors, and atropine should be administered systemically.

- Carotid artery stenting
  - Renal injury: pre- and post-procedural hydration is essential for renal failure patients and sodium bicarbonate is used for renal protection.
  - Intraprocedure hypotension and bradycardia: occurs more frequently with left-sided stenting. Glycopyrrolate and pressors (Neo-Synephrine or dopamine) should be available for intraprocedural bradycardia or hypotension. Most endovascular providers pre-medicate prior to angioplasty with either glycopyrrolate or atropine.
  - Intraprocedural or post-procedural new neurologic deficit: all stenting should be performed with either proximal or distal embolic protection to avoid embolic complications. All patients should be heparinized intraprocedurally. All patients should be on both aspirin and Plavix starting 5 days before the procedure if possible. If not started prior to the procedure, the patient should be loaded with aspirin and Plavix after the procedure. Monitoring of platelet function assay to identify antiplatelet nonresponders may also be helpful in avoiding embolic complications. Intraoperative cerebral angiogram should be performed to evaluate for intracranial large vessel embolus. If a postoperative deficit occurs after closure of the arterial puncture, parenchymal brain imaging and vascular imaging of the head and neck should be performed non-invasively if possible. If a large vessel occlusion is present, endovascular intervention should be considered. If the lumen of the stent is compromised by encroachment through the stent by lipid-laden plaque in the immediate postoperative period, consider placement of a second stent. If neointimal hyperplasia occurs in a delayed fashion, consider cutting balloon angioplasty under embolic protection.

KEY PAPERS

Carotid endarterectomy for asymptomatic carotid stenosis: asymptomatic carotid surgery trial. *Stroke*. 2004;35:2425-2427.

Endarterectomy for asymptomatic carotid artery stenosis. *JAMA*. 1995;273(18):1421-1428.

Endovascular versus surgical treatment in patients with carotid stenosis in the Carotid and Vertebral Artery Transluminal Angioplasty Study (CAVATAS): a randomised trial. *The Lancet*. 2001;357(9270):1729-1737.

Randomised trial of endarterectomy for recently symptomatic carotid stenosis: final results of the MRC European Carotid Surgery Trial (ECST). *The Lancet*. 1998;351(9113):1379-1387.

The North American Symptomatic Carotid Endarterectomy Trial (NASCET) Collaborators. *Stroke*. 1999;30:1751-1758.

Case 18

Ischemic Stroke Management

Joel R. Martin, MD ● J. Scott Pannell, MD ● Scott E. Olson, MD ●
Alexander A. Khalessi, MD

Presentation

An overweight 69-year-old male with diabetes, coronary artery disease, and hypertension presents with acute onset altered mental status, right-sided weakness, and aphasia. Patient was last normal 4 hours ago.

- PMH: type II diabetes, coronary artery disease, and hypertension
- Exam:
  - Hemiplegia of the lower right half of the contralateral face
  - Hemiplegia of the right upper and lower extremities
  - Speech impairments and aphasia
  - Left gaze preference

Differential Diagnosis

- Vascular
  - Cerebrovascular ischemia
    - Thromboembolic stroke
    - Intracranial atherosclerotic disease
  - Transient ischemic attack
  - Intracranial hemorrhage
    - Hypertension
    - Tumor
    - Amyloid angiography
    - AVM
    - Aneurysm
    - Reperfusion injury
    - Coagulopathy
    - Infection
    - Trauma
  - Hypertensive encephalopathy
- Other
  - Partial complex seizure
  - Hypoglycemia or hyperglycemia – can often mimic ischemic stroke
  - Migraine aura

Initial Imaging

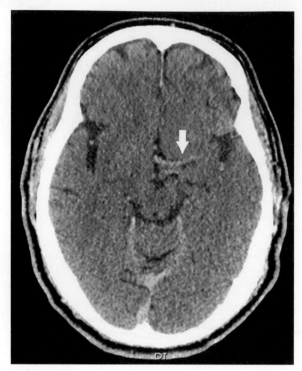

FIGURE 18-1

Imaging Description

- Noncontrast CT scan of the head shows a left dense MCA, suggesting a left MCA thrombus and infarct. Mild loss of posterior left insular cortical ribbon but largely the left. Mild smudging of the left putamen. No other definite signs of acute infarct are demonstrated in the left cerebrum. Head CTA shows acute thrombus and a meniscus sign at the origin of the left MCA, but a lack of opacification of almost the entire left MCA territory.
- Differential: acute thrombus or embolus, atherosclerotic plaque

Further Workup

- Laboratory
  - Serum glucose, BMP, CBC, and serum coagulation studies
  - ESR, CRP, cardiac enzymes, an ECG, toxicology screen, lipid profile, Hb1AC, and TTE with bubble
- Imaging
  - Noncontrast CT of the head
  - CTA of the head and neck
- Consultants
  - Neurology for stroke
  - Interventional neuroradiology

Pathophysiology

Stroke can be divided into two main types: ischemic and hemorrhagic. Ischemic stroke is the most common type, making up about 80% to 90% of all strokes. During an ischemic stroke, blood supply to a vascular territory of the brain is reduced, leading to dysfunction of the brain tissue in that area (Figure 18-2). Ischemic stroke can be caused by four general conditions: thrombosis, an embolism, systemic hypoperfusion, or venous thrombosis. Decreased cerebral blood flow, usually <10 mL/100 g of tissue/min, can lead to cell death.

TABLE 18-1

IV TPA AND MECHANICAL THROMBECTOMY GUIDELINES—cont'd

All patients should receive endovascular therapy with a stent retriever if they meet all the following criteria:
- Pre-stroke modified Rankin score (mRS): 0-1
- Acute ischemic stroke receiving IV rtPA within 4.5 hours of onset according to guidelines above
- Causative occlusion of the internal carotid artery or proximal middle cerebral artery (M1)
- Age 18 years and over
- NIHSS score of 6 or greater
- Alberta Stroke Program Early Computed Tomography Score (ASPECTS) of 6 or greater
- Treatment can be initiated (groin puncture) within 6 hours of symptom onset

Patients with similarly presenting symptomatic basilar and left-sided M2 occlusions should also be considered for mechanical thrombectomy; however, no randomized controlled data are available to support this practice.

Interventional Technique

Digital subtraction angiography (DSA) is the angiographic gold standard for assessing the vasculature of the brain. First, it requires an arterial puncture with a wide-bore needle and the introduction of a flexible catheter into the carotid arteries and injection of a contrast agent to visualize vasculature. Next, angiography of the anterior circulation, by injection of the left common carotid artery, which demonstrates occlusion of the left M1 segment.

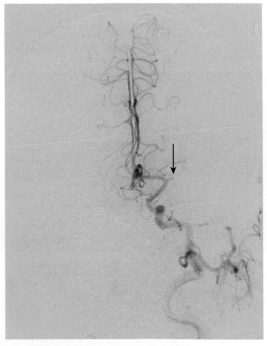

FIGURE 18-3 Angiogram of the anterior circulation, demonstrating occlusion of the left M1 segment of the MCA (black arrow).

Under roadmap/overlay guidance, the left M1 segment, beyond the level of the occlusion to the inferior trunk of the MCA, is catheterized next. Once the catheter is across the level of the occlusion, an angiogram of the distal MCA is performed and demonstrates normal MCA branches and persistent occlusion of the M1 segment.

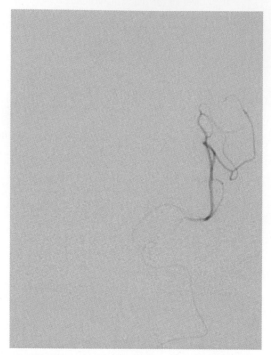

FIGURE 18-4   Angiogram of the distal MCA demonstrating the microcatheter beyond the occlusion in the inferior division of the MCA.

Next, a stent retriever is deployed across the occlusion and withdrawn through an aspiration catheter at the level of the proximal clot face, under direct fluoroscopic observation. Aspiration is performed at the clot face to reduce the probability of conversion to a more proximal occlusion.

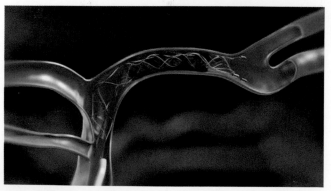

FIGURE 18-5   A stent retriever is deployed across the occlusion and withdrawn through an aspiration catheter. *(Reprinted with permission from Covidien.)*

Next, subsequent angiography is performed, which revealed recanalization of the MCA with irregularity of the proximal M1 segment consistent with a ruptured plaque. Final angiography of the anterior circulation by injection of the left ICA.

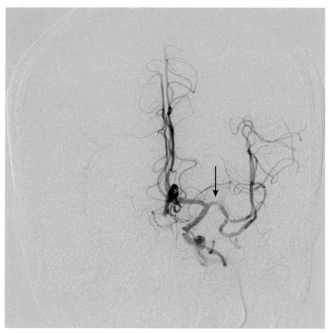

FIGURE 18-6 Final angiography of the anterior circulation by injection of the left ICA demonstrating recanalization of the anterior circulation. There is residual non-flow limiting stenosis of the M1 segment which may be related to vasospasm or intracranial atherosclerotic disease.

After final angiograms were performed, the catheter system is removed, and the right common femoral arteriotomy is closed with a vascular-closure device.

Complication Avoidance and Management

- Groin hematoma
  - The most common complication after cerebral angiogram is a groin hematoma at the site of arteriotomy. The risk of hematoma can be reduced by requiring the patient to maintain a straight leg and avoid hip flexion for several hours after the procedure. Likewise, avoiding heavy lifting (>15 pounds) for the week after the angiogram will mitigate further injury to the arteriotomy.
- Reperfusion injury
  - Hyperperfusion after embolectomy is defined as a major increase in cerebral blood flow that far exceeds the metabolic demand of the brain tissue. It is a rare, but serious, complication after revascularization. Ensuring proper blood pressure management, especially control of initial and delayed hypertension, can prevent reperfusion syndrome.
- Renal injury
  - Radiopaque contrast can lead to a usually reversible form of acute kidney injury (AKI). Pretreating patients with prior kidney injury, ensuring postangiogram repletion of fluids, and avoidance of NSAIDs can help mitigate or prevent AKI.

KEY PAPERS

Berkhemer O, et al. A randomized trial of intraarterial treatment for acute ischemic stroke. *N Engl J Med.* 2015;372(1):11-20.

CAST: randomised placebo-controlled trial of early aspirin use in 20,000 patients with acute ischaemic stroke. CAST (Chinese Acute Stroke Trial) Collaborative Group. *Lancet.* 1997;349:1641-1649.

Gupta R, Connolly ES, Mayer S, et al. Hemicraniectomy for massive middle cerebral artery territory infarction: a systematic review. *Stroke.* 2004;35:539-543.

Hemphill J, Bonovich D, Besmertis L, et al. The ICH score: a simple, reliable grading scale for intracerebral hemorrhage. *Stroke.* 2001;32:891-897.

Huttner H, Schwab S. Malignant middle cerebral artery infarctation: clinical characteristics, treatment strategies, and future perspectives. *Lancet Neurol*. 2009;8:949-958.

Mendelow A, Gregson B, et al. Early surgery versus initial conservative treatment in patients with spontaneous supratentorial intracerebral haematomas in the International Surgical Trial in Intracerebral Haemorrhage (STICH): a randomised trial. *Lancet*. 2005;365:387-397.

The International Stroke Trial (IST): a randomised trial of aspirin, subcutaneous heparin, both, or neither among 19435 patients with acute ischaemic stroke. International Stroke Trial Collaborative Group. *Lancet*. 1997;349(9065):1569-1581.

Vahedi K, Hofmeijer J, Juettler E, et al. Early decompressive surgery in malignant infarction of the middle cerebral artery: a pooled analysis of three randomised controlled trials. *Lancet Neurol*. 2007;6:215-222.

Yao Y, Mao Y, Zhou L. Decompressive craniectomy for massive cerebral infarction with enlarged cruciate duraplasty. *Acta Neurochir (Wien)*. 2007;149:1219-1221.

Section II Nontraumatic Cranial Lesions

Case 19

Vestibular Schwannoma

Robert M. Lober, MD, PhD ● Abdulrazag Ajlan, MD

Presentation

A 43-year-old female presents with left-sided nonpulsatile tinnitus and progressive hearing loss for 1 year, causing difficulty using a cell phone. She denies vertigo but has mild loss of balance with quick head movements.

- PMH: otherwise unremarkable
- FH: no family history of hearing loss, brain tumors, or neurofibromatosis
- Exam
  - Neurologic
    - Normal mentation
    - Extraocular muscles intact; no facial hypoesthesia or weakness
    - Weber test lateralizes to the right; air conduction is better than bone conduction on Rinne test bilaterally.
    - Full and symmetric strength in the extremities
    - Normal gait
    - No nystagmus or incoordination; no rotation on Fukuda testing
  - HEENT
    - No dysmorphic features suggestive of syndromic hearing loss
    - Ear canals clear, and normal tympanic membranes
  - Skin
    - No neurocutaneous stigmata (e.g., café au lait spots with neurofibromatosis, albinism with Waardenburg syndrome)

Differential Diagnosis

- Vascular
  - Infarction
- Infectious
  - Conductive hearing loss from otitis externa
  - Tympanic membrane perforation from otitis media
  - Postmeningitis hearing loss
  - Viral labrinthitis (e.g., mumps, measles, rubella, cytomegalovirus, or HIV)
- Neoplastic
  - Vestibular schwannoma
  - Cerebellopontine angle (CPA) meningioma, epidermoid, or neuroma
  - Petrous bone chordoma or chondrosarcoma
  - Glomus tumor of middle ear
  - Osteoma of external auditory canal
  - Paraneoplastic syndrome of the inner ear

- Drug induced (ototoxin exposure)
  - Medications – diuretics, salicylates, aminoglycosides, quinine, or chemotherapy
  - Industrial substances – heavy metals and solvents
- Idiopathic
  - Otosclerosis (fixation of stapes at the oval window)
  - Meniere's disease (endolymphatic hydrops)
  - Presbycusis
  - Neurodegenerative disorders (e.g., Hunter's syndrome)
  - Sensory motor neuropathies (e.g., Friedrich's ataxia or Charcot-Marie-Tooth disease)
- Congenital
  - Cochlear aplasia
  - Congenital cholesteatoma of the middle ear
  - >300 congenital syndromes associated with hearing impairment (1 : 1000)
- Autoimmune
  - Central hearing loss from multiple sclerosis
- Traumatic
  - Sensorineural hearing loss from noise trauma to organ of Corti
  - Perforation of tympanic membrane
  - Posttraumatic acquired cholesteatoma after a tympanic membrane perforation
  - Temporal bone fracture involving the labyrinth
- Endocrine and metabolic
  - Vitamin B_{12} or folic acid deficiency

Initial Imaging

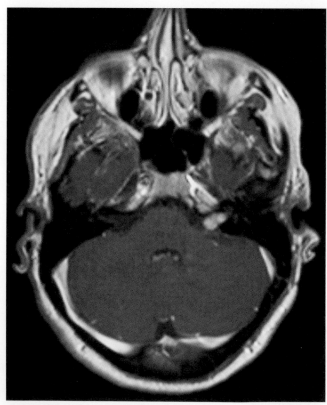

FIGURE 19-1

Imaging Description and Differential

- Enhancing CPA mass along the intracanalicular and extracanalicular portions of the cranial nerve VII/VIII complex with expansion of the internal auditory canal (IAC). There is no compression of the cerebellum.
- Differential: vestibular schwannoma or meningioma

Further Workup

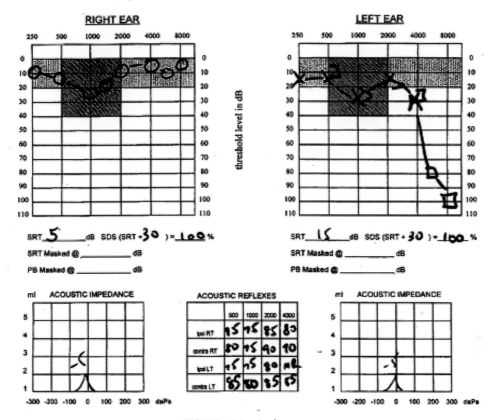

FIGURE 19-2   Audiometry

- Audiometry shows normal right-sided hearing, with a speech reception threshold (SRT) of 5 dB. The patient demonstrates 100% word recognition at 35 dB on the right (reported as the speech discrimination score [SDS]).
- Left-sided hearing increasingly diminishes above 2 kHz, from a threshold of 15 dB at 2 kHz to 30 dB at 4 kHz, and 80 dB at higher frequencies. The average pure tone threshold (for 0.05 kHz, 1 kHz, 2 kHz, and 3 kHz) is about 22 dB. The SRT is 15 dB with an SDS of 100% at 45 dB.
- The Gardner-Robertson hearing scale ranges from grade I to V, with higher grades corresponding to worsening function in pure tone perception and speech discrimination (I is good and V is deaf). Grade III is nonserviceable hearing, corresponding to ≥50 dB pure tone average and <50% speech discrimination. This patient has grade I hearing with a pure tone average of 22 dB and SDS of 100% in the affected ear.
- Acoustic reflex testing removes any bias introduced by a patient's level of cooperation and involves measurement of stapedius contraction in response to a sound stimulus. This has high sensitivity, but low specificity.
- If hearing function is sufficient, but still impaired by a vestibular schwannoma, brainstem audio-evoked responses reliably detect interaural latency prolongation in wave V, which corresponds to a delay in signal reaching the inferior colliculus on the affected side.

- Electronystagmography is used in the assessment of vestibular function and often demonstrates reduced or absent responses on the affected side during bithermal caloric testing. A large tumor without an ipsilateral hypoactive caloric response would be more consistent with other types of cerebellopontine angle tumors (e.g., meningioma).

Pathophysiology

Vestibular schwannomas originate on a vestibular division of cranial nerve VIII. They often arise near the vestibular (Scarpa's) ganglion, just lateral to the junction of central and peripheral myelin. They may expand by eroding the IAC laterally and compressing the brainstem medially. Sporadic tumors are unilateral and more common, whereas tumors associated with neurofibromatosis 2 (NF2) are either bilateral or associated with other tumors. In both cases, schwannoma tumorigenesis results from decreased expression or activity of the protein merlin, encoded by the *NF2* gene on chromosome 22. Microscopically, schwannomas are well circumscribed by a pseudocapsule and contain a biphasic pattern of spindle cells (Antoni A pattern) and loose microcystic areas (Antoni B pattern), along with areas of nuclear palisading (Verocay bodies).

Treatment Options

- Observation
  - During an observation period of 5 years, approximately 2/3 of tumors do not grow, and about 1/2 of patients maintain their hearing.
  - Tumors exceeding 2 cm in maximal dimension have a higher probability of growth.
  - Initial hearing loss predicts a greater chance of hearing loss over time.
  - Additional symptoms may arise, including tinnitus, vertigo, or disequilibrium.
- Stereotactic radiosurgery (SRS)
  - Usually reserved for tumors <3 cm in largest diameter (or <10 cm^3), and without symptomatic brainstem compression.
  - Long-term tumor control rate is over 95%.
  - After 5 years, 60% to 80% of patients maintain useful hearing, leading some authors to recommend SRS as the initial treatment of choice.
  - Malignant transformation after SRS does not appear to be higher than spontaneous transformation in the natural history.
- Surgical
  - Complete resection is often obtained. To preserve facial function, a goal of near total resection may be preferable to gross total resection if an attenuated facial nerve is tightly adherent to tumor such that aggressive dissection would be required to remove all tumor. Intraoperative neurophysiologic monitoring of brainstem auditory evoked potentials and facial nerve function is employed. Adjacent cranial nerves may also be monitored, depending on their proximity to the tumor.
  - Retrosigmoid approach: considered for tumors in the CPA with limited extension into the IAC fundus, especially for patients with useful hearing. Hearing preserved in 20% to 50% of tumors <2 cm and 50% to 80% for tumors <1 cm.
  - Translabyrinthine approach: considered when there is already loss of serviceable hearing, or for tumors >2 cm in which hearing preservation is unlikely. Allows access to the lateral recess of the IAC, as well as identification of the facial nerve at the labyrinthine segment to facilitate its protection.
  - Middle fossa approach: was selected for the current patient; it provides exposure to the IAC contents from a superior trajectory. It is indicated for attempted hearing preservation in tumors with posterior fossa extension of <5 to 10 mm in diameter.

Surgical Technique

Here a middle fossa craniotomy with intraoperative neurophysiologic monitoring was used. The patient is supine, with a shoulder roll and head turned contralaterally, parallel to the floor. An incision is made anterior to the tragus, and temporalis muscle is divided and retracted, preserving the blood supply. A 4 × 4 cm craniotomy is fashioned, 2/3 anterior and 1/3 posterior to the external auditory meatus, limited superiorly by the squamosal suture and inferiorly by the middle fossa floor. Starting from the posterior lateral petrous ridge, the dura is elevated posterior to anterior, and lateral to medial, toward the foramen ovale. The greater superficial petrosal nerve (GSPN) is identified and preserved. The roof of the IAC is drilled on a line bisecting the angle between the GSPN and the arcuate eminence, exposing intracanalicular tumor for resection.

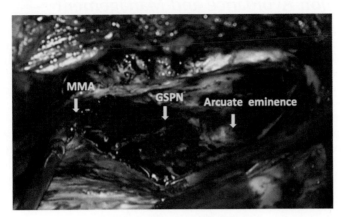

FIGURE 19-3   Dura elevation.

An alternative is the retrosigmoid approach, in which the head is rotated toward the contralateral side. An incision is made approximately two fingerbreadths posterior to the pinna, just medial to the digastric groove, which is generally in line with the sigmoid sinus. Approximately 1/3 of the incision is above the inio-meatal line, which roughly corresponds to the transverse sinus. A 3 × 4 cm craniotomy is fashioned, exposing posterior fossa dura laterally and superiorly to the transverse-sigmoid sinus junction. The durotomy is based on the sigmoid sinus. Arachnoid of the cisterna magna is opened to release cerebrospinal fluid (CSF) for brain relaxation. Cranial nerves are identified for preservation and tumor is debulked centrally before extracapsular sharp dissection to separate nerves from tumor. Extracanalicular tumor is resected and then the posterior rim of the IAC is drilled to expose any intracanalicular portion for resection.

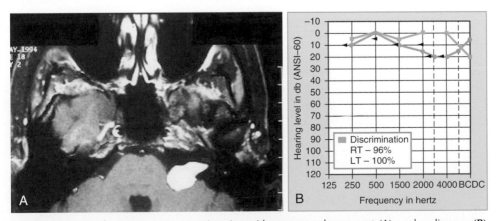

FIGURE 19-4   Axial magnetic resonance imaging with contrast enhancement **(A)**, and audiogram **(B)**, demonstrating an acoustic neuroma in a patient who would be a candidate for hearing preservation surgery. (Winn: Youmans's Neurological Surgery. Fig. 133-3) *(Reprinted with permission from Winn HR. Youmans Neurological Surgery. Philadelphia, PA: Elsevier Limited, Oxford; 2011. Figure 133-3.)*

The translabyrinthine approach was not considered in this case because the patient had serviceable hearing, and the size of the tumor was <2 cm, providing a reasonable likelihood of hearing preservation with alternate methods. This approach begins with a curved incision posterior to the pinna, extending from above the ear to the mastoid tip. A mastoidectomy is performed, exposing the antrum and tip of the incus to determine the position of the facial nerve. Tumor is debulked centrally and then peeled from facial nerve. Closure requires harvesting of an abdominal fat graft to fill the dural and bony defect.

Complication Avoidance and Management

- Middle fossa approach
  - During this approach, brain retraction risks brain contusion or infarction, particularly on the dominant side with a prominent vein of Labbé. Elevation of dura can injure the GSPN, causing eye dryness from lacrimal dysfunction. Care must also be taken in drilling the bone above the labyrinthine segment of the facial nerve, where the vestibule and cochlea may be injured.
- Retrosigmoid approach
  - During this approach, it is preferable to open the arachnoid of the cisterna magna to allow egress of CSF and brain relaxation. The cerebellum can be injured if the dural opening and drainage of CSF from the cisterna magna is not accomplished in a timely manner. Drilling of the IAC should be accompanied by copious irrigation to avoid thermal damage to intracanalicular nerves. Any exposed air cells should be waxed to prevent CSF leakage.
- Translabyrinthine approach
  - The translabyrinthine approach carries a significant risk of CSF leakage, and thus both the middle ear and mastoid air cells must be packed to minimize this risk.

KEY PAPERS

Chamoun R, MacDonald J, Shelton C, et al. Surgical approaches for resection of vestibular schwannomas: translabyrinthine, retrosigmoid, and middle fossa approaches. *Neurosurg Focus*. 2012;33(3):E9.

Gonzalez LF, Lekovic GP, Porter RW, et al. Surgical approaches for resection of acoustic neuromas. *Barrow Quarterly*. 2004;22-32.

Tanriover N, Sanus GZ, Ulu MO, et al. Middle fossa approach: microsurgical anatomy and surgical technique from the neurosurgical perspective. *Surg Neurol*. 2009;71(5):586-596.

Case 20

Sphenoid Wing Meningioma

Omar Choudhri, MD

Presentation

A 40-year-old otherwise healthy female presents with 6 years of worsening headaches and 2 years of memory problems. She had a 2-minute episode of sudden onset of weakness of both legs, without loss of consciousness.

- PMH: prior urinary tract infections, but otherwise unremarkable
- Exam:
  - Awake, alert, and intact speech
  - Cranial nerves and visual fields intact
  - Mild left pronator drift
  - 4+/5 weakness in left leg
  - Gait balanced
  - Mild numbness in left arm and leg

Differential Diagnosis

- Neoplastic
  - Primary tumor
  - Metastatic tumor
- Vascular
  - AVM
  - Cavernous malformation
  - Giant aneurysm with mass effect
  - Stroke/TIA
  - Complex migraine with aura
- Infectious
  - Brain abscess
  - Meningitis
  - Cerebral vasculitis
- Trauma
  - Intracranial hemorrhage/subdural hematoma
- Metabolic
  - Hyponatremia
  - Vitamin deficiencies
  - Sarcoidosis

Initial Imaging

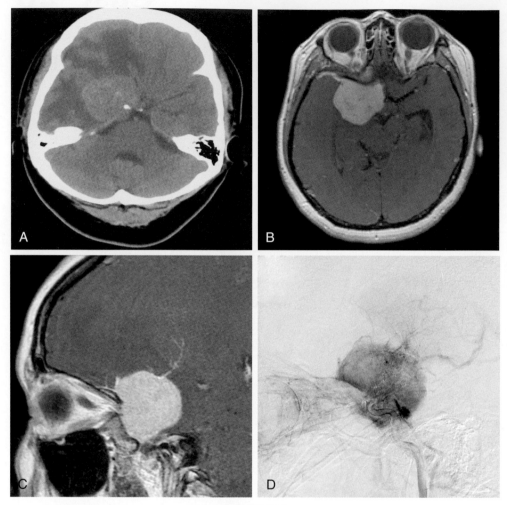

FIGURE 20-1

Imaging Description and Differential Diagnosis

- Noncontrast axial CT head in Figure 20-1A shows an isodense mass along the medial portion of lesser wing of sphenoid. There is associated edema in the right frontal and temporal lobes. The mass has scattered areas of calcification and is causing cisternal/sulcal effacement.
- Postcontrast axial and sagittal MRI in Figure 20-1B and C show an enhanced extraaxial mass along the medial sphenoid wing. The lesion is dural, based along the lesser sphenoid wing, and has a prominent dural tail. It engulfs the right carotid and middle cerebral arteries.
- Differential: sphenoid wing meningioma causing mass effect. Other less likely possibilities include: atypical/malignant meningioma, hemangiopericytoma, solitary fibrous tumor, dural based metastasis, and granuloma.

Further Workup

- Laboratory workup
  - Routine labs
  - ESR, CRP

- Imaging
  - Cerebral angiogram: A cerebral angiogram should especially be done in the case of large meningiomas that may be vascular and benefit from preoperative embolization. Sphenoid wing meningiomas derive vascular supply from the sphenoidal branch of the middle meningeal artery and sometimes from the internal carotid artery. The cerebral angiogram in Figure 20-1D shows a prominent sunburst pattern of vascular blush that persists into the venous phase.
  - CT of the chest, abdomen, and pelvis should be performed when there is suspicion of dural based metastasis.
- Consultants
  - Neurointerventional radiology: for cerebral angiogram, preoperative embolization, balloon test occlusion, and evaluation of the extracranial vessels for vascular bypass if necessary
  - Ophthalmology: Medial and clinoidal lesions may compress the optic nerve, or involve the cavernous sinus, leading to blindness or diplopia.

Pathophysiology

Meningiomas arise from meningothelial arachnoid cap cells and are usually benign, WHO grade I. These are slow-growing tumors that often are asymptomatic until they are large enough to cause mass effect.

Atypical and malignant meningiomas, WHO grade II and III, respectively, have a more aggressive course. Approximately 50% to 60% of meningiomas have 22q allelic loss of the NF2 gene and such meningiomas can be part of the NF2 syndrome.

Sphenoid wing meningiomas, based along the sphenoid ridge, constitute approximately 15% to 20% of all meningiomas. They may be spherical, en plaque along the wing, or both. The lateral cavernous sinus and sphenoparietal sinus are closely related to these meningiomas, and arteriovenous shunting into these venous structures is common.

Management Options

- Serial imaging: Asymptomatic lesions may be followed with serial MRI to document enlargement before treatment.
- Medical: Corticosteroids, such as Decadron, may be useful for symptomatic edema and mass effect before surgery.
- Radiation: Stereotactic radiosurgery and external beam radiation may be useful for small sphenoid wing meningiomas, tumors in patients with contraindications to surgery, or tumor remnants that enlarge after surgery.
- Endovascular: Preoperative embolization of meningiomas may be useful for large sphenoid wing meningiomas. Polyvinyl alcohol particles or liquid embolics (onyx or nBCA glue) are injected through the middle meningeal artery. Blood supply from the internal carotid artery should not be embolized.
- Microsurgical
  - Frontotemporal craniotomy: A frontotemporal craniotomy centered at the pterion and encompassing the sphenoid ridge is the most common approach. Tumor extension into the orbit warrants orbital osteotomy to reduce the brain retraction needed for exposure. Similarly, inferior extension along the middle fossa floor may warrant zygomatic osteotomy.
  - Dolenc approach: For lesions extending into the cavernous sinus, some surgeons use the Dolenc approach to resect the cavernous portion of the sphenoid wing meningioma.

Surgical Technique

The patient is positioned supine; head turned 45 degrees to align the sphenoid ridge vertically along the floor (Figure 20-2A). Mayfield pins, stereotactic MRI guided navigation, intraoperative neuromonitoring (upper and lower extremity SSEPs, MEPs, and cranial nerves (CN) III/IV/VI in cases of cavernous sinus lesions), Decadron, and mannitol are useful.

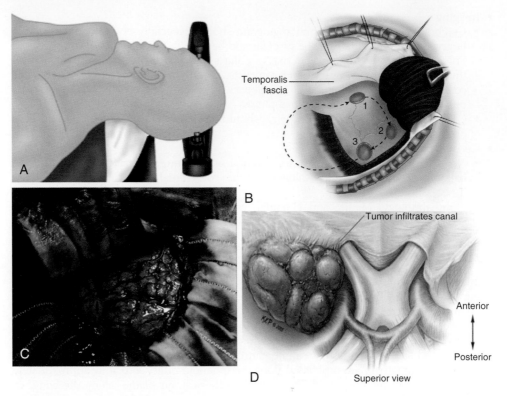

FIGURE 20-2   (A), **(B)**, and **(C)** illustrate the surgical exposure of the sphenoid wing. **(D)** illustrates the tumor infiltrating the dura of the optic canal and the relationship of the tumor with the carotid artery, optic nerve and chiasm. *((A), (B) & (C) reprinted with permission from Jandial R, McCormick P, Black PM. Core Techniques in Operative Neurosurgery. Elsevier; 2011. (D) reprinted with permission from Sughrue ME, Rutkowski MJ, Chen CJ, et al. Modern surgical outcomes following surgery for sphenoid wing meningiomas,* J Neurosurg *119:86–93, 2013.)*

A curvilinear incision behind the frontotemporal hairline usually allows adequate exposure. A standard frontotemporal craniotomy (Figure 20-2B) is completed using burr holes placed at the key hole (1), inferior temporal bone (2), and posterior frontal bone (3). There may be hyperostosis in overlying calvarial bone, especially in large sphenoid wing meningiomas that extend laterally along the sphenoid wing. The dura is often highly vascularized, and early coagulation of the middle meningeal artery is recommended. The sphenoid ridge is then drilled flat. Application of bone wax during drilling of the sphenoid bone can limit blood loss. Dura is tacked up along the craniotomy edges to prevent an epidural hematoma. The dura is then opened in a C-shaped fashion and flapped antero-inferolaterally, toward the orbital and sphenoid ridges (Figure 20-2C).

Using an operating microscope, dissection begins along the anterior sylvian fissure and is continued medially to release cerebrospinal fluid from the arachnoid cistern. Upon encountering the tumor's base, the tumor is disconnected from its dural blood supply by dissecting along the sphenoid ridge, thus devascularizing the tumor as much as possible before debulking. Aggressive bipolar cauterization along the sphenoidal dural surface also allows mobilization of the tumor. Once the tumor is appropriately devascularized, intracapsular debulking is often necessary. The capsule is entered after bipolaring its surface.

Sphenoid wing meningiomas can vary in texture from soft to extremely fibrous. Tools useful for debulking include bipolar and suction (for soft lesions), Cavitron ultrasonic surgical aspirator (CUSA), loop electrocautery, and NICO myriad system. Stereotactic navigation is useful for identification of critical nerves and blood vessels. Once a large portion of tumor is debulked, dissection is continued along the tumor capsule's outer surface, which is often external to the arachnoid. Often, a CSF cleft between the meningioma capsule and the pia-arachnoid aids dissection. Keeping this arachnoid intact and dissecting the tumor away from it helps prevent injury to the internal carotid, middle cerebral, and anterior cerebral arteries; their branches; and the optic nerve. Some tumors traverse the pia and invade cortex. Identification of the optic apparatus, including the optic nerve and chiasm, is extremely important in this dissection (Figure 20-2D).

Complication Avoidance and Management

- Intraoperative bleeding
  - This can be encountered in large tumors with robust dural blood supply. A preoperative cerebral angiogram with embolization is recommended in these cases. Anesthesia should be informed of significant bleeding, and hematocrit monitoring and transfusion should be used as needed.
- Cranial nerve palsies
  - In medial sphenoid wing meningiomas involving the cavernous sinus, injury to CN III/IV and VI can occur during resection. Intraoperative neurophysiologic cranial nerve monitoring is useful in identifying these nerves and avoiding their injury by overly aggressive dissection. Injury from pressure on the optic nerve can be avoided by debulking the tumor before working around the capsule.
- Stroke and large vessel injury
  - Injury to ICA and MCA branches may occur during dissection, leading to an infarct. A micro-Doppler, intraoperative indocyanine green angiography and computer-assisted navigation can help avoid vascular injury. Hemorrhage from the cavernous sinus is usually venous and controllable with pressure and hemostatic agents.

KEY PAPERS

Abdel-Aziz KM, Froelich SC, Dagnew E, et al. Large sphenoid wing meningiomas involving the cavernous sinus: conservative surgical strategies for better functional outcomes. *Neurosurgery*. 2004;54(6):1375-1383, discussion 1383-1384.

Behari S, Giri PJ, Shukla D, et al. Surgical strategies for giant medial sphenoid wing meningiomas: a new scoring system for predicting extent of resection. *Acta Neurochir (Wien)*. 2008;150(9):865-877.

Bikmaz K, Mrak R, Al-Mefty O. Management of bone-invasive, hyperostotic sphenoid wing meningiomas. *J Neurosurg*. 2007;107(5):905-912.

Langevin CJ, Hanasono MM, Riina HA, et al. Lateral transzygomatic approach to sphenoid wing meningiomas. *Neurosurgery*. 2010;67(2 suppl Operative):377-384.

Sughrue ME, Rutkowski MJ, Chen CJ, et al. Modern surgical outcomes following surgery for sphenoid wing meningiomas. *J Neurosurg*. 2013;119(1):86-93.

Case 21

Cerebellar Cystic Hemangioblastoma

J. Dawn Waters, MD ● Griffith R. Harsh IV, MD

Presentation

A 25-year-old woman presents with 2 months of worsening headaches, accompanied by nausea, vomiting, and imbalance. The symptoms are particularly intense in the mornings. She has experienced 2 years of intermittent headaches.

- PMH: none
- Exam:
  - Vital signs, cranial nerves, strength, sensation, and reflexes are all normal.
  - Cerebellar exam demonstrates mild difficulty with tandem gait. No dysdiadochokinesia
  - No papilledema

Differential Diagnosis

The history of morning headaches with nausea is suggestive of increased intracranial pressure, often caused by an intracranial mass or hydrocephalus.

- Neoplastic
  - Metastasis
  - Primary glial tumor
  - Meningioma
- Congenital
  - Chiari malformation
- Vascular
  - AVM
- Autoimmune
  - Tumefactive multiple sclerosis
- Infectious
  - Cerebral abscess
- Other
  - Pseudotumor
  - Pregnancy

Initial Imaging

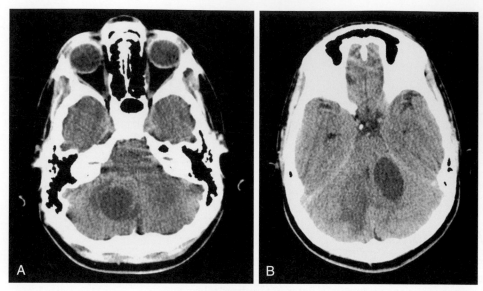

FIGURE 21-1

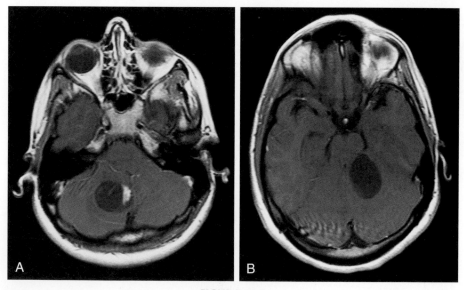

FIGUR E 21-2

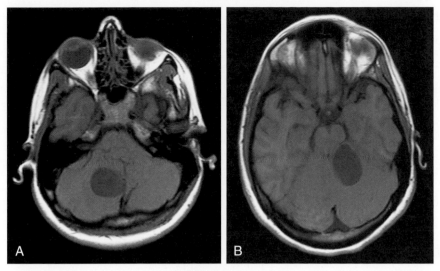

FIGURE 21-3

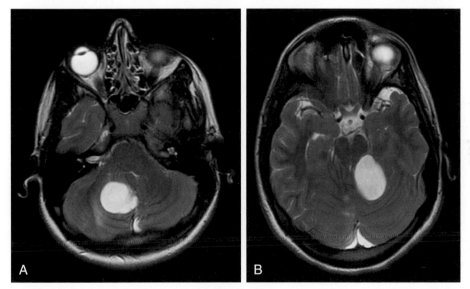

FIGURE 21-4

Imaging Description and Differential

- CT brain: Two cystic lesions in the cerebellum with mild surrounding edema and effacement of the fourth ventricle. Temporal horns appear enlarged (not shown) without significant enlargement of other parts of the lateral or third ventricles.
- MRI brain: Cystic lesions demonstrate fluid signal without restricted diffusion (not shown). Enhancing mural nodule is seen in the medial wall of the right cerebellar cyst (Figure 21-2A).
- Differential:
  - Metastasis
  - Cystic cerebellar hemangioblastoma
  - Cystic glioma (e.g., juvenile pilocytic astrocytoma)

Further Workup

- Laboratory
  - CBC may demonstrate polycythemia.
  - Consider evaluation for catecholamine metabolites if von Hippel-Lindau disease (vHL) associated pheochromocytoma is suspected.
- Imaging
  - Systemic tumor workup may include chest X-ray, CT chest/abdomen/pelvis, and ophthalmic examination.
  - MRI with and without contrast of entire spine to evaluate for multiple hemangioblastomas in the setting of possible vHL
  - Angiography may help characterize vascularity and provide an opportunity for preoperative embolization.
- Consultants
  - Genetic counselor for the patient and her relatives

Pathophysiology

Cerebellar hemangioblastoma may occur sporadically or in association with vHL. Sporadic cases tend to occur in older patients, typically in the fourth decade, as a solitary cerebellar lesion. For patients with vHL, these lesions appear more commonly in the third decade. Close to a third of patients with cerebellar hemangioblastoma have vHL. Conversely, over half of vHL patients develop cerebellar hemangioblastoma.

Cerebellar hemangioblastoma is a benign vascular lesion composed of capillaries lined with endothelial cells, along with pericytes and stromal cells. Cysts are found in about 70% of cases.

In vHL, cerebellar hemangioblastomas demonstrate alternating periods of enlargement and stability. Cystic tumors enlarge more frequently. Untreated tumors sometimes remain stable in size for several years, but they are not known to shrink spontaneously. Patients with symptomatic tumors experience relief after tumor resection in 98% of cases, and preoperative hydrocephalus is cured after tumor resection in over 94% of cases.

Treatment Options

- Medical
  - Corticosteroids provide transient symptomatic relief from edema and mass effect.
- Biopsy and stereotactic drainage of cysts
  - Minimally invasive option is rarely indicated because the diagnostic nodule is hypervascular and a drained cyst often reexpands rapidly.
- Radiation
  - Stereotactic radiosurgery targeting the nodule is effective in controlling the growth of solid tumor.
  - Rarely indicated for cystic tumors causing mass effect
- Interventional
  - Preoperative embolization is rarely useful for large tumors as their blood supply is incompletely segregated from that of surrounding parenchyma.
- Surgical
  - Complete resection is curative and thus preferred for sporadic cerebellar hemangioblastomas.
  - In the setting of vHL, surgery is generally reserved for symptomatic or rapidly growing lesions.

Surgical Technique

Consider using intraoperative image guidance and neuromonitoring. Once under general anesthesia, the patient may be positioned in a standard prone posture for a midline suboccipital approach. Slight head flexion aids the exposure. Follow the avascular plane in the midline muscular raphe to minimize blood loss, muscle injury, and difficulty in closure, while exposing the suboccipital bone and high cervical spinous processes and lamina as needed. Avoid lateral dissection at the foramen magnum and C1 to prevent vertebral artery injury.

Broad openings of bone and dura decompress the cerebellum. Several burr holes permit a suboccipital craniotomy that allows for later reconstruction of the skull. Careful epidural dissection prevents venous sinus injury upon bone removal. Release of CSF from the cisterna magna, or drainage of a tumor cyst, can prevent herniation of a compressed cerebellum. The dura may be opened in a V or Y shape and hinged superiorly at the transverse sinus and torcula. Dural tack-up sutures are useful in controlling epidural bleeding.

The operating microscope is particularly useful for deeper lesions. Once the lesion and cyst are identified, the goal is to remove the enhancing nodule en bloc. Piecemeal removal risks dropped metastasis and excessive bleeding from the vascular lesion. Blocking the subarachnoid space with a cottonoid helps prevent dissemination of tumor debris. The cyst wall distant from the tumor nodule is nonneoplastic and need not be removed; when there is doubt regarding its histology, a frozen section of wall tissue can exclude cystic glioma. Opening the cyst decompresses the cerebellum and exposes the cyst wall and mural nodule. Cerebellar hemangioblastomas are typically orange and well circumscribed. However, great care should be taken if the tumor or cyst is in contact with the brainstem. Dissection of a plane about the nodule should begin in the gliotic plane around the orange vascular lesion. Broadly applying the bipolar electrocautery at low intensity to the lesion's surface will devascularize and shrink the tumor. The tumor's vascular pedicle, once isolated, may be cauterized and cut.

After complete resection and careful hemostasis, the dura should be closed in a watertight fashion. Dural tack-up sutures may provide additional epidural hemostasis. The bone flap may be plated with titanium miniplates to provide at least 3-point fixation. The suboccipital soft tissues should be closed in multiple layers to prevent CSF leak.

Complication Avoidance and Management

- Consider external ventricular drainage for obstructive hydrocephalus, intraoperative cerebellar relaxation, and prevention of postoperative CSF-cutaneous fistula.
- Develop the extracapsular plane around the tumor for an en bloc resection to avoid excessive intraoperative bleeding and dropped metastasis. Block flow of fluids out of the resection cavity to prevent dissemination of tumor cells. Dropped lesions remain benign with treatment options and indications similar to those for the parent lesion.

KEY PAPERS

Catapano D, Muscarella LA, Guarnieri V, et al. Hemangioblastomas of central nervous system: molecular genetic analysis and clinical management. *Neurosurgery.* 2005;56(6):1215-1221.

Jagannathan J, Lonser RR, Smith R, et al. Surgical management of cerebellar hemangioblastomas in patients with von Hippel Lindau disease. *J of Neurosurg.* 2008;108(2):210-222.

Lonser RR, Butman JA, Huntoon K, et al. Prospective natural history study of central nervous system hemangioblastomas in von Hippel-Lindau disease. *J of Neurosurg.* 2014;120(5):1055-1062.

Moss JM, Choi CY, Adler JR, et al. Stereotactic radiosurgical treatment of cranial and spinal hemangioblastomas. *Neurosurgery.* 2009;65(1):79-85, discussion 85.

Poulsen ML, Budtz-Jørgensen E, Bisgaard ML. Surveillance in von Hippel-Lindau disease (vHL). *Clin Genet.* 2010;77(1):49-59.

Case 22

Pituitary Apoplexy

James Wright, MD ● Christina Huang Wright, MD

Presentation

A 30-year-old female with no significant past medical history presents with severe headache, nausea, and blurry vision.

- PMH: otherwise unremarkable
- Vitals: BP 85/40; HR 120; RR 14; Sat 99%; T 100.3
- Exam:
  - Awake, but drowsy
  - Nasal visual fields intact, bilateral temporal visual fields diminished to confrontation
  - Left pupil deviated inferolaterally, dysconjugate gaze, difficulty with adduction of both eyes
  - Full strength and sensation in extremities

Differential Diagnosis

- Neoplastic
  - Pituitary adenoma
  - Brain tumor, primary or metastatic
    - Craniopharyngioma
    - Dermoid/teratoma
- Vascular
  - Stroke
  - Aneurysmal subarachnoid hemorrhage
  - Cavernous sinus thrombosis
- Infectious
  - Intracranial abscess
  - Intrasellar tuberculoma
  - Meningitis
- Other
  - Pituitary apoplexy
  - Hypophysitis
  - Sheehan's syndrome
  - Rathke's cleft cyst
  - Migraine

Initial Imaging

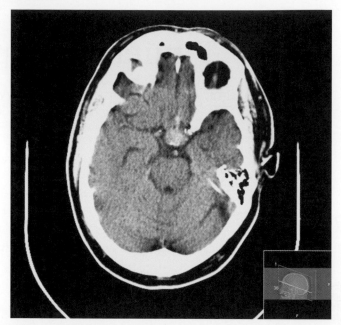

FIGURE 22-1

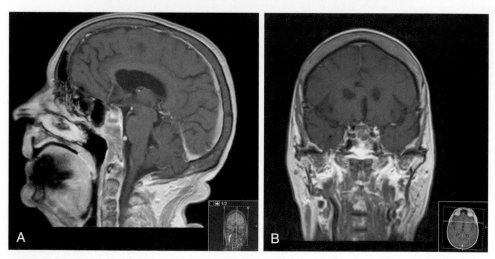

FIGURE 22-2

Imaging Description and Differential

Description: Figure 22-1 represents a noncontrast head CT demonstrating a hyperdensity in the sella, most likely a hemorrhage. Figures 22-2A and 22-2B depict an MRI of the brain with sagittal and coronal images. They demonstrate hemorrhage within a pituitary adenoma, and extension of hemorrhagic products into the cavernous sinus.

Further Workup

- Laboratory
  - Na: 135 mmol/L
  - K: 5 mmol/L

- Glucose: 58 mg/dL
- TSH: 0.1 mIU/L
- Free T4: 0.2 mIU/L
- ACTH: 3 pg/mL
- Cortisol: 2 μg/dL
- FSH: 0.5; LH: 0.2; prolactin: 3.5 μg/L
- Imaging
  - Routine CT has poor sensitivity for diagnosing pituitary apoplexy, unless pure hematoma is present. The mass may be hyperdense and contain fluid. If one is unable to obtain an emergent MRI, a pituitary CT scan is recommended.
  - Urgent MRI is the imaging modality of choice and is most sensitive for hemorrhagic or ischemic injury within the sella. In the case of hemorrhage, the mass will appear hyperintense on T1 due to blood products. Intensity will vary depending on the age of the blood products. In the setting of ischemic apoplexy, DWI and ADC imaging will demonstrate increased signal intensity and restricted diffusion within the mass, indicating infarction of the adenoma or gland.
- Consultants
  - Neuroophthalmology
  - Endocrinology
  - Neurosurgery

Pathophysiology

Pituitary apoplexy is a clinical diagnosis defined by sudden onset headache, vomiting, visual impairment, and decreased consciousness in the setting of hemorrhage or infarction of the pituitary gland or adenoma. It is typically associated with a pituitary adenoma, but may also occur with a nonadenomatous tumor, or normal pituitary gland. About 80% of cases present without a previously diagnosed adenoma.

Pituitary apoplexy can occur spontaneously, or it can be precipitated by trauma, estrogen therapy, dopamine agonists, radiotherapy, anticoagulation, and pregnancy. Hypertension is the most common predisposing factor. Dynamic testing of the pituitary gland is also a risk factor. Patients undergoing cardiac surgery are at increased risk due to anticoagulant therapy coupled with fluctuations in blood pressure.

The mechanism of pituitary apoplexy is still unclear. Theories include ischemic necrosis of adenomatous tissues, compression of the superior hypophyseal artery, or vasculopathy within pituitary tumors. The accumulation of hemorrhagic products and edema produces a sudden increase in pressure within the sella turcica. This compresses surrounding structures and portal vessels, resulting in symptoms and pituitary dysfunction. The earliest and most common symptom is severe headache of rapid onset, which is typically retro-orbital, but may also be diffuse. It is often accompanied by nausea and vomiting. Meningismus results from hemorrhagic products infiltrating the subarachnoid space and contributes to worsening lethargy, photophobia, and pyrexia. Worsening visual acuity and visual field deficits, most commonly bitemporal field cuts, result from chiasmatic compression. Ophthalmoplegia results from compression of the cavernous sinus. Up to 70% of cases demonstrate ocular palsies, with the oculomotor nerve being the most commonly affected. Worsening compression can lead to trochlear and abducens palsies as well as symptoms of stroke from compression of the cavernous segment of the carotid artery.

Treatment Options

- Medical
  - Intravenous fluid and glucocorticoid administration in the acute setting often contributes to symptomatic improvement. Indications for steroid replacement include hemodynamic instability, altered level of consciousness, decreased visual acuity, or worsening visual field defects.
  - An endocrine panel including FSH, LH, ACTH, TSH, FT4, prolactin, IGF-1, GH, testosterone, and estradiol should be drawn before administration of hydrocortisone. Nearly all pituitary hormone levels will be diminished.

- For hemodynamically and neurologically stable patients, the UK guidelines recommend measuring a 9 A.M. cortisol and then initiating replacement for levels <550 nmol/L.
- In patients requiring urgent steroid replacement, an IV hydrocortisone bolus of 100 to 200 mg is recommended after drawing the appropriate labs. After this bolus, a 2 to 4 mg per hour IV infusion or a 50 to 100 mg intramuscular injection every 6 hours should be administered. The dose should then be tapered to a maintenance dose of 20 to 30 mg daily.
- Ophthalmology
  - UK guidelines recommend daily neuroophthalmic assessments in the acute period to evaluate for stabilization or worsening of visual status.
- Surgery
  - Although there are no randomized-controlled trials of surgical intervention for pituitary apoplexy, there is a general consensus that a patient with significant visual deficits, or decreased consciousness, should have surgical decompression.
  - It is recommended that transsphenoidal surgery be performed within the first 7 days of onset of symptoms. In clinically stable patients, semielective transsphenoidal surgery should be considered.
- Observation
  - Observation is recommended for patients without neuroophthalmic deficits. Patients should, however, be closely monitored with formal visual acuity and visual field assessments until improvement is observed. Ocular paresis from III, IV, or VI cranial nerve palsies in the absence of visual field defects or reduced visual acuity is not necessarily an indication for immediate surgery. Case reports and observational studies suggest that resolution of these deficits will typically occur within days or weeks without intervention.

Surgical Technique

A transsphenoidal surgical technique is appropriate and is described in case 23: Cushing's Microadenoma.

Complication Avoidance and Management

- Patient should undergo endocrine and ophthalmic follow-up 4 to 8 weeks after the initial event with assessment of pituitary function and evaluation of visual acuity and visual fields.
- Recurrent apoplexy and tumor regrowth have been documented after both observation and surgery. Long-term follow-up imaging to detect recurrence is indicated.
- Nearly 80% of patients will require some hormone replacement.

KEY PAPERS

Murad-Kejbou S, Eggenberger E. Pituitary apoplexy: evaluation, management, and prognosis. *Curr Opin Opthamol.* 2009;20(6):456-461.

Nawar R, AbdelMannan D, Selman W, et al. Pituitary tumor apoplexy: a review. *J Intensive Care Med.* 2008;23(2):75-90.

Onesti S, Wisniewski T, Post K. Clinical versus subclinical pituitary apoplexy: presentation, surgical management, and outcome in 21 patients. *Neurosurgery.* 1990;26(6):980-986.

Rajasekaran S, Vanderpump M, Baldeweg S, et al. UK guidelines for the management of pituitary apoplexy. *Clin Endocrinol (Oxf).* 2011;74(1):9-20.

Verrees M, Arafah B, Selman W. Pituitary tumor apoplexy: characteristics, treatment, and outcomes. *Neurosurg Focus.* 2004;16(4):1-7.

Cushing's Microadenoma

J. Dawn Waters, MD

Presentation

A 40-year-old woman arrives in the clinic with complaints of hair loss, weight gain, acne, easy bruising, generalized weakness, and facial hair for 5 years; all dramatically worse over the last year. She has lost hair at the top of her head and gained 30 pounds in the past year. Progressive weakness is most notable while climbing stairs or carrying groceries.

- Review of systems: positive for galactorrhea, dysmenorrhea, darkened skin, heart palpitations, frequent oral thrush, and occasional mild headaches
- PMH: hypertension in the past year and hypothyroidism requiring replacement for 8 years
- Physical examination:
  - Marked central obesity with a fatty hump between the shoulders
  - Thin extremities
  - Scattered ecchymoses
  - Facial and back acne
  - 4/5 upper and lower extremity strength with unsteady gait
  - Remainder of the physical examination was normal

Differential Diagnosis

- Neoplastic
  - Cushing's disease/pituitary adenoma
  - Ectopic ACTH secreting tumor (e.g., lung)
  - Adrenal adenoma or carcinoma
- Other
  - Iatrogenic/corticosteroid ingestion

Initial Imaging

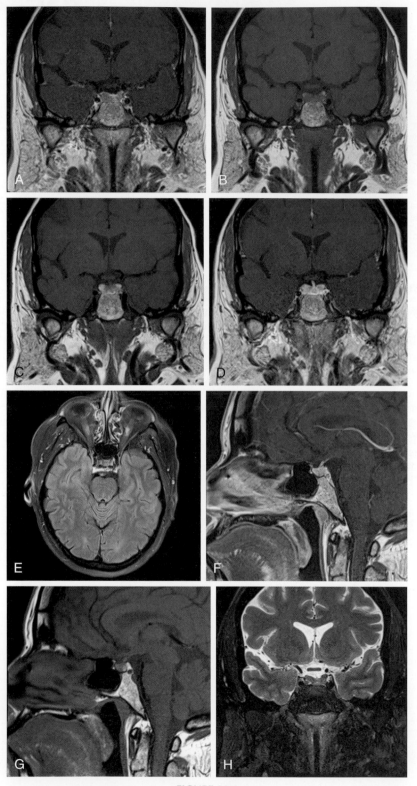

FIGURE 23-1

Imaging Description and Differential

MRI with and without contrast demonstrates a 7 × 7 mm homogeneously enhancing right sellar mass with moderate deviation of stalk toward the left. No compression of optic chiasm.

Further Workup

- Electrolytes
- Endocrine panel
- CT of chest and abdomen
- Low-dose dexamethasone suppression test (abnormal ACTH from pituitary or non-pituitary source fails to suppress)
- High-dose dexamethasone suppression test (nonpituitary ACTH source fails to suppress)
- Inferior petrosal sinus sampling (central versus peripheral ACTH source, right vs left side)
- Results for this case:
  - Morning cortisol: 29 μg/dL (normal range 4–26 μg/dL)
  - ACTH: 120 pg/mL (normal range 10–60 pg/mL)
  - DHEAS: 360 μg/dL (elevated)
  - Prolactin: 8 ng/mL (normal)
  - Electrolytes normal
  - Chest and abdominal CT: 1 cm left adrenal mass consistent with adenoma
  - Inferior petrosal sinus sampling to distinguish source of ACTH (pituitary vs adrenal adenoma):
    - Baseline peripheral (inferior vena cava) ACTH: 125 pg/mL
    - After CRH, peripheral (inferior vena cava) ACTH: 550 pg/mL
    - Baseline right petrosal sinus ACTH: 3200 pg/mL
    - After CRH, right petrosal sinus ACTH: 26,800 pg/mL
    - Baseline left petrosal sinus ACTH: 600 pg/mL
    - After CRH, left petrosal sinus ACTH: 6600 pg/mL
    - Peak baseline petrosal to peripheral ratio: 26 : 1
    - Peak petrosal to peripheral ratio after CRH: 49 : 1

Pathophysiology

Cushing's disease is caused by a pituitary adenoma that secretes ACTH. The resultant elevated cortisol causes significant systemic morbidity, including weight gain, hypertension, diabetes, osteoporosis, generalized muscle atrophy, poor wound healing, and sepsis. These signs and symptoms often prompt an endocrine workup. Thus ACTH-secreting adenomas are often diagnosed when they are still small and before they cause compressive symptoms. In many cases, the lesion is difficult or impossible to see on MRI. In this case an adrenal lesion was also present. Additional tests help localize the source of ACTH secretion to the pituitary. Abnormal pituitary adenoma cells maintain some negative feedback response to high-dose dexamethasone, helping distinguish pituitary adenoma from nonpituitary sources of ACTH secretion that do not suppress secretion in response to dexamethasone. Inferior petrosal sinus testing with a sinus:peripheral ratio of ACTH >2 : 1 before administration of CRH is highly sensitive and specific to a pituitary source. CRH administration yielding a ratio >3 : 1 approaches 100% sensitivity and 100% specificity for a pituitary source.

Treatment Options

- Surgical
  - Transsphenoidal surgery is the treatment of choice for an ACTH-secreting micro-adenoma, and it may be curative.
  - For patients who have failed other surgical and medical options, bilateral adrenalectomy is available to control hypercortisolism.
- Medical
  - Inhibitors of steroid synthesis:
    - Ketoconazole

- Aminoglutethimide
- Metyrapone
- Mitotane
- Radiation
  - Stereotactic radiosurgery
  - External beam radiation therapy

Surgical Technique

An endoscopic approach to the sella is described. After oral endotracheal intubation, an oral-gastric tube is placed, and both are secured to the lower lip or chin. Lumbar drainage, abdominal fat graft harvest, and nasal-septal flap harvest may be considered for control of CSF leak, and preparations should be made if necessary. The patient is positioned supine with the head of the bed up about 10 degrees for drainage. The head is positioned to allow easy access to both nostrils from the surgeon's position at the patient's side, usually bringing the ear toward the shoulder away from the surgeon. The Mayfield pin head-holder can be helpful to maintain this position. Arms are tucked.

The sphenoid sinus is accessed endoscopically through expansion of both sphenoid ostia behind the middle turbinates. The rostrum of the sphenoid sinus and posterior boney septum are removed to provide an adequate working channel. Variable boney septa within the sphenoid sinus, and their relationships to the carotid arteries or optic canals on preoperative imaging, can guide the exposure as they are removed.

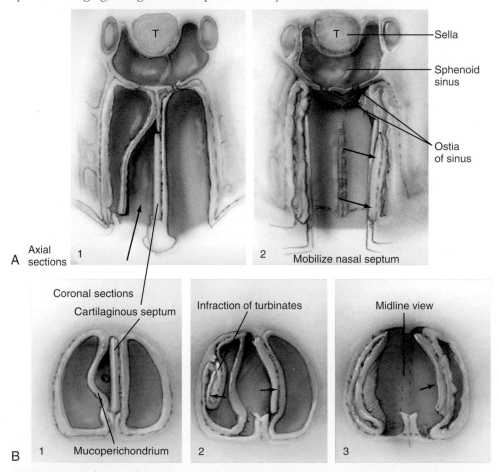

FIGURE 23-2   Submucosal tunnels. A, Axial views: anterior submucosal tunnel (1); septal displacement and posterior submucosal tunnels (2). T, T-tumor. **B,** Coronal views: anterior submucosal tunnel (1); posterior and inferior submucosal tunnels before (2) and after (3) septal displacement. *(From Jane JA Jr, Thapar K, Kaptain GJ, et al. Pituitary surgery: transsphenoidal approach. Neurosurgery. 2002;51:435.) (Reprinted with permission from Winn HR. Youmans Neurological Surgery. 6th ed. Elsevier; 2011.)*

The sella bulges into the sphenoid sinus with the planum sphenoidale above and clivus below. Laterally, thin bone is molded to the contours of the underlying carotid arteries and optic nerves, dipping into an optico-carotid recess at the superior-lateral limits of the sella. The bone of the sellar floor is often thinned or dehiscent. The bone over the face of the sella can be removed with Kerrison rongeurs through a defect in the sella. If necessary, a small high-speed irrigating drill or chisel can be used to create a small defect in the sella.

With the dura exposed, the cavernous and intercavernous sinuses should be visibly blue. The carotid arteries can be localized with Doppler ultrasound. Avoiding these structures, a square of dura can be removed to expose the contents of the sella. The preoperative MRI and inferior petrosal sinus sampling can guide exploration to the abnormal adenoma tissue. Microdissection and suction can be used to develop a plane between the tumor capsule and normal pituitary gland to remove the tumor.

Reconstruction of the sella can be accomplished as needed with any of the following: fat autograft, septal bone, sphenoid mucosa, synthetic bone and dural substitutes, tissue adhesives, and a nasal-septal flap. Debris, blood, and drainage are cleared from the nasopharynx before the conclusion of the case. The oral-gastric tube is suctioned to remove gastric and pharyngeal drainage from the case before extubation.

Complication Avoidance and Management

- Postoperative endocrine management
  - A drop in cortisol levels may be observed postoperatively. The patient should be closely monitored for abnormalities such as diabetes insipidus, SIADH, and hypocortisolism. Insulin requirements for diabetes mellitus may change postoperatively. Consider consulting an endocrinologist.
- CSF leak
  - Observation of CSF leakage intraoperatively usually warrants more extensive reconstruction of the sella to prevent postoperative leakage. A lumbar drain can be placed at the time of surgery to reduce CSF pressure against the reconstruction. If a CSF leak is first detected postoperatively, it should be closely monitored. Slow leaks may be managed by elevating the head of the bed or with a lumbar drain. Larger or persistent leaks may require reoperation to reconstruct the sella.

KEY PAPERS

Berker M, Işikay I, Berker D, et al. Early promising results for the endoscopic surgical treatment of Cushing's disease. *Neurosurg Rev.* [Internet] 2013;105-114. Available from: <http://www.ncbi.nlm.nih.gov/pubmed/24233258>; cited 20.05.14.

Oldfield E, Doppman J. Petrosal sinus sampling with and without corticotropin-releasing hormone for the differential diagnosis of Cushing's syndrome. *N Engl J Med.* [Internet] 1991;(325):897-905. Available from: <http://www.nejm.org/doi/pdf/10.1056/NEJM199109263251301>; cited 20.05.14.

Sheehan JP, Xu Z, Salvetti DJ, et al. Results of gamma knife surgery for Cushing's disease. *J Neurosurg.* 2013;119(December):1486-1492.

Yamada S, Fukuhara N, Nishioka H, et al. Surgical management and outcomes in patients with Cushing disease with negative pituitary magnetic resonance imaging. *World Neurosurg.* [Internet]. Elsevier Inc 2012;77(3–4):525-532. Available from: <http://www.ncbi.nlm.nih.gov/pubmed/22120352>; cited 20.05.14.

Case 24

Pituitary Macroadenoma – Prolactinoma

Melanie G. Hayden Gephart, MD ● YouRong Sophie Su

Presentation

A 47-year-old male was referred for complaints of erectile dysfunction and headaches. He denies recent stress or depression. Headache is not associated with photosensitivity. Patient does report recent loss in peripheral vision.

- PMH: negative for cardiovascular disease, diabetes, liver disease, and kidney disease
- No medications
- Exam:
  - General: no acute distress; gynecomastia; skin normal, no striae
  - HEENT: normocephalic, atraumatic; no lesions or palpable masses
  - Neuro: decreased peripheral visual acuity; pupils reactive; extraocular movements intact
  - GU: testicular atrophy

Differential Diagnosis

- Neoplastic
  - Pituitary adenoma
  - Craniopharyngioma
  - Meningioma
  - Pituicytoma
  - Metastasis
- Inflammatory
  - Lymphocytic hypophysitis
- Vascular
  - AVM of cavernous sinus
  - Aneurysms
- Other
  - Cysts
  - Abscesses
  - Pharmacy (antidepressants and antipsychotics)

Initial Imaging

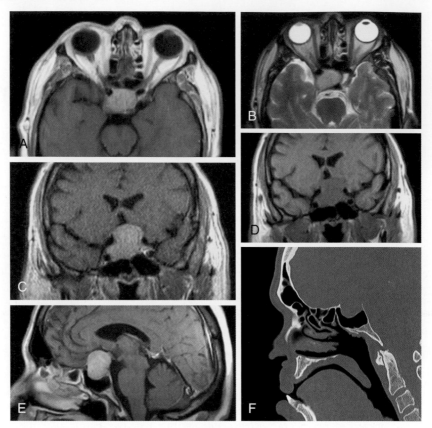

FIGURE 24-1

Imaging Description and Differential

- Figure 24-1A demonstrates a contrast enhancing lesion on T1 MRI. Figure 24-1B shows a T2 image of the same lesion. Figures 24-1C and D demonstrate coronal T1 MRI views, with and without contrast enhancement. Figure 24-1E is a sagittal T1 with contrast. Together, the brain MRI images demonstrate a moderately enhancing sellar mass extending upward to impinge on the optic nerves. Enhancing images suggest invasion into the right cavernous sinus.
- Figure 24-1F is a midsagittal CT demonstrating boney remodeling and enlargement of the sella into the sphenoid sinus.
- Differential: pituitary macroadenoma, pituitary carcinoma, metastasis, hyperplasia (e.g., from primary thyroid deficiency), meningioma, craniopharyngioma, or Rathke's cleft cyst

Further Workup

- Laboratory
  - Serum prolactin (PRL), TSH, free T4, growth hormone, cortisol, LH, FSH, testosterone: patient has elevated PRL and decreased LH, FSH, and testosterone levels
  - If prolactin levels are low, a repeat prolactin level with dilutions to exclude a false-negative result due to the Hook effect
  - CBC

- Imaging
  - MRI with and without gadolinium contrast is the imaging of choice. Most macro-adenomas will be either isointense or hyperintense on T1-weighted imaging, compared with the normal pituitary tissue. The adenoma usually enhances less avidly than the pituitary gland.
  - CT may be useful to define the bones of the sella turcica and sphenoid sinus.
- Consultants: endocrinology, ophthalmology

Pathophysiology

Somatic mutations in progenitor cells lead to monoclonal expansion of lactotrope cells.

Treatment Options

- Medical
  - Dopamine agonists: to help normalize prolactin levels, restore reproductive function, and decrease tumor size
    - Cabergoline: high affinity and selectivity for D2 receptor; preferred medication because has fewer side effects compared to bromocriptine
    - Bromocriptine: D2 receptor agonist and D1 antagonist; has many side effects such as nausea, vomiting, and postural hypotension that many patients find intolerable
  - Gonadal steroid replacement therapy: used if hormone levels remain low, despite maximal treatment with dopamine agonists
- Surgical: reserved for patients who are unresponsive to medication, have intolerable side effects, or for visual deficits
  - Transsphenoidal surgery: endoscopic versus microscopic
  - Craniotomy
- Radiation: rarely required as an adjunct for residual tumor or lack of endocrinologic response to surgery, may be indicated for rare malignant prolactinoma
  - Stereotactic radiosurgery

Surgical Technique

A transsphenoidal surgical technique is appropriate, as described in Case 23: Cushing's Microadenoma.

Surgical Complication Avoidance and Management

- Transsphenoidal surgery: Identification and avoidance of the carotid arteries, optic nerve, and optic chiasm. Ideally, the normal pituitary gland and pituitary stalk will be identified and preserved. It is important to systematically examine the surfaces to minimize recurrences. Use of a 30-degree scope can be helpful.
- Radiation therapy: Generally reserved for recurrent or anaplastic tumors. Maximum dose of 60 Gy to avoid optic neuropathy, endocrine dysfunction, or necrosis.
- Patients must be carefully monitored for both efficacy of treatment (decrease in prolactin levels) and mitigation of complications (hypopituitarism – cortisol, diabetes insipidus)

KEY PAPERS

Casaneuva FF, Molitch ME, Schlechte JA, et al. Guidelines of the Pituitary Society for the diagnosis and management of prolactinomas. *Clin Endocrinol (Oxf)*. 2006;65(2):265-273.
Iglesias P, Diez JJ. Macroprolactinoma: a diagnostic and therapeutic update. *QJM*. 2013;106(6):495-504.
Klibanski A. Prolactinomas. *N Engl J Med*. 2010;362:1219-1226.
Mah PM, Webster J. Hyperprolactinemia: etiology, diagnosis, and management. *Semin Reprod Med*. 2002;20(4):365-374.

Case 25

Craniopharyngioma

Matthew G. MacDougall, MD ● David D. Gonda, MD ●
Michael L. Levy, MD, PhD

Presentation

A 61-year-old female presents with 10 weeks of progressive blurring of vision and headache.

- PMH: otherwise unremarkable
- Exam: extraocular movements normal
  - Visual acuity worsened from most recent ophthalmologic exam
  - Bitemporal visual field defect
  - Other aspects of exam normal

Differential Diagnosis

- Neoplastic
  - Pituitary adenoma
  - Meningioma
  - Craniopharyngioma
  - Optic pathway glioma
  - Hypothalamic glioma
- Developmental
  - Rathke's cleft cyst
  - Arachnoid cyst
- Vascular
  - Giant aneurysm
  - Carotid cavernous fistula
- Infectious/inflammatory
  - Pituitary abscess
  - Langerhans cell histiocytosis
  - Sarcoidosis

Initial Imaging

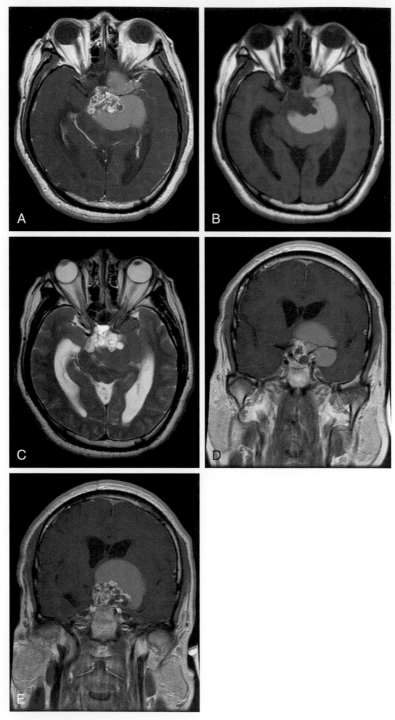

FIGURE 25-1

Imaging Description and Differential

- Axial and coronal MRI demonstrate a large cystic contrast-enhancing mass arising from the sella. The optic chiasm is not distinguishable. The third ventricle is obliterated, and obstructive hydrocephalus is evident in the lateral ventricles. Figure 25-1D demonstrates flow voids of the carotid and middle cerebral arteries within the mass.
- Differential: craniopharyngioma, Rathke's cleft cyst, pituicytoma, or lymphocytic hypophysitis

Further Workup

- Laboratory
  - Electrolytes
  - Pituitary hormones: prolactin, TSH, FSH, ACTH, and GH
- Imaging
  - MRI brain, with and without contrast
- Formal evaluation
  - Visual fields
- Consultants
  - Endocrinology
  - Medical oncology
  - Ophthalmology

Pathophysiology

Craniopharyngiomas are rare histologically benign tumors that typically arise in the suprasellar region. They exhibit a bimodal age distribution, but no gender preference. Peak incidence occurs between ages 5 to 14 and 65 to 74. They usually have symptoms related to mass effect and endocrine disruption. Children often display disruptions in puberty and/or growth, and adults often suffer from diabetes insipidus. Due to the proximity of craniopharyngiomas to the optic apparatus, visual loss is a very common complaint; it occurs in half of all patients. Craniopharyngiomas near the third ventricle can cause obstructive hydrocephalus if mass effect becomes marked (Figure 25-2).

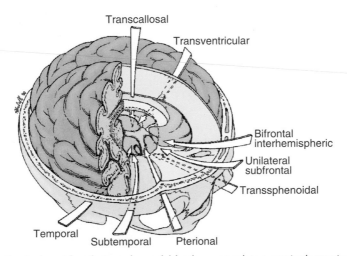

FIGURE 25-2 Surgical corridors that may be useful for the approach to a craniopharyngioma, depending on the size and pattern of the tumor and preference of the surgeon. *(Reprinted with permission from Winn HR. Youmans Neurological Surgery. 6th ed. Elsevier; 2011.)*

These tumors are graded in several ways: by histology; as adamantinomatous or papillary; according to their relationship to the optic chiasm, as prechiasmatic, subchiasmatic, or retrochiasmatic; and in relation to the sella, as intrasellar, suprasellar, or both. A scale grading the tumors' vertical extent has been proposed as well, with grade I being intrasellar or intradiaphragmatic, grade II indicating a tumor within the cistern, but not the sella, grade III in the lower half of the third ventricle, grade IV in the upper half, and grade V in the lateral ventricles or septum pellucidum.

Treatment Options

- Medical
  - Endocrine replacement tailored to the patient's deficits
  - Corticosteroids to reduce cerebral edema
  - Osmotic agents to reduce elevated intracranial pressure may be indicated.
- Biopsy
  - Biopsy may be useful for definitive diagnosis before radiation, if it is believed that a significant resection cannot be accomplished.
  - Depending on tumor composition, cyst drainage may be appropriate.
- Radiation
  - Radiation is useful in adult patients with subtotal resection or tumor recurrence.
- Surgical
  - CSF diversion may be required for hydrocephalus.
  - Pterional craniotomy
  - Transsphenoidal approach
  - Orbitozygomatic craniotomy
  - Interhemispheric/transcallosal craniotomy
  - Subfrontal/transbasal craniotomy
  - Combination approach using the above methods (Figure 25-2)

Surgical Technique

We believe that the appropriate approach is based upon tumor grade. Our primary goal is to maximize resection and minimize hypothalamic, pituitary axis, and visual compromise. For Yasargil grade IV and V tumors, we prefer an orbitozygomatic approach. For grade I to III tumors, many surgeons prefer the standard pterional craniotomy. Given the increased familiarity with pterional approaches, we will discuss that approach here. It will be presented in such a way that allows conversion to an orbitozygomatic approach, should greater access to the tumor be required.

For a pterional craniotomy, the patient is positioned with the cranium fixed in pins, the neck slightly extended, and the malar eminence at the highest point of the field. A curvilinear incision is planned proceeding superiorly from the posterior root of the zygomatic arch, 1 cm anterior to the tragus, and terminating just across midline behind the hairline. The superficial temporal fascia and its fat pad are separated and reflected anteriorly and the pericranium, above the temporalis, is preserved and reflected anteriorly. The temporalis muscle is divided and reflected inferiorly. The zygomatic arch may be removed if necessary to achieve adequate exposure of the pterion (Figure 25-3).

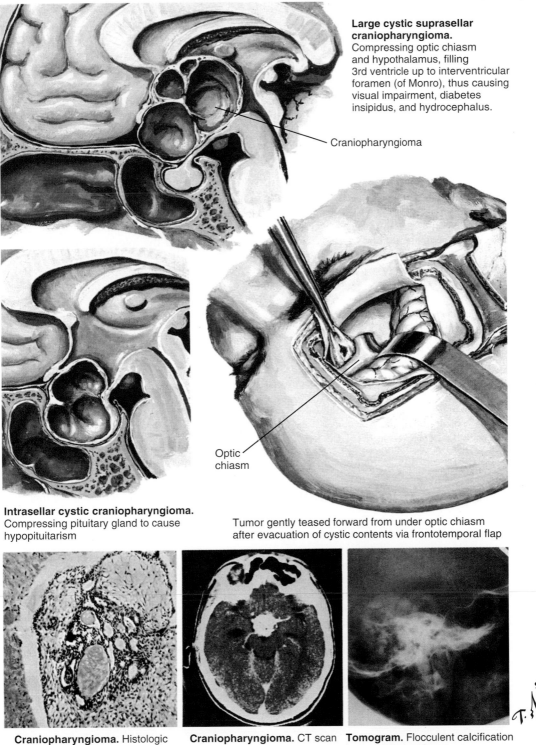

Large cystic suprasellar craniopharyngioma.
Compressing optic chiasm and hypothalamus, filling 3rd ventricle up to interventricular foramen (of Monro), thus causing visual impairment, diabetes insipidus, and hydrocephalus.

Craniopharyngioma

Optic chiasm

Intrasellar cystic craniopharyngioma.
Compressing pituitary gland to cause hypopituitarism

Tumor gently teased forward from under optic chiasm after evacuation of cystic contents via frontotemporal flap

Craniopharyngioma. Histologic section: (H and E stain, ×125)

Craniopharyngioma. CT scan

Tomogram. Flocculent calcification in craniopharyngioma

FIGURE 25-3 An illustration of the view through a pterional craniotomy for resection of craniopharyngioma. *(Reprinted with permission from Netter, FH. Atlas of Human Anatomy. 5th ed. Elsevier, Saunders; Copyright 2011.)*

The bony opening is undertaken with a keyhole burr hole, and another on the other side of the sphenoid wing. Additional burr holes are variably made per the surgeon's preference. The bone between the sphenoid burr holes may be thinned to facilitate fracturing during craniotomy flap elevation. A drill with a footplate is used to connect the burr holes. The bone flap is elevated using careful blunt dissection to release the dura from the underside of the flap. The sphenoid wing may be drilled or rongeured down as deep as the superior orbital fissure to facilitate exposure of the deep sylvian structures. The superior lateral aspect of the supraorbital fissure can be incised to maximize exposure.

A C-shape dural incision is made over the lateral aspect of the frontal and temporal lobes, crossing the sylvian fissure. Dura is fixed to the bony edges using suture to prevent epidural bleeding. The sylvian fissure is opened and CSF is drained from the basal cisterns.

Craniopharyngiomas are often intimately intertwined in a dense network of internal carotid artery, optic nerve, and other critical structures. As such, maximal resection requires a significant understanding of the baseline anatomy, in addition to the relationships of the arachnoid planes to salient structures. Additionally, understanding the nature of involvement of the hypothalamus, and the response of the hypothalamus to surgical manipulation, is an absolute.

Cyst contents are usually drained initially, shrinking the bulk of the tumor. Utilizing sharp dissection, tumor capsule is freed from all vascular adhesions initially. Care must be taken to preserve the integrity of the third nerve. Tumor that extends posterior and inferior to the posterior clinoid process can usually be removed safely, given that a leaf of the membrane of Liliequist will separate tumor from the basilar vasculature. Tumor can additionally be sharply dissected from the underside of the optic nerves and chiasm. The more direct the visualization of the underside of the optic nerves, the less risk of injury to the optic apparatus. Tumors with third ventricular involvement will usually require entry into the lamina terminalis for complete resection.

Arachnoid overlying the tumor is incised, and the tumor capsule is cauterized and incised to facilitate repetitive resection of small soft pieces of tumor through the available anatomic corridors. As tumor bulk is reduced, arachnoid planes between tumor and vital structures may enable removal of the capsule via gentle retraction. Care must be taken to cauterize capsular feeding arteries during this process.

Complication Avoidance and Management

Excessive retraction on the optic apparatus must be avoided. Leaving a small amount of adherent tumor on the optic nerves or carotid artery is preferable to a complete resection, which will result in deficit.

It takes a thorough understanding of the relationship of the hypothalamus to the invasion by craniopharyngioma to minimize hypothalamic injury. In the absence of such, adherent hypothalamic tumor should remain untouched.

Postoperative endocrine complications are extremely common and should be closely managed by an endocrinologist. Visual loss after surgery is also unfortunately very common, and patients ought to be followed by an ophthalmologist.

KEY PAPER

Yaşargil MG, Curcic M, Kis M, et al. Total removal of craniopharyngiomas. Approaches and long-term results in 144 patients. *J Neurosurg.* 1990;73(1):3-11.

Case 26

Glioblastoma

Kevin K.H. Chow, MD, PhD

Presentation

A 55-year-old previously healthy male presents with 2 weeks of generalized headaches, 2 days of weakness of his left arm, and nausea and vomiting associated with abrupt changes in position. He endorses poor memory.

- PMH: otherwise unremarkable
- Exam:
  - Headaches reproducible by bending over or coughing
  - Cranial nerve exam demonstrates left homonymous hemianopsia and subtle left nasolabial flattening. Otherwise cranial nerves II-XII are intact.
  - 4+/5 weakness of extensors in left upper extremity
  - Mild spasticity in left upper extremity

Differential Diagnosis

- Neoplastic
  - Primary brain tumor
  - Metastasis (h/o cancer)
  - CNS lymphoma
- Vascular
  - Intracranial hemorrhage
  - AVM
  - Cavernous malformation
- Infectious
  - Brain abscess (h/o travel, manifestations of infection)
  - Encephalitis
- Other
  - Radiation necrosis

Initial Imaging

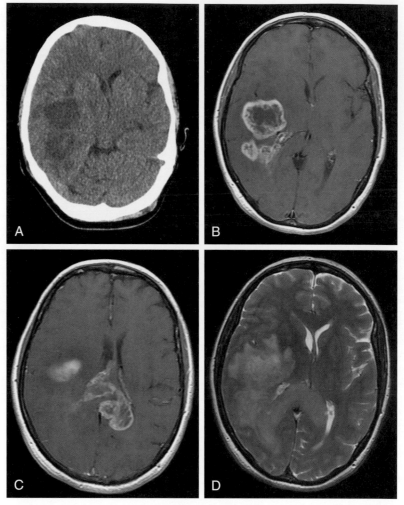

FIGURE 26-1

Imaging Description and Differential

- CT in Figure 26-1A demonstrates multifocal hypodensity of the right frontal and parietal lobes, with mass effect and midline shift.
- Figure 26-1 B and C are T1 MRIs with contrast showing multiple rim-enhancing lesions within deep white matter of the right frontal and parietal lobes, and the corpus callosum.
- Figure 26-1D T2 is an MRI showing a hyperintense lesion with irregular margins surrounded by vasogenic edema within the white matter.
- Differential: glioblastoma, metastasis, or an abscess

Further Workup

- Laboratory
  - Routine labs
  - Metastatic workup
    - Fecal occult blood
    - Prostate-specific antigen

- Imaging
  - Metastatic workup
    - Chest X-ray
    - Mammogram in women
    - CT of chest, abdomen, and pelvis
    - PET scan
  - Operative risk assessment and planning
    - Consider functional MRI and diffusion tensor imaging.
- Consultants
  - Neuro-oncology
  - Radiation oncology

Pathophysiology

Glioblastoma multiforme (GBM) is the most common primary brain tumor. These WHO grade IV lesions are characterized histologically by cellular atypia, anaplasia, mitotic activity, microvascular proliferation, and necrosis. Most arise de novo (primary GBM), and a minority develop by malignant degeneration from WHO II or III astrocytomas or oligodendrogliomas (secondary GBM). The vast majority of GBM are supratentorial. They are highly infiltrative and spread along white matter tracts and blood vessels. Primary GBM is often characterized by EGFR amplification and PTEN mutations, and secondary GBM by TP53 mutations. MGMT promoter methylation prevents repair of the effects of alkylating chemotherapeutic agents, including temozolomide. MGMT promotor methylation is thus associated with greater response to temozolomide, and therefore improved survival.

Treatment Options

- Biopsy – indications
  - Poor medical condition
  - Tumor location prevents safe gross total resection
  - Equivocal imaging characteristics – suspicion of CNS lymphoma or abscess
- Surgical
  - Resection: great extent of resection correlates with increased time to progression and median survival; however, surgery is not curative. The goal is to maximize extent of resection and minimize neurologic injury.
  - Careful patient selection for resection can avoid unnecessary risks where benefits of surgery are uncertain. Risks of surgical debulking may outweigh the benefits for tumors that are multicentric, bilateral, or in eloquent cortex. Additionally, there is limited survival benefit with surgery in elderly patients and patients with a Karnofsky score <70.
- Radiation
  - Involved field radiation therapy of 60 Gy is the standard of care after biopsy or surgical resection.
  - Given the infiltrative nature of GBM, the involved field is generally defined radiographically as the area of the tumor plus a 2 cm margin.
  - Radiation therapy is given with concurrent, and then adjuvant, temozolomide chemotherapy.
- Medical
  - Corticosteroids are indicated for symptoms caused by mass effect from vasogenic edema.
  - Chemotherapy – temozolomide, an oral alkylating agent, is given concurrently with radiation therapy and as an adjuvant after completion of RT. This is the current standard of care.
  - Treatment of recurrent disease – bevacizumab, a monoclonal antibody that binds vascular endothelial growth factor (VEGF)

Surgical Technique

This patient was informed that significant portions of tumor (deep bilateral white matter) could not be safely removed. A stereotactic biopsy of the lesion within the right frontal lobe was performed to confirm the diagnosis and establish the tumor's genetic signature, and further surgery was not recommended.

In cases where resection is pursued, consider preoperative functional MRI and diffusion tensor imaging to map suspected involvement of language areas and motor tracts. MRI image-guidance, intraoperative MRI, intraoperative mapping (e.g., awake craniotomy if speech is threatened), and neuromonitoring are tools to be considered in planning the resection.

The precise positioning and approach used for a craniotomy in the resection of a GBM will depend on the location and size of the tumor. Neuronavigation may be useful to localize the tumor for planning of the incision and craniotomy.

Upon opening the dura, a corticectomy is planned to minimize distance to the underlying tumor and avoid damage to eloquent cortex. The pia, over the intended corticectomy, is cauterized with a bipolar device and cut sharply. Suction and bipolar electrocautery are used to dissect through the parenchyma down to the tumor. GBM grossly appears grayish-pink, friable, and hemorrhagic compared with normal white matter. The surrounding white matter may be boggy with edema. GBM is infiltrative and lacks a true margin with the surrounding parenchyma. For noneloquent cortex, a strategy including a full or partial lobectomy may be pursued to avoid the abnormal friable tumor vessels and the difficulty of controlling bleeding. Near eloquent cortex, a strategy of internal debulking along the rim of tumor pseudocapsule, for maximal safe resection, is often pursued.

Complication Avoidance and Management

- Patient selection, detailed anatomic knowledge, and intraoperative awareness are critical for maximizing quality of life and survival. Useful tools include fMRI and tractography, intraoperative cortical and subcortical mapping, image guidance, and intraoperative MRI.
- Subtotal resection of this highly vascular tumor often results in postoperative bleeding. Gross total resection should be pursued without compromising function.

KEY PAPERS

Hegi ME, Diserens AC, Gorlia T, et al. MGMT gene silencing and benefit from temozolomide in glioblastoma. *N Engl J Med.* 2005;352(10):997-1003.

Ryken TC, Frankel B, Julien T, et al. Surgical management of newly diagnosed glioblastoma in adults: role of cytoreductive surgery. *J Neurooncol.* 2008;89(3):271-286.

Stupp R, Mason WP, van den Bent MJ, et al. European Organisation for Research and Treatment of Cancer Brain Tumor and Radiotherapy Groups; National Cancer Institute of Canada Clinical Trials Group. Radiotherapy plus concomitant and adjuvant temozolomide for glioblastoma. *N Engl J Med.* 2005;352(10):987-996.

Case 27

Anaplastic Oligodendroglioma

Christine K. Lee, MD, PhD ● Melanie G. Hayden Gephart, MD

Presentation

A 60-year-old female with a history of chronic headaches.

- PMH: noncontributory
- Exam: mild memory impairment, no focal neurologic deficits

Differential Diagnosis

- Neoplastic
  - Glioma
  - CNS lymphoma
  - Meningioma
  - Metastases
- Vascular
  - AVM
  - Ischemic stroke
- Infectious
  - Cerebral abscess
  - Encephalitis
  - Toxoplasmosis
- Other
  - MS
  - Radiation necrosis

Initial Imaging

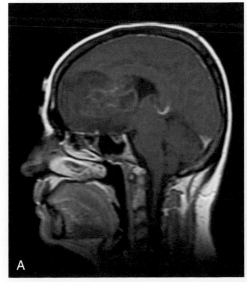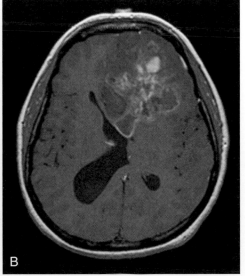

FIGURE 27-1

Imaging Description and Differential

- Brain MRI in Figure 27-1A and B show sagittal and axial contrast-enhanced T1 images, in which a large, irregular, and heterogeneously enhancing mass is seen in left frontal lobe, crossing midline and extending into corpus callosum, with significant mass effect and ventriculomegaly.
- Differential: glioblastoma, anaplastic astrocytoma, mixed glioma, oligodendroglioma, or metastatic disease.

Further Workup

- Laboratory
  - Routine laboratory analysis (CBC, BMP, INR, and UA)
- Imaging
  - MRI, with and without gadolinium contrast. For operative planning, include stereotactic sequences and, in eloquent locations, consider diffusion tensor imaging (DTI) and functional MRI (fMRI).
- Consultants
  - Neuro-oncology
  - Radiation oncology

Pathophysiology

Anaplastic oligodendrogliomas (AOs) are WHO grade III oligodendrogliomas that account for <5% of all primary brain tumors. The mean age at diagnosis is 45 years. These tumors generally arise in the cerebral white matter and are typically supratentorial, most commonly in the frontal lobes, and often have significant calcifications. Patients have the following symptoms: seizures, headaches, focal neurologic deficits, and cognitive changes.

The natural history of oligodendrogliomas is progression from well-differentiated low-grade tumors to high-grade anaplastic lesions; although, some patients with AOs have no evidence of prior low-grade lesions. Both AOs and low-grade oligodendrogliomas frequently have loss of genetic material from Ch 1p and Ch 19q ("1p/19q codeletion"), resulting from an unbalanced translocation. AOs with this codeletion are more sensitive to radiotherapy and alkylating chemotherapy, and thus carry a significantly better prognosis.

Treatment Options

- Surgical
  - Stereotactic resection of tumor with image guidance. Minimizing volume of residual tumor increases time to tumor progression and median survival.
  - If tumor is near eloquent areas of cortex, preoperative DTI and fMRI may help guide resection. Consider intraoperative neuromonitoring or an awake procedure.
  - If tumor is bilateral or multifocal, resection is unlikely to provide significant cytoreduction. Consider biopsy instead.
  - Test for 1p/19q codeletion.
- Medical
  - Most AOs respond to chemotherapy. Temozolomide (also has some efficacy for recurrent AOs), PCV (procarbazine, lomustine, vincristine)
  - Anticonvulsants for seizure control if symptomatic (not for prophylaxis)
  - Corticosteroids for reduction of peritumoral edema before and after surgery
- Biopsy
  - Stereotactic biopsy to determine tumor grade and treatment plan, if not amenable to surgical resection
- Radiation
  - Frequent adjuvant to surgery, regardless of extent of resection
  - Combining with chemotherapy significantly prolongs survival for tumors containing 1p/19q codeletion

Surgical Technique

Supine positioning for frontal lobe glioma, prepare neuromonitoring, place in three-point pin fixation such that tumor is at highest location, and register patient with stereotactic navigation for marking incision. Craniotomy size and position are chosen based on optimal trajectory for radical removal of tumor with preservation of normal brain.

For frontal craniotomy, either perform unilateral craniotomy through curved skin incision taken anteriorly to the hairline, or bifrontal or ¾ bifrontal skin incision if necessary to have low approach to one or both frontal fossa.

Resection is performed with the goal of maximal safe removal of tumor. For a frontal lobe tumor, respect the posterior and deep extension of the tumor, keeping in mind motor cortex, white matter tracks, and Broca's area. Intraoperative cortical mapping can help locate motor and sensory cortex. Transsulcal approach may be used for deep-seated lesions to expose periphery of tumor and preserve normal brain. Strive for maximum debulking of obvious tumor without causing neurologic deficit. After the resection, achieve hemostasis and water-tight dural closure. Carefully reconstruct scalp for maximal integrity and optimal healing, especially if planning postoperative radiation therapy.

Complication Avoidance and Management

- The most common complications include postoperative hematoma and infection. Immaculate hemostasis should be achieved after the resection. Meticulous sterile technique, closure, and prophylactic antibiotics help reduce the risk of infection. During the resection, care should be taken to preserve cortical veins draining toward major sinuses and respect functional anatomic regions to ensure no worsening of the preoperative neurological exam from venous stroke or parenchymal injury. Take postoperative precaution against venous thromboembolism, which is a frequent complication in patients with high-grade gliomas.

KEY PAPERS

Cairncross G, Wang M, Shaw E, et al. Phase III trial of chemoradiotherapy for anaplastic oligodendroglioma: long-term results of RTOG 9402. *J Clin Oncol*. 2013;31:337-343.

Laws ER. Management of (malignant) intracranial gliomas. In: Sindou M, ed. *Practical Handbook of Neurosurgery*. New York: Springer Wien; 2009.

Roth P, Wick W, Weller M. Anaplastic oligodendroglioma: a new treatment paradigm and current controversies. *Curr Treat Options Oncol*. 2013;14:505-513.

Case 28

Low-Grade Glioma

Christina Huang Wright, MD ● James Wright, MD

Presentation

A 35-year-old male presents with an initial generalized tonic-clonic seizure and 3 months of headache.

- PMH: otherwise unremarkable
- Exam:
  - Awake, alert, and oriented
  - Cranial nerves intact
  - Motor exam with full strength, except for mild left arm pronator drift

Initial Imaging

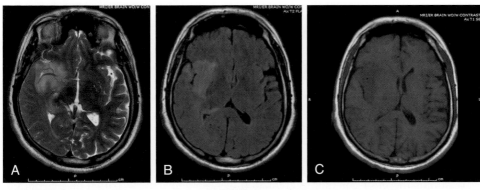

FIGURE 28-1

Imaging Description and Differential Diagnoses

- MRI findings: T2 hyperintensity (Figure 28-1A and B) and T1 hypointensity (Figure 28-1C) within the right insula, right temporal pole, uncus, and inferior right frontal lobe. No associated enhancement or diffusion restriction identified (images not shown).
- Differential diagnosis
  - Low-grade glioma (LGG)
  - Infarction or hemorrhage
  - Cerebritis or encephalitis
  - Ependymoma
  - Multiple sclerosis
  - Other cerebral neoplasms

Further Workup

- Laboratory
  - CSF sampling for cytology and flow cytometry to rule out CNS lymphoma

- Imaging
  - CT scans are often the first images obtained and typically show a hypodense lesion.
  - MRI is the gold standard for noninvasive identification and classification of LGG.
    - On T1-weighted imaging, LGG are typically hypointense to isointense.
    - On T2-weighted sequences, the lesions are hyperintense.
    - LGG rarely have contrast enhancement, but it is somewhat more common in oligodendroglioma (25%–50%).
  - Diffusion tensor imaging (DTI) is invaluable for preoperative planning and intraoperative navigation and often will dictate the limits of resection.
  - PET usually demonstrates reduced fluorodeoxyglucose relative to normal brain tissue, signifying a hypometabolic state.
  - MR spectroscopy: peak levels of certain markers (choline, lactate, lipid, creatine, N-acetylaspartate) may indicate specific areas of malignant transformation and inform biopsy targeting and prognosis.
- Consultants
  - Neuro-oncology

Epidemiology and Pathophysiology

LGG account for approximately 15% to 20% of primary brain tumors in adults. Gliomas are classified by the primary cell type. Other factors such as necrosis, anaplasia, and mitotic figures may increase the grade of a glioma. The classification of LGG remains controversial due to the variety of subtypes with distinct cell lineages and histopathologies. WHO grade 1 gliomas include: pilocytic astrocytoma and subependymal giant cell astrocytoma. WHO grade 2 gliomas include: pilomyxoid astrocytoma, pleomorphic xanthoastrocytoma, diffuse astrocytomas (fibrillary, protoplasmic, gemistocytic), oligodendroglioma, oligoastrocytomas, gangliogliomas, gangliocytomas, and dysembryoplastic neuroepithelial tumors. Fibrillary astrocytoma is the most common subtype and gemistocytic is the most prone to progress to grade IV.

Generally, LGG occurs more frequently in white males and in the younger age group (fourth decade) than high-grade gliomas (sixth decade) do. There are no known hereditary factors associated with LGGs, although they do occur more commonly in patients with neurofibromatosis type 1 and tuberous sclerosis. The etiology of LGG is unknown, thought to be multifactorial, and to include genetic, immunologic, and infectious factors.

Anatomically, LGG has a predilection for the temporal, posterior frontal, and anterior parietal lobes, and specifically the supplementary motor cortex and the insula. The rare LGG involving multiple lobes of the brain is termed gliomatosis cerebri. As LGGs grow slowly, vasogenic edema is uncommon.

Seizure is the most common presentation of LGG and may be partial or generalized. Seizures occur in over 90% of LGG cases. They are most frequent in cortically based tumors.

Chang et al (2008) proposed a preoperative grading scale for LGG that assigns a point to adverse prognostic factors including: age over 50 years, a KPS <80, location in eloquent brain, and a diameter of >4 cm. The lower the score, the greater the 5-year survival rate and the progression-free survival rate (PFS).

Patients with oligodendroglioma have a better prognosis compared to those with astrocytoma or oligoastrocytoma. Chromosomal 1p deletion (with or without 19q deletion) is a favorable prognostic factor in oligodendrogliomas with a longer PFS after adjuvant chemotherapy and radiation. MGMT promoter methylation predicts a shorter time to progression in untreated patients, but longer PFS and overall survival (OS) in patients treated with temozolomide (TMZ).

Treatment Options

- Medical
  - In patients with seizures, antiepileptics should be initiated. However, prophylactic antiepileptics are not indicated.
  - Steroids are often used for symptomatic peri-tumoral edema or mass effect.

- Chemotherapy
  - Although the exact role of chemotherapy remains undefined, multiple recent studies suggest the value of adjuvant chemotherapy.
  - Two regimens are utilized commonly for LGG – temozolomide and a combination of procarbazine, lomustine, and vincristine (PCV).
- Radiation therapy (XRT)
  - XRT after surgery lengthens PFS, but not OS.
  - Higher doses of XRT do not improve outcome and have higher toxicity, including radiation necrosis.
  - Whole-brain XRT has a higher incidence of leukoencephalopathy and cognitive deficits than does stereotactic radiosurgery.
    - Stereotactic radiosurgery
      - Stereotactic radiosurgery may be used as primary, adjuvant, or salvage treatment. It may be particularly useful for small tumors in deep or eloquent brain regions.
- Surgical
  - Literature suggests that more extensive resection improves long-term outcomes, including longer OS and lower rates of malignant transformation.
  - In patients with WHO grade I lesions, long-term remission is possible in both children and adults.
  - Many clinical series have associated more extensive resection GTR and longer survival.

Surgical Technique

- Total resection improves seizure control especially for insular tumor. Stereotactic image guidance is helpful in planning the craniotomy and in guiding the resection of tumors lacking a distinct margin. Brain mapping of tumors near eloquent structures can increase the extent of resection and decrease the risk of new postoperative neurologic deficits.
- Surgical resection is highly recommended for pilocytic astrocytomas when herniation is threatened by tumor or cysts, CSF flow is obstructed, seizures are refractory, or in children for whom adjuvant therapy should be eschewed.
- Surgery is less useful for widely disseminated tumors, multifocal tumors, and tumors invading eloquent brain.
- Craniotomy technique is adapted for each tumor location. The technique for low-grade glioma is similar to that described in Case 27: Anaplastic Oligodendroglioma.

Complication Avoidance and Management

- Complications of resection include new neurologic deficit secondary to stroke or hemorrhage, the risk of which can be minimized by meticulous hemostasis and preservation of draining cortical veins.
- More aggressive resection can entail greater risk of functional loss which can be reduced by intraoperative navigation with DTI. Because LGG often does not enhance with gadolinium, T2 sequences may be more useful for intraoperative navigation.
- The rates of transformation of LGG to higher grades range from 17% to 73% and intervals to progression vary from 2 to 10 years. Delaying surgery and adjuvant chemotherapy is associated with increased risk of malignant transformation.

KEY PAPERS

Chang E, Clark A, Jensen R, et al. Multi-institutional validation of the University of California at San Francisco low-grade glioma prognostic scoring system: clinical article. *J Neurosurg.* 2009;111(2):203-210.

Chang EF, Smith JS, Chang SM, et al. Preoperative prognostic classification system for hemispheric low-grade gliomas in adults. *J Neurosurg.* 2008;109(5):817-824.

Pedersen C, Romner B. Current treatment of low grade astrocytoma: a review. *Clin Neurol and Neurosurg.* 2013;115:1-8.

Recht L, Lew R, Smith T. Suspected low-grade glioma: is deferring treatment safe? *Ann of Neurol.* 1992;31:431-436.

Sanai N, Chang S, Berger M. Low-grade gliomas in adults: a review. *J Neurosurg.* 2011;115(5):948-965.

Soffietti R, Baumert B, von Deimling A, et al. Guidelines on management of low-grade gliomas: report of an EFNS-EANO Task Force. *Euro J Neuro.* 2010;17:1124-1133.

Case 29

Radiation Necrosis versus Tumor Recurrence

Derek Yecies, MD ● J. Dawn Waters, MD

Presentation

A 60-year-old male with a history of glioblastoma (GBM) has new enhancement on follow-up surveillance MRI. He was initially diagnosed with a right frontal-parietal GBM 4 months ago when he was evaluated for left-facial weakness, left arm numbness, and headaches. He underwent a craniotomy at that time. Figure 29-1 demonstrates his imme-diate postoperative scan with a gross total resection and blood products in the resection cavity. Histology confirmed GBM that was negative for EGFRvIII mutation and MGMT promotor methylation. He tolerated a course of chemoradiation with temozolomide, and has continued with monthly temozolomide.

- ROS: generalized weakness, worsening left upper and lower extremity weakness, and paresthesias; denies headaches, nausea, or visual problems
- PMH: hypertension, diabetes, and environmental allergies
- Exam:
  - Afebrile, vitals within normal limits
  - Cranial nerve exam is normal.
  - Motor exam demonstrates 4/5 weakness throughout left upper and lower extremities.
  - Sensory, coordination, and reflexes are normal.

Imaging

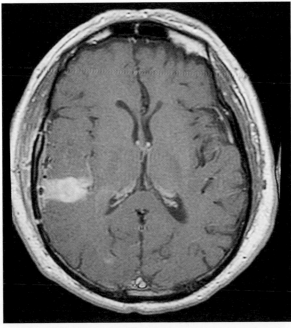

FIGURE 29-1

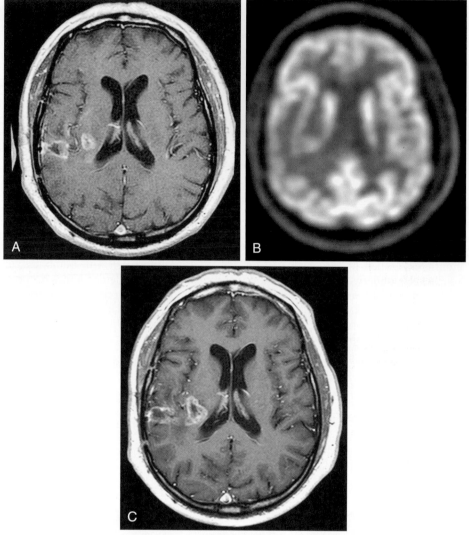

FIGURE 29-2

Imaging Description and Differential

- Figure 29-1 is an axial T1 postgadolinium MRI of the brain performed immediately after the patient's initial craniotomy. It demonstrates a gross total resection and blood products in the resection cavity.
- Figure 29-2A is an axial T1 postgadolinium MRI of the brain obtained 4 months postoperatively and shows enhancement along the resection cavity and a new area of enhancement deep to the original lesion in the periventricular white matter.
- Figure 29-2B is an FDG PET-CT obtained 4 months postoperatively and demonstrates decreased FDG uptake in the right frontal-parietal gray matter, more consistent with treatment effects. No increased uptake was demonstrated in the area of new enhancement.
- Differential for Figure 29-2B and C: tumor recurrence, radiation necrosis, infection, demyelination
- Figure 29-2C is an axial T1 postgadolinium MRI of the brain obtained 7 months postoperatively and demonstrates that the deeper enhancing lesion has enlarged, which is suggestive of recurrent tumor.

Further Workup

- Laboratory
  - Routine labs
  - ESR, CRP, blood cultures
- Imaging
  - No imaging modality has sufficient specificity to replace histology as the standard for distinguishing radiation necrosis from recurrent glioma. Imaging features are more suggestive of recurrence rather than radiation reaction, such as homogeneously enhancing nodularity and perinodular edema, as opposed to more diffuse, less homogeneously intense enhancement and edema occurring preferentially in deep white matter. This supports earlier biopsy and excludes recurrence, rather than continued MRI surveillance..
  - FDG-PET lacks specificity to distinguish between radiation necrosis and recurrent glioma; however, increased uptake is more suggestive of recurrent tumor.
  - MRI spectroscopy is of limited utility because recurrent tumor cells are often mixed within areas of radiation necrosis.
  - Advanced MRI modalities such as diffusion imaging and MR perfusion modalities, including DSC-MRI and DCE-MRI, may differentiate tumor progression from radiation necrosis more accurately in the future.

Pathophysiology

The pathophysiology of delayed radiation necrosis is complex and not fully understood. Higher radiation doses, exposure to systemic chemotherapy, and intrinsic deficits in DNA repair mechanisms, such as those in Fanconi's anemia and ataxia telangiectasia, are associated with higher rates of radiation necrosis. Radiation necrosis is likely mediated by a combination of endothelial damage, direct injury to glial cells, and immune-mediated mechanisms.

Radiation directly damages glial cells and induces myelin loss. Reactive astrocytes in the injured region release hypoxia-inducible factor 1 alpha and vascular endothelial growth factor (VEGF), which incite inflammation and promote pathologic neovascularization. Endothelial damage compromises the blood-brain barrier, leading to vasogenic edema. Radiation-induced apoptosis of endothelial cells induces oxygen free radical formation, VEGF up-regulation, inflammatory cytokine release, and migration of neutrophils and fibroblasts to the affected area. Endothelial cell death is followed by abnormal proliferation of endothelial cells, which further compromises the blood-brain barrier. Ultimately, narrowing of the effected vessels, often associated with fibrinoid necrosis of the vessel wall, induces further ischemia, edema, and cell death in adjacent tissues, resulting in radiation necrosis.

Treatment Options

- Medical
  - Corticosteroids for symptomatic relief
- Biopsy
  - Pathologic analysis of the tissue in question is the gold standard for distinguishing radiation necrosis from tumor recurrence.
  - Given the invasive nature and inherent risk of biopsy, PET-CT or advanced MRI imaging modalities are often used to support the decision to biopsy. Equivocal lesions are often monitored with serial MRI imaging, and those that continue to grow are considered more likely to represent tumor recurrence and warrant biopsy.
- Surgical
  - Resection is indicated for symptomatic mass effect from either tumor recurrence or radiation necrosis. Benefits of craniotomy must be considered in the context of the patient's overall prognosis, functional status, and the location of the lesion.

- Treatment for biopsy-proven radiation necrosis
  - Options include observation, corticosteroids, surgical resection, stereotactic drainage of associated cysts, heparin, warfarin, pentoxyfilline, hyperbaric oxygen, bevacizumab, and laser interstitial thermal therapy.
- Treatment for biopsy-proven recurrent glioma
  - Options include repeat resection, additional radiation therapy (including stereotactic radiosurgery), and chemotherapy (e.g., CCNU, bevacizumab).

Surgical Technique

Stereotactic biopsy of the deep enhancing lesion retrieves scattered tumor cells within a field of radiation necrosis.

The surgical technique for stereotactic biopsy is presented in Case 30: CNS Lymphoma.

The surgical technique for craniotomy is described in Case 26: Glioblastoma.

Complication Avoidance and Management

- The risk of radiation toxicity increases with the total radiation dose, the frequency and dose of each fraction of treatment, and the volume treated. The Medical Research Council Brain Tumor Working Party found that 60 Gy given in 30 fractions over 6 weeks was well tolerated and provided a survival benefit compared with 45 Gy in 20 fractions. A survival benefit of doses beyond 60 Gy has not been demonstrated. Risks of reirradiation include radiation necrosis and dementia.

KEY PAPERS

Bleehen NM, Stenning SP. A Medical Research Council trial of two radiotherapy doses in the treatment of grades 3 and 4 astrocytoma. The Medical Research Council Brain Tumour Working Party. *Br J Cancer.* 1991;64(4):769-774.

Hingorani M, Colley WP, Dixit S, et al. Hypofractionated radiotherapy for glioblastoma: strategy for poor-risk patients or hope for the future? *Br J Radiol.* 2012;85(1017):e770-e781.

O'Connor MM, Mayberg MR. Effects of radiation on cerebral vasculature: a review. *Neurosurgery.* 2000;46:138-151.

Rock JP, Hearshen D, Scarpace L, et al. Correlations between magnetic resonance spectroscopy and image-guided histopathology, with special attention to radiation necrosis. *Neurosurgery.* 2002;51(4):912-919, discussion 919-920.

Shah AH, Snelling B, Bregy A, et al. Discriminating radiation necrosis from tumor progression in gliomas: a systematic review what is the best imaging modality? *J Neurooncol.* 2013;112(2):141-152.

CNS Lymphoma

Zachary Medress ● Kai Miller, MD ● Li Gordon, MD

Presentation

A 45-year-old male presents with a 3-month history of left arm numbness and headaches.

- PMH: renal transplant
- Exam: decreased sensation to light touch in distal left arm
  - Alert and oriented × 3
  - Visual fields intact
  - Full strength bilaterally

Differential Diagnosis

Differential diagnosis for an intracranial mass lesion in an immunocompromised patient:
- Neoplastic
  - Glioma or glioblastoma (GBM)
  - Meningioma
  - Brain metastasis
  - Central nervous system (CNS) lymphoma
- Infectious
  - Abscess
  - Parasitic infection (toxoplasmosis)
  - Fungal infection (aspergillosis)
  - Tuberculosis
- Inflammatory/Demyelinating
  - MS
  - Sarcoidosis

Initial Imaging

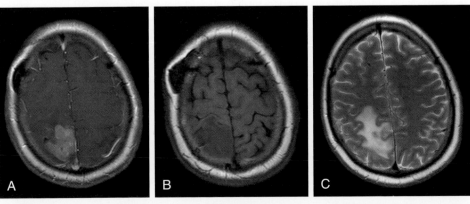

FIGURE 30-1

Imaging Description and Differential

- Brain MRI shows solitary right parietal homogenously enhancing mass (Figure 30-1A) that is hypointense on T1 FLAIR (Figure 30-1B) and hyperintense on T2 (Figure 30-1C).
- Differential: metastasis, primary brain tumor, infection, or lymphoma

Further Workup

- Laboratory
  - Immunodeficiency workup, including HIV
  - CSF with cell counts, protein, glucose, cytology, flow cytometry, IgH rearrangement PCR imaging
  - LDH
  - MRI spine
  - PET-CT to evaluate for extra-CNS lymphoma
  - Routine preoperative labs, including CBC and coagulation profile
- Consultants
  - Hematology/oncology for medical management and bone marrow biopsy
  - Ophthalmology for bilateral slit-lamp examination to evaluate for ocular lymphoma

Pathophysiology

CNS lymphoma is a rare malignant lymphoma heavily associated with immunocompromised hosts, including HIV/AIDS, solid organ transplant (in particular EBV mismatch), and inherited immunodeficiencies including common and combined variable immunodeficiencies, Wiskott-Aldrich syndrome, and ataxia telangiectasia. However, primary CNS lymphoma can also occur in immunocompetent patients. EBV infection has been associated with CNS lymphoma in both immunocompromised and immunocompetent hosts and may underlie malignant transformation and clonal expansion of CNS B-cells. Autoimmune diseases, such as rheumatoid arthritis and SLE, may also predispose one to CNS lymphoma. Pathology most commonly shows diffuse large B-cell lymphoma.

Treatment Options

- Surgery
  - Stereotactic biopsy: the procedure of choice to establish tissue diagnosis of CNS lymphoma if CSF cytology fails to make the diagnosis
  - Surgical resection: typically contraindicated in CNS lymphoma as these tumors are highly invasive and recurrence is common. Surgical resection is confined to patients with no lesion amenable to biopsy, or with acute decompensation secondary to herniation requiring emergent decompression.
- Medications
  - Steroids: in stable patients, corticosteroids should not be administered before biopsy as they interfere with histologic analysis. If a patient is unstable due to brainstem compression or elevated intracranial pressure, steroids may be temporizing as surgical decompression is arranged.
  - Chemotherapy:
    - With or without radiation, offers the best chance for remission, although the prognosis of CNS lymphoma remains poor
    - High-dose methotrexate is the first-line treatment for CNS lymphoma. Carmustine, emozolomide, topotecan, arabinoside, and rituximab have also been used.
- Radiation
  - Whole brain radiation is preferred for CNS lymphoma given its diffuse infiltrative nature. It is associated with a complete response rate of up to 90%, but offers poor long-term disease control. Whole brain radiation, combined with high-dose methotrexate, offers better long-term disease control and has become standard therapy at many centers for CNS lymphoma.

Surgical Technique

Surgical intervention for CNS lymphoma is usually limited to stereotactic biopsy. Frameless systems are now the standard of care for brain biopsy procedures; however, frame-based systems may be used for lesions that are smaller than 5 to 10 mm or located within deep structures. The patient is placed supine with the head fixated using the Mayfield clamp. The entry point is selected using neuronavigation, and several core biopsies are taken from multiple regions of the tumor. The biopsies are sent for frozen and permanent section, and closure is delayed until frozen sections confirm adequate tissue sample and diagnosis. If frozen section confirms CNS lymphoma, resection is not pursued.

Complication Avoidance and Management

- Stereotactic biopsy
  - Complications include intratumoral hemorrhage, intraparenchymal hemorrhage, and extension of hemorrhage into the ventricles. Patients should be carefully screened for coagulopathy or platelet dysfunction. A trajectory should be chosen preoperatively that minimizes the risk of bleeding and neurologic deficit by avoiding sulci, ventricles, and eloquent brain regions. If bleeding occurs from the biopsy site, a cannula should be left in place until the bleeding stops, and a postoperative head CT should be ordered to evaluate for intraparenchymal hematoma.
- Chemoradiation
  - Leukoencephalopathy and neurotoxicity may complicate combination high-dose methotrexate and radiation and have synergistic toxic effects. Neurotoxicity may present as rapidly progressing dementia, gait ataxia, and urinary incontinence and is more common in older patients. There is no standard treatment of methotrexate-induced neurotoxicity, although data suggest that administration of aminophylline and folinic acid, in addition to removing an Ommaya catheter, if present, may improve outcomes.

KEY PAPERS

Owen CM, Linskey ME. Frame-based stereotaxy in a frameless era: current capabilities, relative role, and the positive- and negative predictive values of blood through the needle. *J Neurooncol.* 2009;93(1):139-149.

Thiel E, Korfel A, Martus P, et al. High-dose methotrexate with or without whole brain radiotherapy for primary CNS lymphoma (G-PCNSL-SG-1): a phase 3, randomised, non-inferiority trial. *Lancet Oncol.* 2010;11(11):1036-1047.

Weller M, Martus P, Roth P, et al. Surgery for primary CNS lymphoma? Challenging a paradigm. *Neuro Oncol.* 2012;14(12):1481-1484. [Epub 2012/09/18. eng]; PubMed PMID: 22984018. Pubmed Central PMCID: PMC3499010.

Case 31

Brain Metastases

Kevin K.H. Chow, MD, PhD

Presentation

A 55-year-old male smoker with history of small cell lung cancer (SCLC), in remission s/p chemotherapy and lung radiation, presents with early morning headaches and memory problems for the past 3 weeks.

- PMH: SCLC and hypertension
- SH: 30 pack/year smoking history
- Exam:
  - Diminished breath sounds in RLL
  - No focal neurologic deficits
  - 24/30 on Folstein mini-mental status exam

Differential Diagnosis

- Neoplastic
  - Metastasis
  - Primary brain tumor (e.g., GBM)
- Vascular
  - Cerebral hemorrhage or infarct
- Infectious
  - Cerebral abscess
- Other
  - Progressive multifocal leukoencephalopathy
  - Demyelination
  - Inflammatory process
  - Radiation necrosis

Initial Imaging

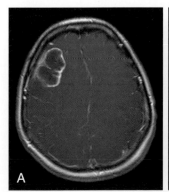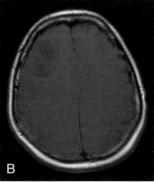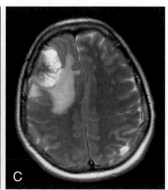

FIGURE 31-1

Imaging Description and Differential

- Figure 31-1 A and B depicts an MRI brain, with and without contrast. Figure 31-1C is the corresponding T2 image. These demonstrate a peripherally enhancing right frontal lesion with surrounding T2-bright edema. Features that are generally suggestive of brain metastases include localization at gray-white junction, circumscribed margins, significant vasogenic edema, and multiple lesions.
- Differential: brain metastasis, primary brain tumor, abscess, cerebral infarct, progressive multifocal leukoencephalopathy, or radiation necrosis

Further Workup

- Laboratory
  - Routine labs
  - Fecal occult blood test, PSA in men
- Imaging
  - Incremental studies only as needed
  - MRI brain with contrast is the imaging modality of choice for diagnosis of brain metastasis.
  - CXR
  - CT chest/abdomen/pelvis
  - Radionuclide bone scan
  - Full body PET scan
  - MR spectroscopy
  - Mammogram for women
- Consultants
  - Neuro-oncology
  - Medical oncology
  - Radiation oncology

Pathophysiology

The true incidence of brain metastasis is likely underestimated, as patients often die of their systemic disease before they become symptomatic from brain lesions. This is corroborated by the fact that brain metastases are often first detected postmortem. Brain metastases comprise up to half of all brain tumors and occur in up to 30% of cancer patients. Of patients with brain metastases, the most common sites of the primary tumor are lung (30%–40%) and breast (20%–30%) due to higher incidence of these tumors in general. Melanoma, however, has the highest propensity to metastasize to the brain – up to 70% of patients with melanoma will develop brain metastases. Metastasis to the brain generally occurs via hematogenous spread, and thus brain metastases are usually located at the gray-white junction, or watershed areas, where the vessels narrow and tumor cells are thought to become trapped and accumulate. Metastases are also often multifocal, particularly with lung cancer and melanoma.

Treatment Options

- Medical
  - Chemotherapy
  - Palliative care and symptom management for patients with poor prognosis
    - Corticosteroids for control of peritumoral edema
    - Antiepileptics for treatment or prevention (optional) of seizures
  - Prophylaxis for venous thromboembolic disease
- Radiation
  - Whole brain radiation therapy (WBRT) – may be given prophylactically (for SCLC), or as treatment for metastases not amenable to surgical resection
  - Stereotactic radiosurgery (SRS) – generally reserved for three tumors or fewer and lesions smaller than 3 cm in size. May be used to deliver higher radiation dose than

WBRT to radioresistant tumors. Focal radiation avoids neurocognitive deficits seen with WBRT.
- Radiation-sensitive cancers: SCLC, breast, lymphoma, and multiple myeloma
- Radiation-resistant cancers: melanoma, renal cell, NSCLC, and colon
- Biopsy
  - Indications include the need for diagnosis of metastatic disease:
    - Uncertain diagnosis (e.g., unknown primary, no other site to biopsy, single lesion concerning for new primary)
    - Poor surgical candidates for craniotomy
  - Lesions not amenable for resection due to eloquent/deep location
- Surgical resection
  - The decision about whether or not to offer surgery will depend on the patient's functional status, medical comorbidities, presence of systemic disease, and the characteristics of the brain metastases themselves, including size, location, and number of lesions. Patients with poor prognosis and functional status from extensive systemic disease are unlikely to benefit from surgery unless they are having significant symptoms, or the lesions are life threatening due to mass effect.
  - Of the patients with good functional status and well-controlled systemic disease, surgery is often beneficial when the lesion(s) can be completely resected. A relatively healthy patient with a solitary lesion in an accessible location should undergo surgical resection, potentially followed by focal or WBRT.

Surgical Technique

The surgical planning and technique for a cerebral metastasis shares many similarities with the technique described for glioblastoma (GBM, Case 26). Please refer to that case for an overview of surgical considerations for a lobar tumor. Differences related to brain metastasis will be highlighted here.

Many metastases are well demarcated within the cerebrum, in contrast to infiltrative primary brain tumors. The color and texture of tumor may vary based upon the primary, but is usually readily distinguishable from surrounding brain parenchyma, which may be boggy with edema. A gross total resection can often be achieved by developing the plane around the tumor capsule. Seeding of the subarachnoid space with tumor cells and fragments can be lessened by removal of intact tumor as a single specimen. Dissection within the tumor may cause bleeding from friable tumor vessels that may be difficult to control until the lesion is completely resected.

Complication Avoidance and Management

- Multidisciplinary management of brain metastases is critical for avoiding the complications of poor management decisions. The multidisciplinary team for a patient with brain metastases should include neurosurgery, neuro-oncology, medical oncology, and radiation oncology.
- Postoperative complications that result in neurologic deficits can significantly decrease survival by affecting the patient's functional status and ability to undergo subsequent treatments. Strategies to decrease the risk of postoperative complications include careful preoperative planning and imaging, and the use of intraoperative neuronavigation or MRI to guide resection in complex cases.

KEY PAPERS

Eichler AF, Loeffler JS. Multidisciplinary management of brain metastases. *Oncologist.* 2007;12(7):884-898.

Kalkanis SN, Kondziolka D, Gaspar LE, et al. The role of surgical resection in the management of newly diagnosed brain metastases: a systematic review and evidence-based clinical practice guideline. *J Neurooncol.* 2010;96(1):33-43.

Owonikoko TK, Arbiser J, Zelnak A, et al. Current approaches to the treatment of metastatic brain tumours. *Nat Rev Clin Oncol.* 2014;11(4):203-222.

Case 32

Intraventricular Colloid Cyst

Arjun V. Pendharkar, MD ● Melanie G. Hayden Gephart, MD

Presentation

A 41-year-old male presents with an episode of confusion, slurred speech, and syncope. Symptoms resolved without intervention. Head CT is concerning for a mass in the third ventricle.

- PMH:
  - Chronic lower back pain
  - Obesity
- PSH:
  - Cervical spine discectomy
- Exam: no neurologic deficits
  - Mental status: alert and oriented to self, time, location and situation, briskly follows commands, speech fluent and appropriate
  - Remainder of the neurologic exam is normal

Differential Diagnosis

- Developmental
  - Colloid cyst
  - Ependymal cyst
  - Neoplastic
  - Glioma
  - Lymphoma
  - Meningioma
  - Metastasis (h/o cancer)
- Vascular
  - Intracranial aneurysm of the posterior circulation
  - Vertebrobasilar dolichoectasia
- Infectious
  - Neurocysticercosis

Initial Imaging

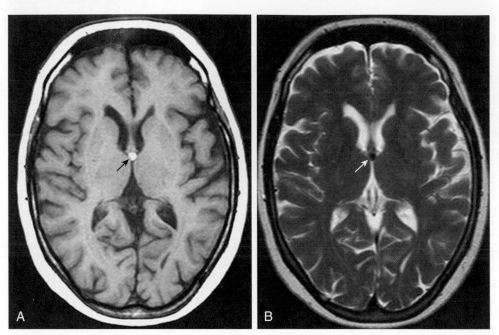

FIGURE 32-1   *(Reprinted with permission Daroff RB.* Neurology in Clinical Practice. *6th ed. Elsevier. 2000.)*

Imaging Description and Differential

- Figure 32-1A is an axial T1-weighted MRI demonstrating a spherical hyperintense mass in the anterior portion of the third ventricle at the level of the foramen of Monro. Figure 32-1B is an axial T2-weighted MRI showing a corresponding hypointense lesion.
- Differential: colloid cyst; less likely an ependymal cyst or neoplastic lesion

Further Workup

- Laboratory
  - Routine preoperative labs
- Imaging
  - MRI planning for frameless stereotactic navigation

Pathophysiology

Colloid cysts, although rare, represent 0.5%–2% of primary developmental, or neoplastic, brain masses and are the most common of such masses in the third ventricle. These benign lesions are considered congenital. Nonetheless, they often do not present until the third to fifth decades. There is no gender predilection. Colloid cysts arise from ectopic endodermal cells in the velum interpositum. Almost all arise in the third ventricle and are attached to its roof immediately dorsal to the foramen of Monro. The classic presentation of paroxysmal headache, associated with changes in head position, is rare and these lesions are most often identified incidentally. Patients can be considered cured after complete resection of the cyst. Even though complete resection relieves obstruction, CSF diversion by third ventriculostomy, or shunting, may be necessary. Cysts may recur if incompletely resected.

Treatment Options

Patients with acute symptomatic obstruction of CSF outflow require emergent ventricular drainage. Intermittent symptoms, or enlargement of a large cyst threatening obstruction, are indications for surgical treatment of the colloid cyst.

- Surgical
  - Open transcallosal: this approach is preferred to the transcortical route when ventricles are not enlarged by hydrocephalus. It also provides access to the third ventricle and both foramina of Monro. It carries a risk of cortical venous infarction and damage to the cingulate gyrus.
  - Open transcortical: this approach avoids interhemispheric retraction and callosal sectioning. It may be difficult unless the ventricles are enlarged. It carries an approximate 5% risk of epilepsy. The contralateral foramen of Monro is not readily accessible via this route.
  - Endoscopic approach: this approach follows a transcortical route, but requires a smaller craniotomy, shorter cortical incision, and less retraction. Rates of complete resection are lower than with open microsurgical resection.
  - Stereotactic aspiration: generally limited to symptomatic patients unable to tolerate an open or endoscopic operation.

Surgical Technique

The patient is placed supine with the head secured in Mayfield pins; neuronavigation is registered and confirmed for accuracy. Kocher's point is identified on the nondominant side. After sterile skin preparation and draping, a linear incision is created using a number 10 blade. Bovie electrocautery is used to dissect to the bone, and the scalp is retracted using a self-retaining retractor. A burr hole is created using a high-speed drill. The dura is coagulated using bipolar electrocautery and opened sharply.

Stereotactic navigation is used to guide a 19 Fr peel-away catheter into the frontal horn of the right lateral ventricle (Figure 32-2). CSF return is confirmed. The sheath is peeled away and the leaflets are securely stapled to the scalp. The endoscope is connected to a

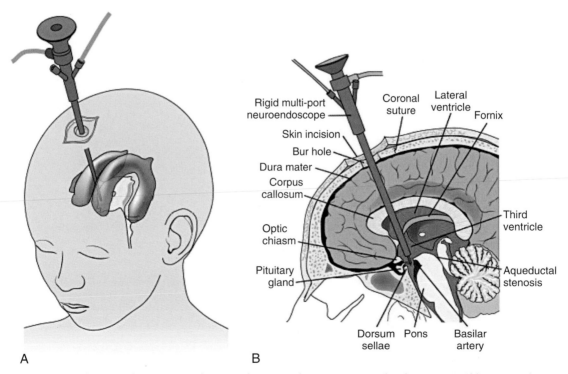

A   B

FIGURE 32-2   Schematics demonstrating the surgical trajectory for ETV using a rigid endoscope. **(A)** Oblique view showing the endoscope passing through the lateral ventricle, foramen of Monro, and into the third ventricle. **(B)** Sagittal view depicting the perforation of the floor of the third ventricle. It is important to understand the close relationship of the floor of the third ventricle to the anterior structures (optic chiasm, infundibulum, and clivus) and posterior structures (basilar artery and brainstem) to avoid undesired complications. *(Reprinted with permission from Quiñones-Hinojosa A. Schmidek and Sweet Operative Neurosurgical Techniques. 6th ed. Elsevier. 2012.)*

light source, irrigated, video towered, and white balanced before its placement through the peel-away sheath.

After identification of anatomic landmarks, the endoscope is carefully advanced toward the foramen of Monro. The colloid cyst is identified, opened, and entered using monopolar cautery advanced through the endoscope. The proteinaceous contents of the cyst are removed using suction and irrigation. After successful decompression, graspers are used to remove the cyst wall en bloc. When resection is complete, the cavity is irrigated through the endoscope until the CSF is clear. The endoscope is removed and an external ventricular drain is placed. The wound is irrigated and closed in layers.

Complication Avoidance and Management

- Endoscopic/open transcortical
  - This approach may be difficult in patients without enlarged ventricles. Frameless stereotactic neuronavigation may facilitate ventricular access. In endoscopic cases, ample irrigation is usually sufficient to control injury to a small vessel or choroid plexus. Ensure outflow of irrigation throughout the case to avoid dangerous elevation of intracranial pressure. Endoscopic electrocautery can be used in cases of uncontrolled bleeding. Cyst wall adherent to the fornix, thalamus, or ependymal veins should be left *in situ* to avoid neurologic and cognitive injury.
- Transcallosal approach
  - A transchoroidal approach dividing the choroid plexus of the floor of the lateral ventricle at the foramen of Monro can improve access to cysts located more posteriorly. A septum pellucidotomy should also be performed in case postoperative hydrocephalus requires ventricular drainage.

KEY PAPERS

Cappabianca P, Cinalli G, Gangemi M, et al. Application of neuroendoscopy to intraventricular lesions. *Neurosurgery*. 2008;62(suppl 2):575-597.

Hellwig D, Bauer BL, Schulte M, et al. Neuroendoscopic treatment for colloid cysts of the third ventricle: the experience of a decade. *Neurosurgery*. 2003;52:525-533.

Kondziolka D, Lunsford LD. Microsurgical resection of colloid cysts using a stereotactic transventricular approach. *Surg Neurol*. 1996;46:485-490.

Case 33

Cerebral Abscess

Aatman Shah ● Henry Jung, MD

Presentation

A 58-year-old African American male presents with a 1-week history of headache, vomiting, and memory difficulty. He was in his normal state of health until 1 week ago. He denies IV drug abuse, recent trauma, and smoking.

- PMH: none
- ROS: otherwise negative
- Travel history: unremarkable
- Exam:
  - Temperature of 39°C
  - Moderate confusion
  - Normal left-sided upper and lower extremity strength
  - 4/5 weakness of right upper and lower extremity
  - Normal sensation to light touch

Differential Diagnosis

- Infection
  - Bacterial abscess
  - Neurocysticercosis
  - Toxoplasmosis
  - Tuberculoma
- Neoplastic
  - Glioblastoma multiforme or other primary brain cancer
  - Metastatic brain cancer
- Other
  - Hemorrhage

Initial Imaging

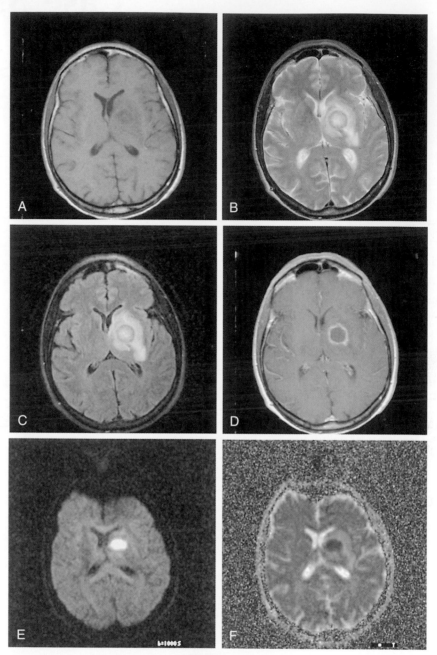

FIGURE 33-1

Imaging Description and Differential

MRI in Figure 33-1 A-F demonstrates a 2.2 × 2.6 cm ring-enhancing lesion in the left globus pallidus with edema and mass effect. DWI demonstrates a hyperintense lesion with low ADC.

(**A**) Unenhanced T1-weighted MR image demonstrates a hypointense lesion in the left globus pallidus with edema and mass effect. (**B**) Corresponding T2-weighted image shows a hyperintense lesion surrounded by a hypointense ring. (**C**) Signal in the lesion does not suppress on FLAIR MRI. (**D**) Enhanced T1-weighted MRI shows peripheral enhancement of the lesion. (**E**) Diffusion-weighted MRI shows hyperintense signal in the lesion. This is usually present in brain abscess, but is nonspecific. (**F**) Diffusion coefficient map confirms restricted diffusion.

- Differential: intracerebral abscess, tumor, or hemorrhage

Further Workup

- Lab work: elevated WBC, ESR, C-reactive protein, and blood cultures
- Chest X-ray to rule out pneumonia and tuberculosis

Pathophysiology
Brain Abscess

The signs/symptoms of an abscess are usually nonspecific. Symptoms often include altered level of consciousness, vomiting, and seizures. Infection may enter the intracranial compartment directly or indirectly via three routes: (1) direct extension, (2) hematogenous dissemination, or (3) trauma.

Direct Extension (20%–50% of Cases)

Sources of contiguous infection include the middle ear, paranasal sinuses, dental root, osteomyelitic bone, or an emissary vein. The most common pathogen is *Streptococcus milleri*.

Hematogenous Spread from a Distant Focus (20%–35% of Cases)

These abscesses are commonly multiple and multiloculated; they carry a higher mortality rate than abscesses from contiguous foci. Hematogenous spread is associated with cyanotic heart disease, pulmonary arteriovenous malformations, endocarditis, chronic lung infections, bronchiectasis, cystic fibrosis, and HIV infection. The most common pathogen is *Streptococcus viridans*.

Trauma (10% of Cases)

Traumatic open skull fractures that pierce dura can contaminate the brain. Brain abscesses can result from penetrating foreign bodies, such as pencil tips, bullets, and shrapnel, or from intracranial surgery. The most common pathogens are *Staphylococcus aureus* and *S. epidermidis*.

Four Histologic Stages of Abscess Formation

- Early suppurative cerebritis (days 1–2) – characterized by endothelial swelling and neutrophil infiltration. CT findings may show hypodensity with patchy enhancement
- Late suppurative cerebritis, with central necrosis (day 3–7) – characterized by central necrosis and infiltration of macrophages, lymphocytes, and plasma cells. CT findings demonstrate central hypodensity with a thick surrounding enhancing ring.
- Early capsule stage (days 8–14) – characterized by capsular vascularization, fibroblast infiltration leading to collagen deposition, and edema. CT findings demonstrate a central core with a thinner surrounding enhancing ring.
- Late capsule stage (day 14 and onward) – characterized by central necrosis, thin collagen capsule, and lymphocytes. CT findings demonstrate a hypodensity surrounding a thin enhancing ring.

Treatment Options

- Medical options
  - Diuretics and steroids may be used to reduce swelling of the brain.
  - Antibiotics: broad-spectrum antibiotics, most commonly vancomycin, ceftriaxone, and metronidazole, may be prescribed initially. Antifungal medications may also be prescribed if fungal infection is likely. Antibiotic therapy should be guided by culture results. Often 6 to 8 weeks of IV antibiotics are required.

- Antibiotics without surgery may be considered for patients with:
  - Several abscesses
  - A small abscess <2 cm
  - A preexisting shunt for hydrocephalus
  - *Toxoplasma gondii* in the setting of HIV
  - An inaccessible abscess in eloquent brain or brainstem
  - Meningitis
- Surgical options
  - Surgery is generally indicated for:
    - Significant mass effect or elevated intracranial pressure
    - Risk of abscess rupture into the ventricles
    - Removal of an associated foreign body
    - Fungal abscesses
    - Abscesses containing gas
    - Failure of antibiotic therapy
  - Techniques include:
    - Stereotactic drainage – needle aspiration can be guided by CT or MRI
    - Open surgical excision – the surgical procedure used depends on the size and location of the abscess

Surgical Technique

Simple aspiration may be performed stereotactically with prior CT or MRI to locate the abscess. With the patient appropriately registered using a stereotactic guidance system, an entry point and trajectory are planned to avoid vascular structures and eloquent cortex. After a small burr hole is created and the dura is incised, the biopsy needle is guided to the abscess and the pus is then drained. Cultures are obtained so that more specific antibiotics or antifungal drugs can be given.

In this case the patient underwent MR-guided aspiration of yellow purulent material. Gram staining demonstrated gram positive cocci, and cultures grew *Streptococcus viridans, S. constellatus,* and *S. intermedius.*

Complication Avoidance and Management

- Complications of brain abscess
  - Sudden worsening of headache accompanied by meningismus may indicate rupture of a brain abscess into the cerebral ventricles. This condition is associated with high mortality; aggressive intervention may be required. Due to the increased vasculature of the cortical gray matter, the lateral part of the abscess is thicker than the medial, periventricular part. As a result, subcortical abscesses are prone to rupture medially, into a ventricle. Antimicrobial therapy should be administered quickly in patients exhibiting prodromal symptoms or with abscesses adjacent to the ventricular system.

KEY PAPERS

Muzumdar D, Jhawar S, Goel A. Brain abscess: an overview. *Int J Surg.* 2011;9(2):136-144.

Nath A, Berger J. Brain abscess and parameningeal infections. In: Goldman L, Schafer AI, eds. *Cecil Medicine.* 24th ed. Philadelphia, Pa: Saunders Elsevier; 2011 [chap 421].

Tunkel AR. Brain abscess. In: Mandell GL, Bennett JE, Dolin R, eds. *Principles and Practice of Infectious Diseases.* 7th ed. Philadelphia, Pa: Elsevier Churchill Livingstone; 2009 [chap 88].

Chiari I Malformation

Henry Jung, MD ● Aatman Shah

Presentation

A 39-year-old female presents with longstanding neck pain and occipital headaches. Her headache is exacerbated with neck flexion, coughing, or sneezing. She also has intermittent numbness in her fingers, and she believes her grip strength has weakened over the past few years.

- PMH: otherwise unremarkable
- Exam:
  - Normal upper and lower extremity strength, with the exception of her right and left grip strength, which were 4+/5
  - Normal sensation to light touch
  - Normal reflexes and negative Hoffmann's reflex
  - Normal gait

Differential Diagnosis

- CSF flow aberrations
  - Chiari malformation
  - Syringomyelia
  - Hydrocephalus
- Degenerative
  - Cervical spine spondylosis
- Neoplastic
  - Tumors of the cervicomedullary junction or cervical spine
- Other
  - MS
  - Vitamin B_{12} deficiency

Initial Imaging

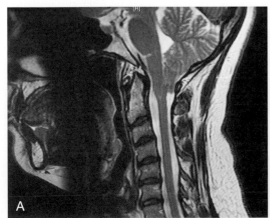
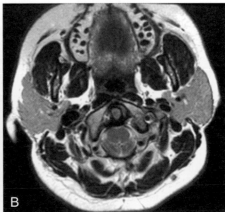

FIGURE 34-1

Imaging Description and Differential

- Brain/cervical spine MRI in Figures 34-1A and B show T2 sagittal and axial images, which demonstrate cerebellar tonsillar herniation. The tonsils have descended more than 5 mm through the foramen magnum, and there is crowding at the cervicomedullary junction. No hydrosyringomyelia is present.
- Differential: Chiari I malformation

Further Workup

- Imaging
  - MRI brain
  - MRI cervical spine (to rule out cervical myelopathy and to screen for syrinx)
  - Myelography in patients who cannot receive MRI

Pathophysiology
Chiari I Malformations

Chiari I malformations involve cerebellar herniation at least 5 mm below the level of the foramen magnum. Chiari I malformations may be congenital or acquired. Congenitally, mesodermal defects during development can lead to a small posterior fossa, which causes compression of the neural elements and herniation through the foramen magnum. The crowding at the foramen magnum causes aberrant CSF flow across the craniocervical junction.

Causes of acquired Chiari I malformations include: repetitive lumbar punctures, lumbar drainage, chronic CSF leaks, lumboperitoneal shunting, and traumatic pseudomeningoceles. A cranial-spinal pressure gradient across the foramen magnum, in which the spinal compartment has a lower pressure than the intracranial compartment, can cause a "sump effect," pulling the cerebellar tonsils into the foramen magnum. This is thought to promote formation of a Chiari malformation.

Syringomyelia

A number of theories have been proposed to explain the development of syringomyelia in Chiari I malformations. Gardner's "hydrostatic theory" proposes that, due to delayed embryonic opening of the fourth ventricle's outlets, there are exaggerated CSF pulsations into the central canal, which then lead to hydromyelia formation.

Williams' "craniospinal pressure dissociation" theory notes that there is difficulty in rapidly equilibrating CSF pressure wave during a Valsalva maneuver. During this delay, a pressure differential between intracranial and intraspinal spaces exists, which pulls the cerebellar tonsils downward. The resultant obstruction of CSF flow between the posterior fossa and the cervical subarachnoid space causes continued fluid flow into the central canal from the fourth ventricle.

Oldfield's theory proposes that CSF pulsation pressure, generated during the cardiac cycle, drives spinal CSF into the cord. This leads to diffusion of CSF through the perivascular space of the spinal cord and formation of a central syrinx.

Treatment Options

- Observation
  - Recommended for asymptomatic patients
- Surgery
  - Patients respond best to surgery within 2 years of symptom onset, thus early surgery is recommended for symptomatic patients.
- Posterior fossa decompression (suboccipital craniectomy), with or without cervical laminectomy of C1 (occasionally further levels); this is the most frequently performed

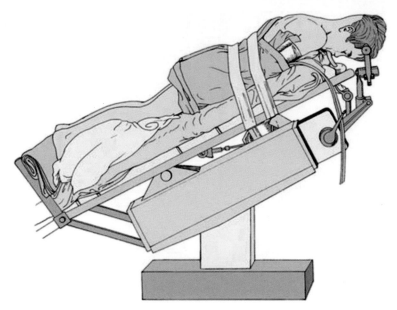

FIGURE 34-2   Positioning for the decompression of a Chiari malformation. *(Reprinted with permission from Winn HR. Youmans Neurological Surgery, 6th ed. Elsevier. 2011.)*

surgery for Chiari I malformation. The goal is to decompress the brainstem and restore normal CSF flow at the craniocervical junction.
• In patients with concomitant hydrocephalus or elevated ICPs, the hydrocephalus should be treated first with either VP shunting or third ventriculostomy. If symptoms or associated syrinx persist despite treatment of hydrocephalus, then a posterior fossa decompression should be considered.

Surgical Technique

The patient is placed prone with the head flexed and secured in a Mayfield head holder. The neck is flexed to open the interspace between the occiput and posterior arch of C1. Figure 34-2 illustrates the customary positioning.

A midline incision is made from the inion to the C2 spinous process. Staying in the midline avascular plane minimizes blood loss and postoperative pain.

The foramen magnum and the C1 posterior arch are exposed for the width of the cervical dura. The bone above the foramen magnum (about 3 cm high by 3 cm wide) is removed; removal of too much occipital bone can lead to cerebellar sag and herniation. A C1 laminectomy is performed. A C2 laminectomy is rarely needed.

Generally, the dura is then opened in a Y-shaped fashion. Many surgeons open only the dura with the thought that restoration of CSF flow may be accomplished with a greater expansion of basal arachnoid cisterns. The tonsils may be gently separated to inspect for adhesions covering the outlets of the fourth ventricle. To help restore CSF flow, some surgeons use bipolar cautery to shrink the tonsillar tips or lyse the subarachnoid adhesions. Figure 34-3 illustrates the operative exposure of a Chiari decompression with the cerebellar tonsils separated to reveal the floor of the fourth ventricle.

A dural graft is then sewn in to enlarge the lower posterior fossa and craniocervical junction. Artificial dural graft, harvested pericranium, or fascia lata may be used for the graft.

In cases involving a syrinx, the first line treatment is to perform the suboccipital craniectomy as previously described. If the syrinx persists, a syringosubarachnoid or syringopleural shunt may be required.

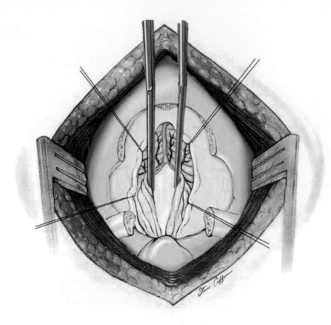

FIGURE 34-3 Operative exposure in a Chiari decompression. The floor of the fourth ventricle can be visualized by spreading apart the cerebellar tonsils. *(Reprinted with permission from Winn HR. Youmans Neurological Surgery, 6th ed. Elsevier. 2011.)*

Complication Avoidance and Management

- Suboccipital craniectomy, with or without cervical laminectomy of C1:
  - Risks of Chiari decompression include CSF leak, pseudomeningocele, vascular injury (especially PICA), and meningitis. Although occipital-cervical instability is a potential complication, cervical kyphosis or postoperative instability is rarely seen. CSF leaks developing in the postoperative period may indicate hydrocephalus, which may require treatment with VP shunting.
  - A posterior fossa craniectomy that is extended too widely has a risk of the cerebellum herniating through the craniectomy defect ("cerebellar slump"). This may cause headaches unlike the typical Chiari headaches. Cranioplasty to return the cerebellum to its correct position may be required.

KEY PAPERS

Milhorat TH, Chou MW, Trinidad EM, et al. Chiari I malformation redefined: clinical and radiographic findings for 364 symptomatic patients. *Neurosurgery*. 1999;44:1005-1017.

Oldfield EH, Muraszko K, Shawker TH, et al. Pathophysiology of syringomyelia associated with Chiari I malformation of the cerebellar tonsils. Implications for diagnosis and treatment. *J Neurosurg*. 1994;80:3-15.

Tubb RS, Pugh JA, Oakes WJ. Chiari malformations. In: Winn RH, ed. *Youmans Neurological Surgery*, Vol. 1. Philadelphia, PA: Saunders; 2011:1918-1927.

Case 35

Ependymoma

Zachary Medress ● Melanie G. Hayden Gephart, MD

Presentation

A 6-year-old boy has a 4-month history of headache, lethargy, nausea, vomiting, and worsening performance at school. He was born at full term by an uncomplicated delivery.

- PMH: type 1 diabetes
- Exam:
  - Right lateral gaze palsy
  - Papilledema on fundoscopic exam
  - Visual fields intact
  - Full strength in bilateral upper and lower extremities
  - Positive Romberg test

Differential Diagnosis

- Neoplastic
  - Medulloblastoma
  - Pilocytic astrocytoma
  - Ependymoma
  - Diffuse pontine glioma
  - Atypical teratoid/rhabdoid tumor
  - Hemangioblastoma
  - Chordoma/chondrosarcoma
- Infectious
  - Meningitis
  - Lyme disease
  - Cerebral abscess
- Developmental
  - Hydrocephalus
- Toxic/Metabolic
- Autoimmune
- Vascular
  - Vasculitis
  - Arteriovenous malformation
  - Dural arteriovenous fistula

Initial Imaging

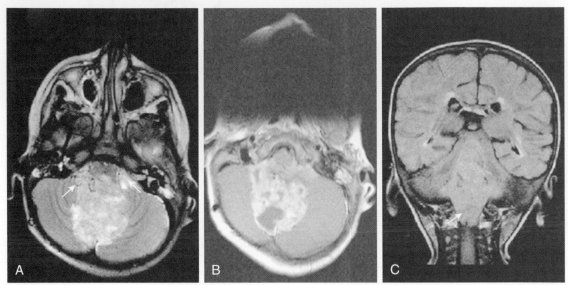

FIGURE 35-1   *(Reproduced from Adam A, Dixon AK, eds.* Grainger & Allison's Diagnostic Radiology. *5th ed. Elsevier; 2008.)*

Imaging Description and Differential

- Figure 35-1 shows an irregular, contrast-enhancing, posterior fossa tumor (B) that is hyperintense on T2. This mass involves the foramina of Luschka (A) and Magendie, with extension through the foramen magnum (C).
- Differential: medulloblastoma, pilocytic astrocytoma, AT/RT, choroid plexus papilloma (adults), or PNET

Further Workup

- Laboratory
  - CBC, BMP, INR
- Imaging
  - MRI of the full spine to rule out disseminated CNS disease, as ependymoma can be widely metastatic
  - On MRI, ependymomas are iso to hypointense on T1, hyperintense on T2, and avidly contrast enhancing. They may contain calcification, hemorrhage, or multiple cysts.
  - CT is frequently used to screen for intracranial lesions. On CT, ependymomas are homogenously contrast enhancing isodense lesions.
- Consultants
  - Neuro-oncology
  - Radiation oncology

Pathophysiology

Ependymomas arise from ependymal cells within the ventricular system and central canal of the spinal cord. They show a bimodal age distribution with peak incidence at 6 years of age and within the third decade. In children, ependymomas are the third most common posterior fossa tumor; most arise from the floor of the fourth ventricle and involve the foramina of Luschka or Magendie. In adults, 60% of ependymomas are located in the spinal cord where they can cause syrinx formation.

Histologically, ependymomas have monomorphic ovoid cells and perivascular pseudo-rosettes. World Health Organization (WHO) classification includes grade 1 tumors (subependymoma and myxopapillary ependymoma), grade 2 (papillary, clear cell, tany-cytic, and mixed ependymoma), and grade 3 (anaplastic ependymoma). Myxopapillary ependymomas are indolent extramedullary tumors that involve the filum terminale or conus medullaris. Clear cell ependymomas are predominantly found in the pediatric population and are located supratentorially. Tanycytic ependymoma is a rare, slow-growing ventricular tumor with histology similar to that of astrocytoma and schwannoma. Ana-plastic ependymoma is an aggressive variant with high mitotic activity, necrosis, and poor clinical prognosis. Ependymomas are associated with NF2, loss of chromosomes 12 or 14q, and a high expression of HOX genes. Overall, the prognosis for children with epen-dymomas is poor, with only 40% surviving 5 years. Prognosis is improved if gross total resection is achieved.

Treatment Options

- Biopsy
  - Biopsy is reserved for cases where surgical resection is not possible.
- Surgery
  - Gross total resection is the gold standard of treatment for ependymomas and should be pursued whenever safe, as incompletely resected ependymomas have a high rate of regrowth. Extent of resection is the most important prognostic indicator. En bloc removal is preferred when possible, to prevent dissemination of cancerous cells. Restoration of CSF pathways is critical when operating on ependymomas that arise in the fourth ventricle.
- Radiation
  - Radiation depends on tumor grade and subtype, but in general is reserved for subtotal resection, metastases, or recurrence. Radiation to the spinal cord is used to treat drop metastases.
- Chemotherapy
  - Chemotherapy is reserved for tumors that are inoperable and not amenable to radia-tion, such as those involving the brainstem. Commonly used agents include carbo-platin, cisplatin, and etoposide.

Surgical Technique

When resecting posterior fossa ependymomas, the patient is positioned prone with the head flexed. Intraoperative neurophysiologic monitoring of cranial nerves VI-XII is recom-mended. In cases with severe hydrocephalus, gradual release of CSF through a ventricu-lostomy is recommended. A suboccipital craniotomy is performed with removal of the foramen magnum in order to optimize access to the tumor. A C1 laminectomy may be required for tumors that extend caudally into the spinal canal. A Y-shaped incision is made in the dura and the cerebellar tonsils are elevated laterally. Vascular supply to the tumor comes primarily from the posterior inferior cerebellar arteries; feeding vessels are carefully isolated from the parent arteries and cerebellum, coagulated, and divided. The tumor's lateral surface is carefully dissected and its center is decompressed with suction and ultra-sonic aspiration. Small fragments invading the floor of the fourth ventricle may need to be left to avoid injury to underlying brainstem nuclei and tracts. After tumor resection, hemostasis is achieved using bipolar cautery and hemostatic agents, and the dura is closed in a watertight fashion. The craniotomy flap may be secured with titanium miniplates, and the incision is closed in layers.

Complication Avoidance and Management

- Posterior fossa ependymomas may involve cranial nerves VI-XII at their nuclei in the brainstem, and cranial nerve palsy is a possible complication of tumor resection. If there is concern for vagus nerve or nucleus damage intraoperatively, one should consult ENT to assess vocal cord function and undertake measures to prevent aspiration. Tracheos-tomy is required for patients with bilateral vocal cord paralysis. Most young patients with cranial nerve palsies after surgery eventually recover function.

- Ensuring that dural closure is watertight and replacing the bone flap can reduce the incidence of pseudomeningocele and CSF leak. Dural grafts and dural sealants may help ensure a watertight closure. Pseudomeningocele formation may indicate underlying hydrocephalus, which may require CSF diversion through a ventriculoperitoneal shunt.

KEY PAPERS

Grundy RG, Wilne SA, Weston CL, et al. Primary postoperative chemotherapy without radiotherapy for intracranial ependymoma in children: the UKCCSG/SIOP prospective study. *Lancet Oncol.* 2007;8(8):696-705.
Mack SC, Witt H, Piro RM, et al. Epigenomic alterations define lethal CIMP-positive ependymomas of infancy. *Nature.* 2014;506(7489):445-450.

Case 36

Normal Pressure Hydrocephalus

Robert C. Rennert, MD ● Vincent J. Cheung, MD ● J. Dawn Waters, MD

Presentation

A 70-year-old male with a history of hypertension and rheumatoid arthritis presents to clinic for evaluation of long-standing difficulty walking, urinary incontinence, and memory problems. His prior workup included a high-volume lumbar puncture, which documented an opening pressure of 15 cm H_2O and a normal laboratory profile. The patient and his wife reported transiently improved gait after the lumbar puncture.

- PMH: HTN and RA
- Exam:
  - Alert, oriented to self and city, but not date
  - CNS II-XII intact
  - 5/5 strength in all major muscle groups, and sensation intact
  - Mild dyskinesia on finger to nose
  - Shuffling, unsteady gate, and requires a walker

Differential Diagnosis

- Neurodegenerative
  - Alzheimer's disease
  - Lewy body dementia
  - Vascular dementia
- Other hydrocephalus etiologies
  - Aqueductal stenosis
  - Obstructive hydrocephalus
- Infectious
  - AIDS dementia complex
  - Lyme neuroborreliosis
- Urologic
  - Urinary tract infection
  - Benign prostatic hypertrophy (BPH)
- Other
  - Hypothyroidism
  - Vitamin B_{12} deficiency

Initial Imaging

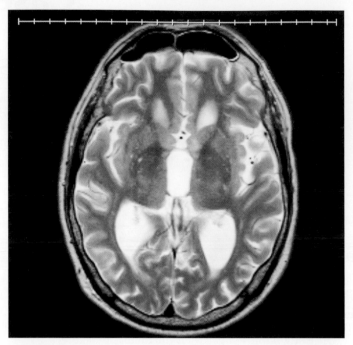

FIGURE 36-1

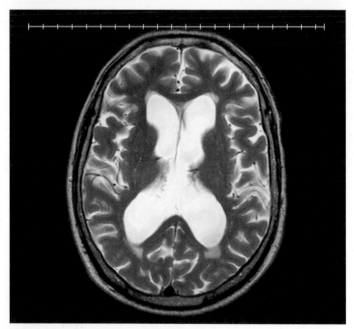

FIGURE 36-2

Imaging Description

- Figure 36-1: axial T2-weighted MRI demonstrating a rounded third ventricle, consistent with hydrocephalus
- Figure 36-2: axial T2-weighted MRI demonstrating anterior and posterior transependymal flow, consistent with hydrocephalus

Further Workup

- Laboratory
  - Routine labs
  - HIV/Lyme serology, thyroid function, and vitamin B_{12} level
- Imaging
  - CT brain (looking for ventricular enlargement with no CSF obstruction)
  - MRI brain, with and without contrast (gold standard imaging to assess for white matter lesions and other lesions)
- Other tests
  - High-volume lumbar puncture or lumbar drainage to assess opening pressure. Symptomatic improvement after CSF removal predicts an increased likelihood of response to shunting.
- Consultants
  - Neurology (may assist with dementia workup)

Pathophysiology

The etiology of normal pressure hydrocephalus remains speculative but in most cases is thought to result from impaired absorption of CSF. Specifically, occult infections or hemorrhages may cause fibrosis of arachnoid granulations, leading to a buildup of CSF and dysfunction of periventricular white matter tracts secondary to local pressure effects (despite the normal pressure classically seen on lumbar puncture). Other proposed mechanisms in patients without previous infections, trauma, or hemorrhage include hypertension-induced periventricular white matter atrophy causing decreased ventricular compliance, or underlying retrograde jugular venous flow impairing CSF absorption.

Treatment Options

- Medical
  - There are no definitive medical therapies for NPH, although reducing CSF production with acetazolamide may be tried.
- Surgical
  - CSF shunting is the treatment of choice for NPH. Ventriculo peritoneal (VP) shunting is preferred; lumbo-peritoneal shunting is an option.

Surgical Technique

For VP shunts, the right lateral ventricle is typically targeted for catheterization. Usually image guidance is not needed for catheterizing enlarged ventricles in NPH, but may be considered for ventricular catheterization in general based on ventricular size and surgeon's preference. Adjustable valves are commonly used, and a model should be selected that is appropriate for lower pressures seen with NPH.

The cranial entry point to catheterize the lateral ventricle is typically based on surgeon's preference. A familiar option is Kocher's point, which is located 3 cm from midline (or the midpupillary line) and 1 cm anterior to the coronal suture. From this point, the catheter is directed perpendicular to the surface of the brain, through the frontal lobe, and into the right frontal horn. Alternatively, Keen's point is located 2.5 to 3 cm above and 2.5 to 3 cm behind the posterior pinna. From this point, the catheter traverses the posterior parietal lobe into the trigone of the lateral ventricle. In placing a shunt, Keen's point has the advantage of a shorter and more direct course for the distal catheter to the abdomen.

The patient is positioned supine with the head turned such that the cranial access point, abdominal incision, and the intervening pathway along the posterior cranium, neck, and chest are accessible. The neck should be in a relaxed position to avoid jugular obstruction. The entire planned course of the shunt is prepped and draped so the tunneling device can be seen as it passes in the subcutaneous layer.

A "J" curvilinear cranial incision, with the base of the flap posterior, avoids placing the incision directly over the burr hole or catheter upon closing, minimizing wound breakdown and infection. A subgaleal pocket is created to receive the valve of the shunt. A burr hole is made at the cranial access point. The bone edges are waxed. The dura is cauterized and opened sharply. A cortical entry point free of large veins is identified and the pia is cauterized with bipolar electrocautery. It is advisable to catheterize the ventricle only after the peritoneal access and cranial-to-abdominal tunneling is complete.

A general surgeon may be helpful in providing laparoscopic abdominal access. For an open abdominal approach, the entry point is often based on surgeon's preference. The right upper quadrant is common and convenient. Here, the abdominal incision is made 2 cm below the rib cage. Dissection is carried down through the subcutaneous fat to the anterior rectus sheath. This may be incised to reveal the underlying muscle fibers. Generally, the fibers are split vertically instead of being cut horizontally. The posterior rectus sheath fascia may be grasped with small Kelly clamps and elevated off the underlying bowel. The clamps may be left in place on the fascia for easy identification upon closure. With the fascia elevated, it is opened with scissors to avoid heat injury to nearby bowel. Preperitoneal fat may be encountered here. If herniating preperitoneal fat is obstructing visualization, reverse Trendelenburg position may ease the intraabdominal pressure in the superior abdomen to allow better visualization. The peritoneum is grasped under direct visualization and elevated off of the underlying bowel. After ensuring there is no adherent bowel, scissors are used to create a small cut in the peritoneum. A purse-string suture loosely placed at the access site, and small Kelly clamps at the edges, may be used to easily find the opening later. Bowel peristalsis, or other intraperitoneal structures, should be positively identified.

The specific process of passing the catheter from the cranial site to the abdominal site may vary based on equipment. In general, a catheter passer is tunneled from the cranial pocket to the abdominal incision. Relaxing incisions may be used along the course as needed if the tunneling device is stuck. Carefully pass the device over the clavicle, avoiding the subclavian vessels and pleural space. The stylet is removed and the shunt's distal catheter is passed through. Suction and irrigation may help float the catheter through the hollow passer. If a hollow passer is not available, a strong silk suture may be secured to the catheter to pull it through the tract. The shunt valve is then primed and secured to the catheter.

The ventricular catheter is then inserted and its stylet is removed. Once CSF flow is confirmed, the ventricular catheter is cut to an appropriate length and attached to the valve with a silk tie. A right-angled catheter guide may be used to secure the catheter and prevent kinking at the edge of the burr hole. After ensuring flow of CSF to the distal end of the system, the distal catheter is placed in the peritoneum. The peritoneal purse-string suture is tied without obstructing the catheter. Fascia of the abdominal wall should be closed in anatomic layers.

Complication Avoidance and Management

- Patient selection is key, as improperly selected patients, or those with dementia alone, will not benefit from shunting.
- Care must also be taken when tunneling over the clavicle to avoid a pneumothorax or injury to subclavian vessels.
- Consider involving a general surgeon if the patient has had multiple prior abdominal surgeries or infections.
- Subdural hematomas may develop from overdrainage. If an adjustable valve is used, a higher resistance setting is advisable in the beginning to avoid overdrainage. Headaches that occur during an upright position may be a symptom of overdrainage. If these headaches develop, instruct the patient to lie flat and consider setting the valve to a higher resistance.

KEY PAPERS

Bradley WG. Cerebrospinal fluid dynamics and shunt responsiveness in patients with normal-pressure hydrocephalus. *Mayo Clin Proc.* 2002;77:507-508.

Bradley WG Jr. Idiopathic normal pressure hydrocephalus: new findings and thoughts on etiology. *AJNR Am J Neuroradiol.* 2008;29:1-3.

Shprecher D, Schwalb J, Kurlan R. Normal pressure hydrocephalus: diagnosis and treatment. *Curr Neurol Neurosci Rep.* 2008;8:371-376.

Case 37

Arachnoid Cyst

J. Dawn Waters, MD

Presentation

A 29-year-old woman presents to the emergency department after a helmeted bicycle accident with brief loss of consciousness.

- PMH: depression
- Review of systems: nonfocal headache and right shoulder pain. Otherwise negative.
- Exam: neurologically intact with pain-related limitation of right shoulder movement

Differential Diagnosis

- Traumatic
  - Concussion
  - Subarachnoid, subdural, or intraparenchymal hemorrhage

Initial Imaging

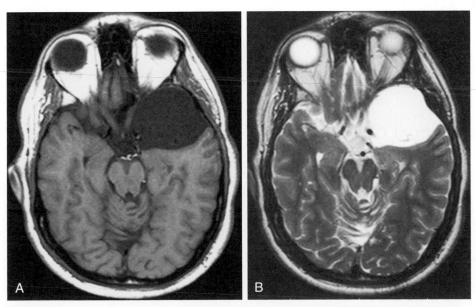

FIGURE 37-1 *(Reprinted with permission Daroff RB. Neurology in Clinical Practice. 6th ed. Elsevier; 2000.)*

Imaging Description and Differential

- Nonenhanced T1 (Figure 37-1A) and T2 (Figure 37-1B) MRI of the brain demonstrate a right anterior middle fossa mass with signal characteristics similar to those of CSF. The temporal lobe is displaced and the basal cisterns remain patent. There are no signs of hemorrhage.
- Radiographic differential diagnosis includes:
  - Cystic neoplasm, including metastasis
  - Porencephalic cyst
  - Epidermoid cyst

Further Workup

- Imaging
  - CT of head is useful for screening.
  - Cranial ultrasound: useful for screening infants
  - MRI with diffusion-weighted images; arachnoid cysts show no diffusion restriction
  - MRI with contrast; arachnoid cysts show no contrast enhancement
  - Cine phase-contrast MRI to characterize flow dynamics related to the fluid collection
  - CT cisternogram is rarely necessary; delayed or lack of contrast filling is characteristic of arachnoid cysts
- Electroencephalogram
  - Indicated for supratentorial arachnoid cysts if seizures or other cortical dysfunctions are suspected
- Neurocognitive evaluation

Pathophysiology

Arachnoid cysts are nonneoplastic intraarachnoid collections of CSF-like fluid typically arising near CSF cisterns, but isolated from normal subarachnoid or intraventricular CSF flow. They are diagnosed in children and adults and account for about 1% of intracranial masses. Commonly found in the middle fossa, they also occur in interhemispheric, suprasellar, posterior fossa, and spinal cisterns. Primary cysts are congenital, and less common secondary cysts may develop after trauma, meningitis, or surgery. Theories regarding the origin of congenital arachnoid cysts include abnormal splitting of the arachnoid membrane during development.

Most arachnoid cysts are asymptomatic and stable on serial imaging; some cysts spontaneously shrink. Signs and symptoms may develop due to local mass effect, increased intracranial pressure, hydrocephalus, or hemorrhage into a cyst after trauma. Hypotheses regarding cyst enlargement include CSF flow thorough a one-way valve, osmotic gradients, and active fluid production from the cyst wall.

Treatment Options

- Observation
  - Asymptomatic or mildly symptomatic cysts may be observed. Though controversial, it may be preferable to initially manage some symptoms, such as headaches or seizures, medically. In asymptomatic adults, a single repeat MRI of the brain at an 8-month interval to rule out an enlarging cyst is usually sufficient. In children, observation until adulthood with serial MRI is preferable to CT, which involves radiation exposure.
- Surgical
  - Surgical management is typically reserved for symptomatic or enlarging lesions. Surgical options include:
    - Endoscopic fenestration
    - Open fenestration
    - Burr hole drainage
    - Shunting of cyst

Surgical Technique

Endoscopic fenestration of the cyst wall into an adjacent CSF cistern is a minimally invasive procedure that permits visual inspection of the cyst and collection of a specimen for pathologic examination. Advantages of endoscopic fenestration include avoiding the need for a permanent shunt and lower recurrence rates than simple burr hole drainage without fenestration into a CSF cistern. Oertel et al reported a 90% rate of clinical improvement and an 8% recurrence rate after endoscopic arachnoid cyst fenestration. Cyst shunts should be considered for patients with hydrocephalus or failures of endoscopic fenestration.

The endoscopic fenestration technique varies with cyst location. In planning endoscopic cyst fenestration, consider image guidance for optimal burr hole placement to allow access through the cyst to the adjacent CSF cistern. Once the neuroendoscope has been introduced into the cyst through the burr hole and dural opening, the wall of the cyst can be grasped to initiate the fenestration. Sections of the cyst wall may be removed with care to avoid injuring blood vessels and nerves in the cistern. The fenestration may be enlarged with a small Fogarty balloon.

Complication Avoidance and Management

- Cyst recurrence may require repeat fenestration or shunting.
- Avoidance and management of postoperative subdural hygroma or hematoma requires careful preoperative screening for coagulopathy, intraoperative hemostasis, and postoperative observation. Symptomatic collections often require open drainage.

KEY PAPERS

Oertel JMK, Wagner W, Mondorf Y, et al. Endoscopic treatment of arachnoid cysts: a detailed account of surgical techniques and results. *Neurosurgery*. 2010;67(3):824-836.

Raffel C, McComb G. To shunt or to fenestrate: which is the best surgical treatment for arachnoid cysts in pediatric patients? *Neurosurgery*. 1988;23:338-342.

Westermaier T, Schweitzer TR-IE. Arachnoid cysts. Neurodegenerative diseases. *Landes Bioscience*. 2012;37-50.

Section III
Neurosurgical Trauma

Case 38

Penetrating Head Injuries

Vincent J. Cheung, MD   ● Brandon C. Gabel, MD   ●
Joseph D. Ciacci, MD

Presentation

A 32-year-old previously healthy man presents to the trauma bay after suffering a gunshot wound to the head. Paramedics estimated that 1 liter of blood was lost at the scene. The patient was a GCS 3 after arrival. However, after initial resuscitation, he began withdrawing with his right leg and localizing to pain with his right arm. On exam, patient moans but does not follow commands or have comprehensible speech. His left pupil is 6 mm fixed. His right pupil is 4 mm and briskly reactive to 2 mm.

Differential Diagnosis

- Other retained foreign bodies, or penetrating injuries

Initial Imaging

Imaging Description and Differential

CT scan with left frontal extraaxial hyperdensity consistent with epidural hematoma.

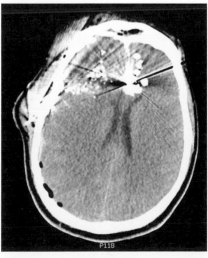

FIGURE 38-1

Further Workup

- Advanced trauma life support (ATLS) protocol to assess for other injuries
- Basic preoperative labs
- Coagulation panel

Pathophysiology

Gunshot wounds initially produce temporary cavitation of tissue as the bullet passes through the brain. This results in pressure waves that injure both adjacent and distant tissue. After the initial cavitation, tissue quickly collapses into the cavity. Hemorrhage into the cavity occurs, resulting in a space-occupying hematoma along the tract. Higher velocity projectiles have a higher kinetic energy and therefore usually cause more damage. Open penetrating wounds also cause contamination of the intracranial cavity.

BOX 38-1   Surgical Recommendations for Penetrating Brain Injury

1. Avoid use of the entry/exit wound when planning scalp incision.
2. Identify global/hemispheric injuries and role for large decompressive craniectomy.
3. Separate cranial-facial-orbital compartments with autologous bone, or titanium mesh, for support and watertight repair with dural substitutes.
4. Initiate early repair and fixation of the orbital bandeau to support future cranial vault reconstruction.
5. Perform conservative debridement of the trajectory path and imbedded fragments.
6. Consider intraoperative cerebral angiography in patients with combined penetrating neck and brain injury.

(Reprinted with permission from Ellenbogen RG, Abdulrauf SI, Sekhar LN. Principles of Neurological Surgery. 3rd ed. Elsevier; 2012.)

BOX 38-2   Criteria for Intracranial Fragment Removal

1. Fragment movement
2. Abscess formation
3. Vascular compression
4. Ventricular obstruction (hydrocephalus)
5. Heavy metals identified in cerebrospinal fluid

(Reprinted with permission from Ellenbogen RG, Abdulrauf SI, Sekhar LN. Principles of Neurological Surgery. 3rd ed. Elsevier; 2012.)

BOX 38-3   Criteria for Intracranial Angiography Following Penetrating Brain Injury

1. Penetrating injury through pterion, orbit, or posterior fossa
2. Penetrating fragment with intracranial hematoma
3. Known cerebral artery sacrifice or pseudoaneurysm at the time of initial exploration
4. Blast-induced penetrating injury with Glasgow Coma Scale score <8
5. Transcranial Doppler or computed tomography angiographic evidence of severe vasospasm

(Reprinted with permission from Ellenbogen RG, Abdulrauf SI, Sekhar LN. Principles of Neurological Surgery. 3rd ed. Elsevier; 2012.)

Treatment Options

- Medical management
  - Upon arrival, initial evaluation and management was initiated per ATLS protocol. The patient was intubated for airway protection and bolused with IV fluids to avoid hypotension. Pulse oximetry was used to monitor and prevent hypoxia. The patient was examined for evidence of associated spinal injuries, and spinal precautions were maintained. Prophylactic antibiotics and antiepileptics were administered. The patient was bolused with 3% hypertonic saline and started on a continuous infusion. The patient was hyperventilated to target an $EtCO_2$ of 25 mmHg (corresponding with a $PaCO_2$ of 30 mmHg).
- Surgical management
  - After initial resuscitation, the patient was brought to the operating room for an emergent right-sided decompressive hemicraniectomy. An arterial line and central venous catheter were placed. The patient was positioned supine with a wedge under his right side so that the right side of his head could be oriented up during maintenance of spinal precautions. A standard trauma flap was turned. A pericranial flap was preserved in anticipation of repairing the frontal sinus. A craniotomy was then performed. At this point, it was evident that the entry wound violated the left frontal sinus. The frontal sinus was cranialized. The sinus mucosa was meticulously debrided with curettes and pituitary rongeur forceps. A small piece of temporalis muscle was used to pack the deep portion of the sinus. The operative field was then debrided. Bone and bullet fragments were carefully removed from the brain surface and bullet tract. After debridement, care was taken to ensure meticulous hemostasis. The previously prepared periosteal flap was then used to cover the cranialized frontal sinus and tucked under the right frontal lobe. A large craniectomy was accomplished, and the wound was closed in standard fashion. At the end of the operation, a contralateral intracranial pressure monitor was placed.

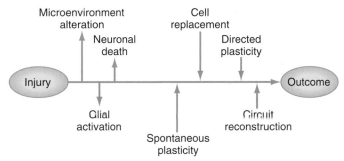

FIGURE 38-2 Schematic overview of the course of treatment. Traditional strategies for treating traumatic brain injury focus on reducing sequelae of the primary brain insult to salvage acutely threatened tissue, whereas restorative strategies introduce interventions that support spontaneous and directed repair of neural circuits to improve functional recovery. *(Reprinted with permission from Winn HR. Youmans Neurological Surgery. 6th ed. Elsevier; 2011.)*

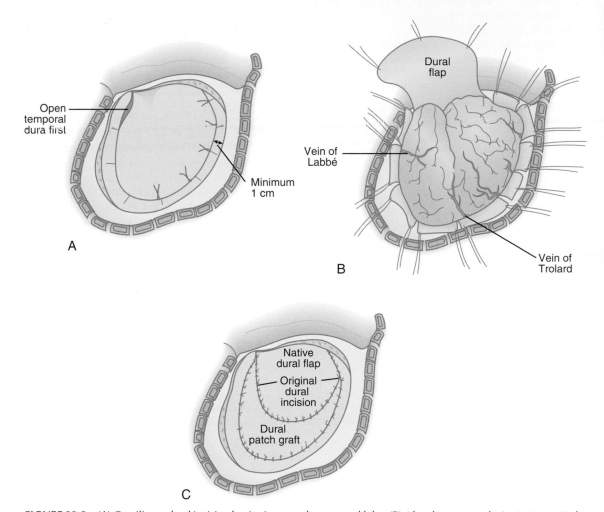

FIGURE 38-3   **(A)** Curvilinear dural incision beginning over the temporal lobe. **(B)** After durotomy, relaxing incisions in the perimeter of the exposure are made for additional relaxation. **(C)** Dural closure incorporating a generous dural patch to allow outward herniation of the brain. *(Reprinted with permission from Winn HR. Youmans Neurological Surgery. 6th ed. Elsevier; 2011.)*

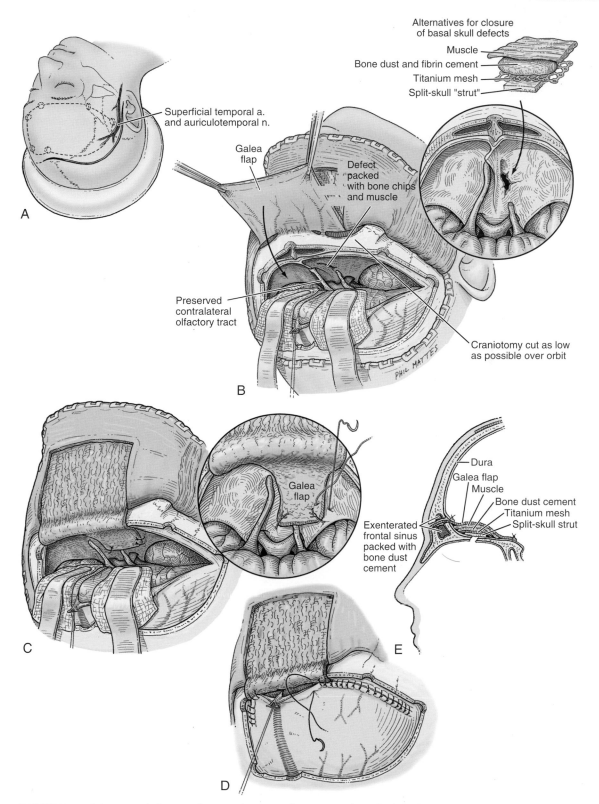

FIGURE 38-4   Schematic of a bicoronal approach to repair fractures involving the frontal sinus and anterior skull base. After cranializing the frontal sinus, a vascularized galeal flap is placed over the sinus **(B)**. If defects in the ethmoid bone are seen, a combination of a split-skull "strut" graft, titanium mesh, bone dust, and fibrin (including muscle) can be used to further reinforce the defect **(B)**. **(E)** Sagittal section after the repair. *(Reprinted with permission from Winn HR. Youmans Neurological Surgery. 6th ed. Elsevier; 2011.)*

Complication Avoidance and Management

- "ABCs" come first. Be sure that the patient's airway is secure and patient is hemodynamically stable. It is critical to avoid hypotension and hypoxia. Mannitol should be avoided in favor of 3% hypertonic saline, or used with caution, as diuresis can result during hypotension in an underresuscitated patient.
- Be cognizant of potential spinal injuries and maintain strict spinal precautions.
- It is important to note any clinical or radiologic evidence of air sinuses being violated. In this particular case, we anticipated the need for frontal sinus repair by preparing a pedicalized periosteal flap. Primary dural closure is preferred and can be achieved with a periosteal, temporalis fascia, or a fascia lata graft.
- Study imaging preoperatively to anticipate any potential venous sinus injuries. Displacement of bone fragments that are tamponading an injured venous sinus can result in voluminous intraoperative bleeding. Be sure to have blood products readily available.
- Transventricular and bihemispheric injuries portend a worse outcome.
- Intracranial pressure monitoring and management is critical for postoperative care.
- Seizure prophylaxis, broad-spectrum antibiotic prophylaxis, and administration of tetanus vaccination are recommended for any patient with a penetrating head injury.
- It is also important to look for other gunshot wounds during your initial physical examination.

KEY PAPERS

Grahm TW, Williams FC Jr, Harrington T, et al. Civilian gunshot wounds to the head: a prospective study. *Neurosurgery*. 1990;27(5):696-700, discussion 700.

Hofbauer M, et al. Predictive factors influencing the outcome after gunshot injuries to the head—a retrospective cohort study. *J Trauma*. 2010;69(4):770-775.

Kaufman HH. Treatment of civilian gunshot wounds to the head. *Neurosurg Clin N Am*. 1991;2(2):387-397.

Kim KA, et al. Vector analysis correlating bullet trajectory to outcome after civilian through-and-through gunshot wound to the head: using imaging cues to predict fatal outcome. *Neurosurgery*. 2005;57(4):737-747, discussion 737-47.

Case 39

Intractable Intracranial Hypertension

Vincent J. Cheung, MD ● David R. Santiago-Dieppa, MD ●
Brandon C. Gabel, MD ● Joseph D. Ciacci, MD

Presentation

An 18-year-old male pedestrian with no significant past medical history was struck by a car traveling 25 miles per hour. Upon admission to the trauma bay, he was nonverbal, pupils were 5 mm bilaterally and sluggishly reactive. He withdrew from pain in all four extremities. GCS was 7 on arrival.

Differential Diagnosis

- Epidural hematoma
- Subdural hematoma
- Diffuse axonal injury
- Anoxic brain injury
- Nonconvulsive status epilepticus

Initial Imaging

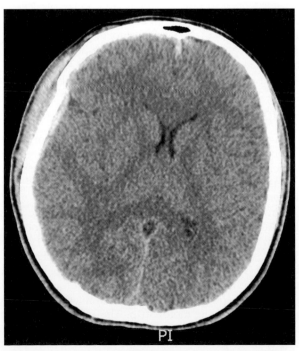

FIGURE 39-1

Further Workup

- Advanced trauma life support (ATLS) workup for other injuries
- Repeat CT scan (after initial stabilization)
- Basic preoperative labs
- Coagulation panel

Pathophysiology

There are two major mechanisms of posttraumatic intracranial hypertension: cerebral edema and disruption of cerebral autoregulation.

Cerebral edema has been classified into two subtypes: cytotoxic and vasogenic edema. Cytotoxic edema occurs when cells suffer an ischemic insult. ATP is rapidly depleted and the cells lose their ability to preserve their transmembrane ionic gradients. Sodium accumulates in the cell, resulting in an osmolar gradient that produces swelling and cell death. Vasogenic cerebral edema results from disruption of the blood-brain barrier. Proteins pass through the blood-brain barrier into the extracellular space, resulting in the accumulation of interstitial fluid.

Cerebral autoregulation is the ability of the cerebrovascular system to maintain a constant cerebral blood flow over a physiologic range in blood pressure. In patients with traumatic brain injury, vasomotor paralysis can result in the compromise of their cerebral autoregulatory capacity. Cerebral blood flow may dramatically increase, resulting in hyperemia. Increased cerebral blood flow results in elevated cerebral blood volume. Consistent with the Monro-Kellie doctrine, as the cerebral blood volume increases and cerebral edema progresses, CSF is displaced, followed by venous blood. If left unchecked, increased intracranial hypertension results in herniation, and potentially death.

Medical Management

The patient was intubated for airway protection and a low-dose propofol drip was initiated for sedation. The head of the bed was kept up at 30 to 45 degrees. The patient's hard cervical collar was inspected and loosened to prevent excessive compression of jugular venous outflow. A right-sided intraventricular drain was placed. Initial ICP was measured at 30. The drain was left open to flow at 15 cm H_2O above the level of the tragus. The patient was bolused with 1 g/kg of mannitol and 300 mL of 3% hypertonic saline, and a 3% hypertonic saline drip was started. Serum osmolality and sodium were checked every 4 to 6 hours. An arterial line was placed and blood pressure was strictly controlled. $EtCO_2$ was monitored and ventilation was titrated to a target $EtCO_2$ of 30 to 35. Seizure prophylaxis was administered. After initiating these interventions, ICPs decreased to the low teens.

Surgical Management

Intraventricular drain placement is an effective intervention for the treatment of ICP through CSF diversion and is the gold standard for ICP measurement. Alternatively, a fiberoptic intraparenchymal ICP monitor may be placed if placement of the external ventricular drain (EVD) is difficult or not possible. Monitoring ICP with either an EVD or an intraparenchymal monitor is recommended for patients who are a GCS of 8 or less with a positive head CT. In trauma patients, EVD placement should be considered when the patient does not have a reliable exam, or if the patient's imaging and neurologic status are suspicious for intracranial hypertension. Kocher's point is the classic site of entry for a frontal EVD and is 10 to 11 cm posterior from the nasion (as measured along the surface of the scalp) and 2.5 to 3 cm lateral to midline at the midpupillary line. Alternatively, Kocher's point can be identified at 1 cm anterior to the coronal suture (can be palpated under the skin) along the midpupillary line. It is recommended to remain in front of the coronal suture to avoid injuring the motor strip. The patient's head of bed is positioned up, or the patient is placed in reverse Trendelenburg if there is suspicion of a coexistent spinal injury. The head is generously shaved and Kocher's point is marked. The skin is prepped and draped in the usual manner, leaving enough room to tunnel the EVD catheter

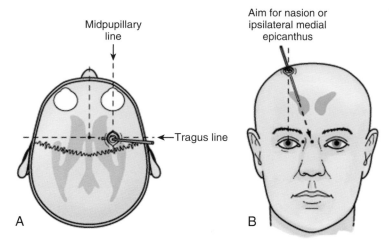

Midpupillary line

←Tragus line

Aim for nasion or ipsilateral medial epicanthus

A

B

FIGURE 39-2   Schematic representation of landmarks used for ventriculostomy catheter placement. **(B)** In the mediolateral plane, one should aim for the ipsilateral medial canthus. *(Reprinted with permission from Winn HR. Youmans Neurologic Surgery. 6th ed. Elsevier; 2011.)*

after placement. Subcutaneous infiltration of lidocaine with epinephrine is performed to assist with scalp hemostasis. A small linear incision centered on Kocher's point is created. A hand-twist drill is used to make a burr hole, and a trochar or spinal needle is used to sharply puncture the underlying dura. The EVD catheter is passed with the stylet in place to 6 cm from the outer table of the skull. The EVD is passed perpendicular to the surface of the skull, aimed toward the ipsilateral medial canthus in the coronal plane, and toward the external auditory meatus in the sagittal plane (Figure 39-2). The stylet is removed and CSF flow is confirmed. The catheter is tunneled laterally under the skin. The incision is closed with nonabsorbable sutures and the EVD is secured to the scalp with sutures. The EVD is then connected to the drainage collection and pressure transduction system. An appropriate ICP pressure waveform and opening pressure are noted.

Complication Avoidance and Management

- Maintain strict sterility during placement of the EVD. This helps prevent infection post procedure.
- We recommend never passing an EVD catheter more than 7 cm from the outer table of the skull. Measuring the distance between the outer table of the skull and the ventricle on a coronal CT can help determine the distance where CSF flow should be encountered.
- If CSF is not obtained after three passages of the catheter, one may consider an alternative means of monitoring intracranial pressure.
- CSF diversion should be used with caution in patients with a mass lesion. CSF drainage can increase the size of an extraaxial hematoma.
- If intracranial hypertension is refractory to maximum medical management (CSF diversion, hyperosmolar agents, and sedation), consider surgical decompression.

KEY PAPERS

Donkin JJ, Vink R. Mechanisms of cerebral edema in traumatic brain injury: therapeutic developments. *Curr Opin Neurol.* 2010;23(3):293-299.
Stocchetti N, Maas AI. Traumatic intracranial hypertension. *N Engl J Med.* 2014;370(22):2121-2130.
Torre-Healy A, Marko NF, Weil RJ. Hyperosmolar therapy for intracranial hypertension. *Neurocrit Care.* 2012;17(1):117-130.
Unterberg AW, Stover J, Kres B, et al. Edema and brain trauma. *Neuroscience.* 2004;129(4):1021-1029.

Case 40

Epidural Hematoma

Vincent J. Cheung, MD ● Brandon C. Gabel, MD ●
Joseph D. Ciacci, MD

Presentation

A 27-year-old male is assaulted with a blow to the head while walking home. He loses consciousness temporarily, but wakes up and goes home to recover. Several hours later, his roommate calls 911 because he notices that the patient is acting confused and has progressively become less responsive.

On physical exam the patient was noted to have a tense subgaleal hematoma that is palpable on the right side of his head. His eyes are closed and he does not open them to command. His left pupil is 6 mm and sluggishly reactive. His right pupil is 4 mm and briskly reactive. He localizes to pain with his left upper extremity and withdraws from pain with his right upper extremity. He withdraws from pain briskly in his lower extremities.

Differential Diagnosis

- Epidural hematoma
- Subdural hematoma
- Meningioma (if no clear history of trauma)
- Tuberculoma (if no clear history of trauma)
- Extramedullary hematopoiesis (if no clear history of trauma)

Initial Imaging

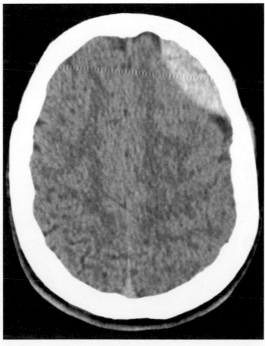

FIGURE 40-1

Further Workup

- Advanced trauma life support (ATLS) workup for additional injuries
- Basic preoperative labs
- Coagulation panel

Pathophysiology

Traumatic epidural hematomas are most commonly caused by injury to the middle meningeal artery, as it runs under the squamosal portion of the temporal bone, resulting in hemorrhage in the fronto-temporal region. However, damage to venous structures can result in epidural hematomas as well. Epidural hematomas may be associated with a skull fracture, but fracture is not necessary for underlying vessels to be damaged. Epidural hematomas may be associated with other intracranial hemorrhages, such as traumatic subarachnoid hemorrhage or subdural hematomas. The classic symptoms of an epidural hematoma are a brief loss of consciousness, followed by a lucid interval, and then delayed neurologic deterioration. However, this presentation is only seen in a minority of patients with epidural hematomas.

Management

The patient is bolused with mannitol and 3% hypertonic saline and is taken emergently to the operating room where he is intubated. The patient is positioned on the operating table in a supine position. The head is turned right so that the left side of his head is up. The head is shaved, prepped, and draped. An incision is made overlying the epidural hematoma. A craniotomy is performed, allowing wide exposure of the epidural hematoma (Figure 40-2). With a combination of irrigation, gentle suction, and forceps, the clot is removed and the dural surface is exposed. The dura is inspected and hemostasis is achieved with bipolar forceps. Dural tack-up sutures are placed to prevent reaccumulation of the hematoma postoperatively. The bone flap is replaced and secured. The scalp is closed in standard fashion.

Discussion

An epidural hematoma can be a neurosurgical emergency. It is critical to rapidly assess the patient and prepare for possible emergent evacuation. Initial evaluation should involve a focused neurologic examination, evaluation of airway protection, hemodynamic stability, and a standard trauma evaluation. Depending on the mechanism of trauma, one should

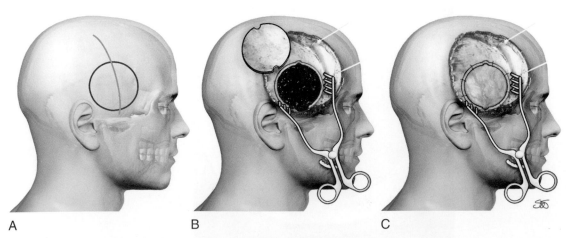

A   B   C

FIGURE 40-2 Acute epidural hematoma. A smaller "slash" incision is used for a more focused craniotomy. *(Reprinted with permission from Winn HR. Youmans Neurologic Surgery. 6th ed. Elsevier; 2011.)*

maintain a high suspicion of other major injuries, such as occult bleeding or spinal fractures. Hyperosmolar agents are helpful in temporizing neurologic injury from intracranial hypertension. Surgical approach is tailored to the size and location of the epidural and to other traumatic intracranial pathology that may be present. Indications for evacuation of an epidural hematoma include: thickness >15 mm, volume >30 mL, midline shift (MLS) >5 mm, GCS <8, anisocoria, and focal neurologic deficit.

KEY PAPERS

Bullock MR, Chesnut R, Ghajar J, et al. Surgical management of acute epidural hematomas. *Neurosurgery*. 2006;58(3 suppl):S7-S15, discussion Si-Siv.

Lee EJ, Hung YC, Wang LC, et al. Factors influencing the functional outcome of patients with acute epidural hematomas: analysis of 200 patients undergoing surgery. *J Trauma*. 1998;45(5):946-952.

Rivas JJ, Lobato RD, Sarabia R, et al. Extradural hematoma: analysis of factors influencing the courses of 161 patients. *Neurosurgery*. 1988;23(1):44-51.

Case 41

Chronic Subdural Hematoma

Erik I. Curtis, MD ● Brandon C. Gabel, MD ● Joseph D. Ciacci, MD

Presentation

- 81-year-old female with a history of increased confusion and difficulty with ambulation for the last month, per family report
- PMH: hypertension, emphysema, and vascular dementia
- Physical exam:
  - AAO × 2, intermittently confused, follows commands
  - PERRLA, EOMI, face symmetric, tongue midline
  - Left-sided pronator drift
  - Motor exam with 5/5 strength in all extremities
  - Normal reflexes

Differential Diagnosis

Chronic subdural hematoma may occur in a setting of:
- Trauma
- Spontaneous subdural hemorrhage
- Brain atrophy
- Subdural hygroma
- Coagulopathy
- Subdural empyema (often associated with signs/symptoms of infection; if this is suspected, a contrast enhanced imaging study is needed)

Initial Imaging

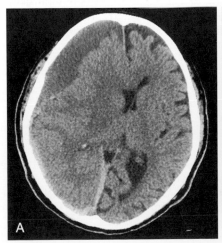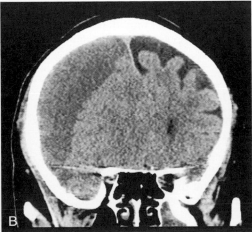

FIGURE 41-1

Further Workup

- Laboratory workup
  - Routine labs (CBC with differential, chemistries)
  - Heme workup with coagulation panel, platelet assay, DIC panel, and TEG
  - CRP, ESR if infection is suspected on imaging
- Preferred imaging diagnostics
  - CT brain, simple noncontrast study sufficient
  - MRI of the brain may assist in identifying relative age of subdural collection; DWI can be helpful in infectious workup.
  - N.B. – contrast studies are usually only necessary when investigating infectious/neoplastic etiologies

Classification

It is important to reconcile radiologic findings with the patient's neurologic examination. Chronic subdural hematomas are common in the elderly population, and their incidence increases with age. Additionally, many of these patients are taking anticoagulants, which increases the risk. Chronic subdural hematomas are bilateral in 20% to 25% of cases. Uncomplicated chronic subdural hematomas (SDHs) should reflect a relatively hypodense and homogenous density/signal intensity, with possibly some layering of blood products. Mixed density or "acute on chronic" SDHs will show layering of acute and chronic blood products in the same extraaxial space. Long-standing chronic SDHs may be loculated and show internal septations and thickening of the arachnoid and dural coverings. Surgical evacuation of chronic subdural hematomas should be considered when there is neurologic deficit, thickness >10 mm, or midline shift >5 mm.

Pathophysiology

Chronic SDHs often occur after shearing of bridging veins, but may also be associated with vascular abnormalities (arteriovenous malformation or aneurysm), coagulopathies, alcoholism, neoplasm, or infection. Classically, an SDH is thought to originate in cases of an enlarged subarachnoid space, such as in cerebral atrophy in an elderly patient with stretching and tearing of a bridging vein. This hematoma then begins the processes of organization and resorption. As the degradation process occurs, the hematoma will become progressively more liquefied, serous, and closely resemble the density of water or CSF. This involves granulation tissue surrounding the hematoma and small neovascularized membranes infiltrating the hematoma. These friable and fragile vessels are prone to rehemorrhage and frequent disruption, leading to chronic loculated subdural hematoma formation. It is thought that rehemorrhage/recurrence occurs in 5% to 10% of chronic SDHs. It is important to note that hemorrhagic products in the subdural space can act as a potent epileptogenic focus, and these patients will benefit from seizure prophylaxis.

Management

Treatment options include close observation and medical management versus surgical evacuation.

- **Burr hole evacuation** – a twist drill or power drill is used to expose the subdural space and allow for chronic subdural "motor-oil" hematoma to be evacuated.
- **Subdural drain placement** – placement of a subdural drain is performed either at the bedside or post-burr hole evacuation in the operative suite. Placement of a drain has been shown to decrease the risk of recurrence.
- **Craniotomy and evacuation of hematoma** – a typical open craniotomy is performed and the dura incised to expose and release the subdural contents and hematoma.

Surgical Technique
Burr-Hole Craniotomy

The head is turned away from the side of the hematoma. Two 1 to 2 cm linear incisions are made directly over the chronic subdural location. Burr holes are then placed underlying the incisions. Bipolar electrocautery is performed over the dura; the dura is then opened sharply. The subdural space is visualized and a rich, liquefied, "motor-oil" appearance of chronic subdural hematoma should be appreciated and evacuated (Figure 41-2). Copious irrigation is performed to ensure complete evacuation of posthemorrhagic blood products. Coagulation of any identifiable sources or hemorrhage should be performed. A subdural or subgaleal drain is placed and tunneled away from the incision line. This drain should be attached to a closed system, such as a bulb or graduated cylinder. The galea and scalp are closed in standard fashion.

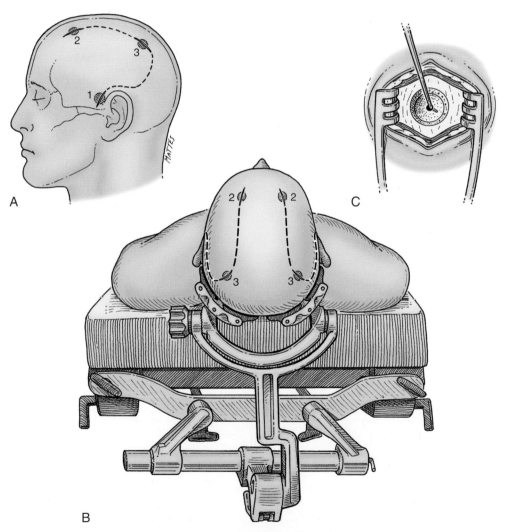

FIGURE 41-2   Placement of exploratory burr holes should begin in the temporal fossa, ipsilateral to the suspected lesion. The patient is positioned in a subdural head holder to expose both sides of the scalp. *(Reprinted with permission from Winn HR. Youmans Neurological Surgery. 6th ed. Elsevier; 2011.)*

Complications

- Recurrence of hematoma, necessitating reevacuation
- Injury of parenchyma, resulting in intracerebral hemorrhage occurring in up 1% to 5% (in some reports)
- Tension pneumocephalus
- Superficial or deep infection
- Seizures
- Wrong-sided or site surgery

KEY PAPERS

Fogelholm R, Heiskanen O, Waltimo O. Influence of patient's age on symptoms, signs, and thickness of hematoma. *J Neurosurg.* 1975;42:43-46.

Hamilton MG, Frizzell JB, Tranmer BI. Chronic subdural hematoma: the role of craniotomy reevaluated. *Neurosurgery.* 1993;33:67-72.

Lee KS, Shim JJ, Yoon SM, et al. Acute-on-chronic subdural hematoma: not uncommon events. *J Korean Neurosurg Soc.* 2011;50(6):512-516.

Lind CR, Lind CJ, Mee EW. Reduction in the number of repeated operations for the treatment of subacute and chronic subdural hematomas by placement of subdural drains. *J Neurosurg.* 2003;99:44-46.

Markwalder TM, Steinsiepe KF, Rohner M, et al. The course of chronic subdural hematomas after burr-hole craniostomy and closed system drainage. *J Neurosurg.* 1981;55:390-393.

Robinson RG. Chronic subdural hematoma: surgical management in 133 patients. *J Neurosurg.* 1984;61: 263-268.

Tabaddor K, Shulman K. Definitive treatment of chronic subdural hematoma by twist-drill craniostomy and closed-system drainage. *J Neurosurg.* 1977;46:220-226.

Weir BK, Gordon P. Factors affecting coagulation, fibrinolysis in chronic subdural fluid collection. *J Neurosurg.* 1983;58:242-245.

Zanini MA, de Lima Resende LA, de Souza Faleiros AT, et al. Traumatic subdural hygromas: proposed pathogenesis based classification. *J Trauma.* 2008;64(3):705-713.

Case 42

Subaxial Cervical Fracture

Erik I. Curtis, MD ● Brandon C. Gabel, MD ● Nicholas Fain ●
Joseph D. Ciacci, MD

Presentation

- A 24-year-old male was involved in a high-speed motor vehicle accident
- PMH: diabetes mellitus type 1
- Physical exam:
  - AAO × 3, sensory deficits in BUE and BLE with a sensory level at C7/T1
  - Motor exam with 5/5 strength in bilateral deltoids/biceps
  - 0/5 in bilateral triceps/wrist flexion/wrist extension and BLE
  - Sensory level at C7 with no sensation below
  - No rectal tone and distended bladder on palpation

Initial Imaging

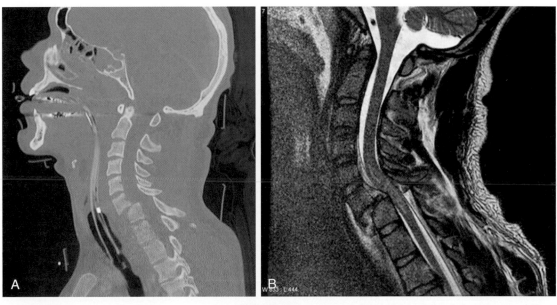

FIGURE 42-1

Differential Diagnosis

Fracture of the cervical vertebrae may occur in the setting of:
- Trauma
- Neoplastic infiltration (either primary or metastatic disease)
- Infectious etiology (e.g., osteomyelitis, Pott's disease)
- Degenerative changes seen in autoimmune disease
- Osteoporosis and metabolic bone diseases

Further Workup

- Laboratory workup
  - Routine labs (CBC w/ diff, chem, and coag panel)
  - CRP, ESR if infection is suspected on imaging
- Preferred imaging diagnostics
  - Plain film AP and lateral views of the C-spine
  - CT cervical spine to assess bony anatomy and/or reconstructions for operative planning
  - MRI cervical spine to assess CSF spaces, spinal cord proper, discs, and ligamentous structures
  - N.B. – contrast studies are usually only necessary when investigating infectious/neoplastic etiologies, or to evaluate scar tissue

Classification

Cervical spine fractures can be described morphologically as compressive, burst, flexion-distraction, or as a fracture dislocation type in the classic way that fractures elsewhere in the vertebral column are described. Several standardized classification systems have been attempted, though none are universally accepted, or used, at this time. The Allen-Ferguson classification system describes subaxial cervical traumas based on the mechanism of injury. The novel Subaxial Cervical Spine Injury Classification System (SLIC), as proposed by Vaccaro et al, is a recent attempt to use a point-based system in the classification of subaxial cervical injuries. It is important to note both the mechanism of injury and the morphology when describing a cervical injury. The determination of vertebral stability and the integrity of the discoligamentous structures are paramount when considering surgical therapy.

Pathophysiology

The subaxial spine is the site of the majority of cervical fractures and dislocations, being accountable for 65% of all cervical fractures and >75% of all cervical dislocations. Numerous types of fractures, or fracture patterns, exist and can result from pathologic stress placed on the bony or ligamentous components of the vertebral column. These can be as a result of hyperextension or hyperflexion, or axial loading or rotational forces, and the morphology of the fracture will often elucidate the mechanism of injury. Trauma accounts for the majority of fractures in younger populations, and ground-level falls account for the majority of fractures in the elderly. Subaxial spine fracture is associated with a high risk of noncontiguous fracture in other areas of the vertebral column and the provider should have a high suspicion of noncontiguous fracture on initial, assessment. Several specific subaxial cervical fractures exist and are described in the literature.

Spinous Process Avulsion

Hyperflexion. Often seen in the context of trauma. Results from shear forces causing sudden strain on muscular attachments to the spinous processes at this level. Avulsion of the C7 spinous process, commonly referred to as "clay-shoveler's fracture," is a result of sudden trapezius contraction in the context of attempting to eject stuck clay from the end of a shovel.

Teardrop Fracture

Hyperflexion + axial loading. Fracture of the anterior, inferior vertebral body, producing a small chip appearing as a teardrop on lateral films. Results from compression in the setting of flexion of the vertebral column. This is an unstable injury with concomitant fracture and disruption of the anterior ligamentous complex. Posterior ligamentous structures are frequently injured as well. Usually accompanied by retrolisthesis of the anterior vertebral body at the level of the fracture. A more benign form of this fracture, called an **avulsion fracture**, results from hyperextension injury. An avulsion will present without malalignment of the vertebral body or soft tissue swelling. An uncomplicated avulsion fracture spares the posterior ligamentous complex and is usually a stable spinal fracture.

Quadrangular

Flexion + compression + axial loading. An obliquely fractured vertebral body from the anterior superior margin traveling to the inferior end plate. Assessment of the ligamentous structures is key to determining stability.

Wedge

Flexion + compression. Fracture of <50% of vertebral body, without disruption of the annulus or posterior ligament. Typically a stable fracture pattern.

Burst

Flexion + compression + axial loading. Fractured vertebral body ranging in degree of comminution. This is an unstable fracture pattern with disruption of the anterior and middle column. Neither anterior nor posterior longitudinal ligaments are intact, and retropulsion of contents into the cord and subsequent disruption are common.

Subluxation

Distraction + flexion. May represent, an anterior or posterior subluxation from fracture of the vertebral body, but is also accompanied by disruption or fracture of at least one facet joint. Results from the studies by White and Panjabi demonstrated that anterior translation of the vertebral body >3.5 mm, or angulation of one vertebral body in relation to the next >11 degrees, indicates mechanical instability.

Facet Fracture

Extension + compression + rotation. Single or multiple fractures through the articulating facet or facets. Represents an unstable pattern.

Traumatic Spondylolisthesis

Extension + axial loading. An anterior displacement of the vertebral body as a result of single or bipedicular fracture and/or pars interarticularis. The anterior elements shift forward, and the posterior elements are disrupted. This is an unstable fracture pattern.

Management

When deciding on a treatment regimen, there are many variables to consider. It is important to consider the neurologic examination of the patient, as well as the type and resultant mechanical stability of the fracture and/or coexisting injury to the discoligamentous complex. A treatment option can range from rigid external immobilization (e.g., halo vest) to surgical fusion, with or without decompression of the neural elements.
- External immobilization (e.g., halo vest):
  - Useful in patients with nondisplaced, stable fractures
  - Useful as a bridge to surgical treatment
- Surgical correction is indicated for unstable fractures, considerations include:
  - Anterior versus posterior approach
  - Decompression of the neural elements if indicated
  - Instrumentation with bony fusion

Surgical Technique
Anterior Cervical Discectomy and Fusion (ACDF)

The patient is placed in the supine position. An intraoperative X-ray or fluoroscopy may be obtained at this time to confirm adequate neutral positioning of the cervical vertebral column. A 3 cm transverse or linear incision is made at the desired cervical level, such that the medial aspect is located at the lateral edge of the trachea and the lateral edge is marked by the sternocleidomastoid (SCM) muscle. Using blunt dissection, the platysma is exposed and dissected through to expose the deeper tissue layers. Once the SCM muscle has been identified laterally, bluntly dissect toward the midline with care to stay medial to the carotid sheath. Use the hand-held Cloward retractor to pull aside the lateral strap muscles, or medial soft tissue as needed. Again, blunt dissection is used to expose the anterior longitudinal ligament (ALL) and anterior cervical spine. Define the ALL, the bilateral longus colli muscles, and the anterior cervical vertebral bodies. Mark the exposed level and confirm the location with intraoperative X-ray or fluoroscopy. Using careful monopolar electrocautery, free the longus colli muscles bilaterally to allow for placement of a radiolucent cervical retractor system (Figures 42-2, 42-3, and 42-4). If necessary, expand the field superiorly or inferiorly to access all relevant levels. After incising the annulus, a series of curettes and rongeur forceps are used to remove the disc in its entirety. The uncinate process should define the lateral limit of the discectomy. Osteophytes should be removed with either a high-speed drill or rongeur forceps. It is important to remove the often adherent cartilaginous superior and inferior end plate, as failure to do so may inhibit bony fusion. Foraminotomy may be considered at this juncture if indicated. Measure the height and width for an appropriately sized interbody device, autograft, and/ or allograft. Care is taken to measure the appropriate length and width for an anterior cervical plate. Place the plate over the interbody implant and bridge the vertebral body above and below. Drill and screw the plate in place, engaging the lock after finishing the insertion of all screws. Ensure hemostasis is achieved. Placement of a postsurgical drain may be considered. Meticulous closure is performed.

Complications

- Recurrent laryngeal nerve injury (may be transient or permanent)
- Postoperative hematoma
- Injury to the carotid sheath or its contents

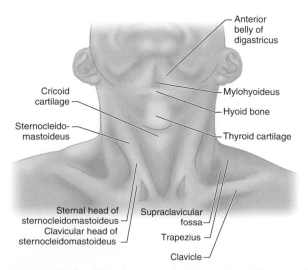

FIGURE 42-2 Use anatomic landmarks to determine the cervical level; the thyroid cartilage localizes C4-C5, and palpation of the carotid tubercle localizes to the C6 level. If it is difficult to ascertain the level accurately, mark the incision slightly superior to the estimated level of pathology; it is easier to expose inferiorly than superiorly. *(Reprinted with permission from Jandial R, McCormick P, Black PM. Core Techniques in Operative Neurosurgery. Elsevier; 2011.)*

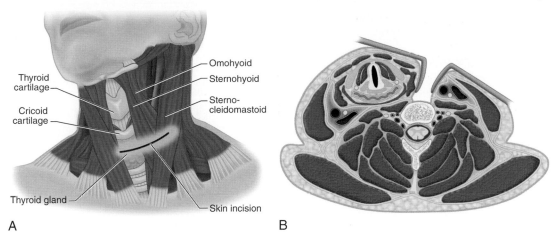

FIGURE 42-3 **(A)** Make a transverse skin incision. Incise the platysma to expose the deep cervical musculature. Use bipolar electrocautery to maintain hemostasis. **(B)** Develop the avascular plane. Use blunt dissection in this plane to expose the vertebral bodies. Dissect the longus colli muscle to the prevertebral fascia laterally using blunt techniques. *(Reprinted with permission from Jandial R, McCormick P, Black PM.* Core Techniques in Operative Neurosurgery. *Elsevier; 2011.)*

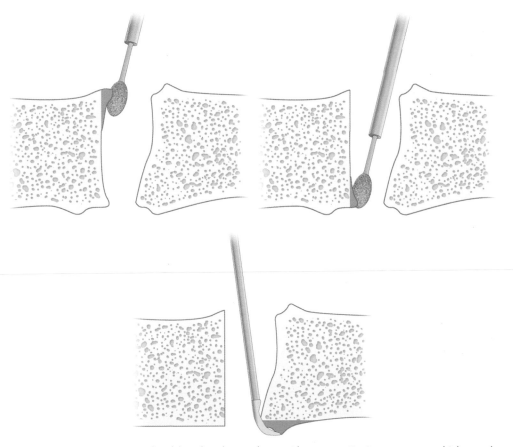

FIGURE 42-4 Remove ventral and then dorsal osteophytes with a curette, Kerrison rongeurs, or high-speed burr. Remove end plates to expose blood-rich cancellous bone. *(Reprinted with permission from Jandial R, McCormick P, Black PM.* Core Techniques in Operative Neurosurgery. *Elsevier; 2011.)*

- Dysphagia, dysarthria, and wound infection
- Long-term subsidence or adjacent level disease

KEY PAPERS

Anderson PA, Moore TA, Davis KW, et al. Spine Trauma Study Group. Cervical spine injury severity score. Assessment of reliability. *J Bone Joint Surg*. 2007;89(5):1057-1065.

Browner BD. *Skeletal Trauma*. 4th ed. MDConsult; 2008.

Canale ST, Beaty JH. *Campbells' Operative Orthopaedics*. 12th ed. MDConsult; 2010.

Denis F. The three column spine and its significance in the classification of acute thoracolumbar spinal injuries. *Spine*. 1983;8:817-831.

Dvorak MF, Fisher CG, Fehlings MG, et al. The surgical approach to subaxial cervical spine injuries: an evidence-based algorithm based on the SLIC classification system. *Spine*. 2007;32(23):2620-2629.

Furlan JC, Noonan V, Singh A, et al. Assessment of impairment in patients with acute traumatic spinal cord injury: a systematic review of the literature. *J Neurotrauma*. 2010;28(8):1445-1477.

Hadley MN, Walters BC, Aarabi B, et al. Clinical assessment following acute cervical spinal cord injury. *Neurosurgery*. 2013;72(3):40-53.

Harris JH Jr, Edeiken-Monroe B, Kopaniky DR. A practical classification of acute cervical spine injuries. *Orthop Clin North Am*. 1986;17:15.

Holdsworth FW. Fractures, common dislocations, fractures-dislocations of the spine. *J Bone Joint Surg*. 1963;45(1):6-20.

Kotani Y, Abumi K, Ito M, et al. Cervical spine injuries associated with lateral mass and facet joint fractures: new classification and surgical treatment with pedicle screw fixation. *Eur Spine J*. 2005;14:69-77.

Vaccaro AR, Hulbert RJ, Patel AA, et al. The subaxial cervical spine injury classification system: a novel approach to recognize the importance of morphology, neurology, and integrity of the disco-ligamentous complex. *Spine*. 2007;32:2365.

Watson-Jones R. The results of postural reduction of fractures of the spine. *J Bone Joint Surg*. 1938; 20:567-586.

White AA, Panjabi MM. *Clinical Biomechanics of the Spine*. 2nd ed. Philadelphia: Lippincott; 1990.

Case 43

Odontoid Fractures

Brandon C. Gabel, MD ● Erik I. Curtis, MD ● Joseph D. Ciacci, MD

Presentation

The patient is a 61-year-old male who presented after a fall from a bicycle. He was brought to the emergency department where he complained of neck pain.

- PMH: mitral regurgitation and hypertension
- Exam:
  - 5/5 strength throughout both upper and lower extremities
  - Sensation intact to light touch throughout
  - Normal reflexes
  - Pain with palpation of posterior cervical spine

Differential Diagnosis

Fracture of the odontoid may occur in the setting of:

- Trauma
- Neoplastic infiltration of the dens (either primary or metastatic tumors)
- Osteomyelitis
- Degenerative changes seen in rheumatoid arthritis
- Osteoporosis and metabolic bone diseases

Initial Imaging

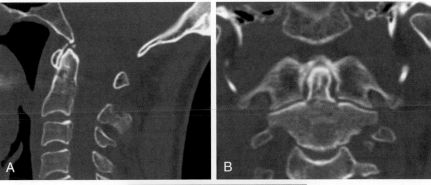

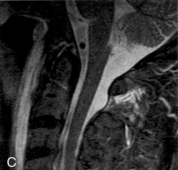

FIGURE 43-1

Imaging Description and Differential

Initial imaging with CT revealed a type II dens fracture, best depicted on sagittal and coronal views (Figures 43-1A and B). MRI imaging showed no evidence of transverse ligamentous injury, but there was evidence of anterior prevertebral swelling and mild C1-C2 interspinous injury (Figure 43-1C).

Differential diagnosis is limited to traumatic fracture of the dens. There are no imaging characteristics that suggest other etiologies for the fracture, especially given the patient's history.

Further Workup

- Laboratory workup
  - Routine labs
  - CRP, ESR if infection is suspected on imaging
- Imaging
  - MRI cervical spine to assess transverse ligament, alternatively, flexion/extension films may be obtained in a neurologically intact patient, or if MRI is not available.
  - CT cervical spine to assess for other fractures at C1 or the subaxial cervical spine
  - AP, lateral, and open mouth odontoid views

Pathophysiology

Using the Anderson and D'Alonzo classification system, dens fractures are usually defined as type 1, 2, or 3. Type 1 fractures involve the tip of the dens and are the rarest form. Type 2 fractures involve the base of the dens, and type 3 fractures extend into the body of C2. Type 2 fractures are the most common, but also the most difficult to manage; type 2 fractures traditionally have the greatest nonunion rate when managed nonoperatively. The most important factors regarding prognosis include: age >65 years, significant angulation, significant displacement/distraction, posterior displacement of the dens, displacement in more than one plane, and delay in diagnosis. Fractures of the dens require a combination of both horizontal shear and vertical compressive forces. In younger patients, high-impact mechanisms are usually required to cause a fracture of the dens. Ground-level falls account for the majority of fractures in the elderly population. It is also important to note that coexistent injury to the atlas or subaxial cervical spine may be present, and should be assessed on imaging and physical examination.

Treatment Options

Treatment options depend on the type of fracture (i.e., type 1, 2, or 3), the degree of displacement, angulation, obliquity, chronicity of the fracture, and whether or not there is a coexisting ligamentous injury. Additionally, consider the patient's body habitus (i.e., barrel chested or short necked). Current treatment options include rigid cervical collars, halo vest immobilization, posterior surgical fixation, and odontoid screw placement.

- Cervical collar or halo vest immobilization
  - Useful in patients with type 1 and type 3 fractures
  - Useful as a bridge to surgical treatment in unstable type 2 injuries or highly comminuted fractures
- Surgical correction is indicated for comminuted or displaced fractures, with or without transverse ligamentous injury.
  - Posterior fusion
    - Sublaminar wiring (Brooks, Gallie, Sonntag)
    - Transarticular C1-C2 screw fixation
    - Segmental screw fixation (Harms)
      - Requires favorable C1 and C2 bony anatomy for screw placement
      - Should be avoided when there is a "high riding" or medially coursing vertebral artery
      - This technique, when feasible, has been shown to have higher fusion rates.

- Anterior fusion
  - Odontoid screws
    - Useful in patients with acute or subacute fractures
    - Contraindications include: barrel chested patients; patients with short necks; comminuted, angulated, or displaced fractures; and coexistent transverse ligament injury

Surgical Technique

For anterior odontoid screw placement, the patient is positioned supine. Before instrumentation, a large radiolucent bite block should be placed by the surgical team. Two C-arms are placed in orthogonal orientation for biplanar visualization of the dens. Lateral and open mouth views of the dens and body of C2 should be easily obtained before skin incision. We perform a standard incision at the C5 to C6 level. Blunt dissection is carried down to the prevertebral fascia. Further blunt dissection with Kittner dissectors is then carried superiorly toward the C2 and C3 disc space. A self-retaining retractor is placed to allow visualization of the C2 and C3 disc space and base of the dens, and to protect soft tissues. Once the C2 and C3 disc space is exposed, a small trough is drilled in the caudal C2 body in the midline. A drill is used to create a hole in the body of the dens (Figure 43-2); this hole is extended across the fracture line into the tip of the odontoid (Figure 43-3). A lag screw is placed through this pilot hole (Figure 43-4). Lag screws provide a compressive force that pulls the fractured fragment toward the base of the dens, enabling fusion to occur across the fracture.

For posterior instrumented fusions, the patient is placed in a Mayfield head holder and turned prone on chest rolls. The patient is placed in slight reverse Trendelenburg with the knees flexed. Before skin incision, lateral fluoroscopy is used to ensure adequate alignment. The incision is centered from the inferior occipital bone to the C3 spinous process. The C1 and C2 posterior elements are then exposed with electrocautery. If screw placement is planned, the medial portion of the C1 lateral masses are exposed and palpated with a 4 Penfield. The C2 nerve root should be mobilized inferiorly, or alternatively, may be sacrificed during placement of C1 lateral mass screws. Judicious use of fluoroscopy should be used during placement of C1 screws. C2 screws may be placed in the pedicle or pars interarticularis, depending on the patient's anatomy on preoperative CT. An alternative to C2 pedicle screws is intralaminar C2 screw fixation. After placement of screws or

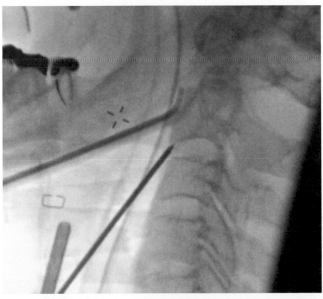

FIGURE 43-2   Lateral intraoperative fluoroscopic film showing placement of K-wire at the caudal border of the C2 vertebral body.

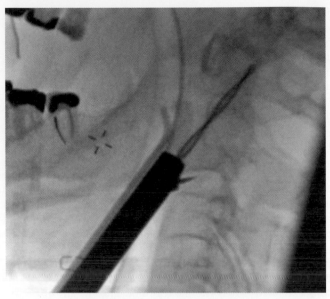

FIGURE 43-3 Lateral intraoperative fluoroscopic film showing drilling of the odontoid processes.

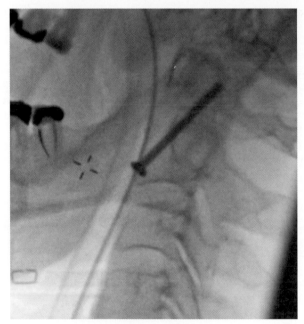

FIGURE 43-4 Lateral intraoperative fluoroscopic film showing placement of odontoid screw across the fracture.

sublaminar wiring, the cortical bone overlying the C1 and C2 region should be decorticated. Autograft and/or allograft are placed over the decorticated regions to achieve bony fusion.

Complication Avoidance and Management

- During placement of C1 screws, it is important to note the length of the screw on lateral fluoroscopy. If the screw is at the depth of the anterior tubercle of C1, an anterior breach is likely.

- High-riding or medially oriented vertebral artery anatomy may make placement of C1 or C2 screws unfeasible. If this is the case, then alternative fixation with intralaminar screws, wiring, or hybrid construct may be considered. If necessary, the construct can be extended from occiput to the subaxial cervical spine.
- Anterior odontoid screw fixation should not be performed in patients with atlantoaxial instability. Preoperative MRI should be used to assess transverse ligament injury. Additionally, significantly displaced fractures that cannot be reduced, or chronic fractures with corticated surfaces, are not candidates for odontoid screw fixation.

KEY PAPERS

Greene KA, Dickman CA, Marciano FF, et al. Acute axis fractures. Analysis of management and outcome in 340 consecutive cases. *Spine.* (Phila PA 1976) 1997;22(16):1843-1852.

Hsu WK, Anderson PA. Odontoid fractures: update on management. *J Am Acad Orthop Surg.* 2010;18(7): 383-394.

Martin MD, Bruner HJ, Maiman DJ. Anatomic and biomechanical considerations of the craniovertebral junction. *Neurosurgery.* 2010;66:A2-A6.

Steinmetz MP, Mroz TE, Benzel EC. Craniovertebral junction: biomechanical considerations. *Neurosurgery.* 2010;66:A7-A12.

White AA, Panjabi MM. *Clinical Biomechanics of the Spine.* Philadelphia: Lippincott; 1990.

Case 44

Hangman's Fracture

Brandon C. Gabel, MD ● Vincent J. Cheung, MD ●
Joseph D. Ciacci, MD

Presentation

The patient is a 23-year-old male who presented after a high-speed motorcycle accident. He complained of pain in his neck but denied numbness, tingling, or weakness.

- PMH: unremarkable
- Exam:
  - 5/5 strength bilateral upper extremities and lower extremities
  - Sensation intact to light touch throughout
  - Tenderness to palpation of posterior cervical spine, with no obvious step-offs

Differential Diagnosis

Hangman's fractures most commonly occur in the setting of trauma. Patients with the following diseases may be at an increased risk after minor trauma:

- Neoplastic infiltration
- Osteomyelitis
- Degenerative changes
- Osteoporosis

Initial Imaging

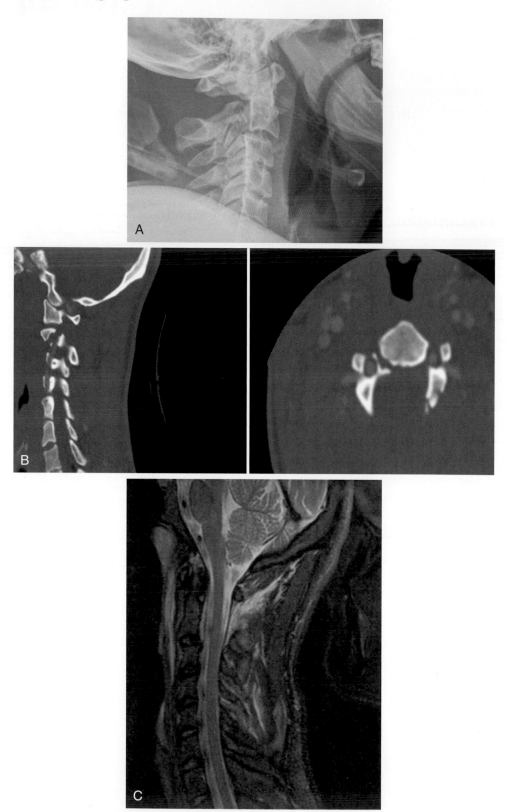

FIGURE 44-1

Imaging Description and Differential

Imaging depicts a traumatic Hangman's fracture (A) through the right C2 pedicle and left C2 pars interarticularis with STIR signal apparent on MRI (C), indicating significant soft tissue injury. In the setting of trauma, there is little differential diagnosis to consider. Concomitant vertebral artery injury should be ruled out with CT angiogram, which in this case was negative for vascular injury (B).

Further Workup

- Laboratory workup
  - Routine labs
- Imaging
  - MRI of the cervical spine to assess ligamentous injury
  - CT imaging to assess for bony anatomy, and to aid in potential operative planning
  - CT or MR angiogram to assess the vertebral arteries
  - Flexion/extension plain films may be useful in select cases.

Pathophysiology

Unlike many of the other cervical vertebrae, the axis has unique anatomic morphology. In order to understand a Hangman's fracture, it is important to better define two bony features of the C2 vertebrae: the pars interarticularis and the C2 pedicle. These two terms are often used interchangeably but are, in fact, distinct bony elements. The C2 pars interarticularis is the bone that lies posterior to the transverse foramen, extending from the superior articulating surface of C2 to the inferior articulating surface of C2. The pedicles of C2 are bony structures that lie medial to the transverse foramen and immediately underneath the C1 and C2 facet joint; they are located and angulated much more medially compared with the pars interarticularis.

A hangman's fracture is better classified as a bilateral fracture extending through the pars interarticularis and/or pedicles of the axis. Most fractures of this type are secondary to a hyperextensive force in combination with an axial load (i.e., hitting your face on the windshield during a high-speed MVA). However, these fracture patterns can also be seen under conditions of flexion and distraction forces.

There are different grading systems used to classify these fractures and are based on the orientation, degree of angulation, and/or displacement of the fracture. In the Effendi system, a type 1 fracture is a hairline fracture extending through the pars/pedicles without significant angulation or displacement, a type 2 fracture has significant displacement of the C2 body relative to the C3 body (i.e., anterolisthesis), and a type 3 fracture is similar to a type 2 fracture, except the body of C2 rests in a flexed position (i.e., angulated position). Levine and Edwards have proposed adding a type 2a, which has no displacement, but severe angulation of the C2 body.

Hangman's fractures rarely cause neurologic injury because of the capaciousness of the canal at this level, but may be considered biomechanically unstable in certain cases. Neurologic injury may occur as a result of vertebral artery injury; any associated posterior circulation abnormalities seen in a patient's history or physical examination should raise suspicion for dissection of the vertebral artery.

Treatment Options

Treatment options depend on the degree of angulation and displacement, as well as the neurologic status of the patient. Additional factors to consider include the presence of any additional cervical spine fractures (i.e., concomitant C1 or subaxial spine fractures).

- Conservative management is indicated for patients without neurologic injury and with anatomic, or near anatomic, alignment of the fracture.
  - External immobilization (i.e., halo vest)
- Surgical management is indicated for those with significant angulation/displacement, or neurologic deficit.

- Anterior approaches
  - C2 and C3 discectomy and fusion
- Posterior approaches
  - C1 and C3 posterior instrumented fusion (constructs may, or may not, "skip" the C2 depending on the degree of bony involvement)

Surgical Technique

For an anterior C2 and C3 discectomy, the patient is positioned supine. Intraoperative fluoroscopy is used to ensure good alignment before skin incision. Intraoperative neuromonitoring may also be used. A combination of blunt and sharp dissection is carried down to the prevertebral fascia. A localizing image is taken to ensure the appropriate level is exposed. A discectomy is then performed. An interbody device, autograft, and/or allograft are then placed in the disc space. Depending on the type of interbody device used, a plate may be secured to the C2 and C3 bodies to prevent graft extrusion and aid in fusion.

For posterior instrumented fusions, the patient is placed in a Mayfield head holder and turned prone on chest rolls. The patient is placed in slight reverse Trendelenburg with the knees flexed. Before skin incision, lateral fluoroscopy is used to ensure adequate alignment. The incision is centered from inferior occipital bone to C3 spinous process. The C1, C2, and C3 posterior elements are then exposed with electrocautery. If screw placement is planned, the medial portion of the C1 lateral masses are exposed and palpated with a no. 4 Penfield. The C2 nerve root should be mobilized inferiorly or, alternatively, may be sacrificed during placement of C1 lateral mass screws (Figures 44-2 and 44-3). Judicious use of fluoroscopy should be used during placement of C1 screws. C2 screws may be placed in the pedicle via the pars interarticularis (Figure 44-4); frequently the C2 level is skipped entirely. C2 intralaminar screws may alternatively be placed. Lateral mass screws are placed at the C3 level. If placement of screws is contraindicated or not feasible, then

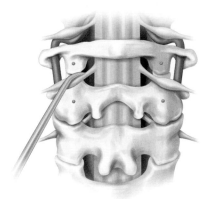

FIGURE 44-2 Curettes are used to define the bony margins of the inferior portion of the posterior ring of C1 out to the lateral masses of C1. Surgifoam is used to stop bleeding from the nearby vertebral venous plexus. The C1 and C2 joint must be exposed and denuded of soft tissue to provide a surface for bone grafting. The starting point for C1 lateral mass screws and C2 pars/pedicle screws is shown. *(Reprinted with permission from Jandial R, McCormick P, Black PM. Core Techniques in Operative Neurosurgery. Elsevier; 2011.)*

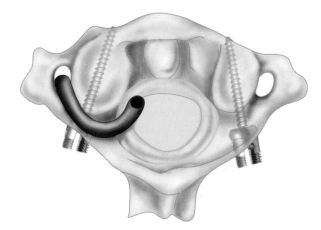

FIGURE 44-3 We perform C1 and C2 fixation using lateral fluoroscopic guidance. Gentle caudal retraction on the C2 dorsal root ganglion is required to expose the C1 lateral mass screw entry point, which lies halfway between the junction of the C1 posterior arch and the inferior posterior part of the C1 lateral mass. A no. 4 Penfield dissector can be used to feel the medial border of the C1 lateral mass. A high-speed burr is used to mark the entry point. We recommend drilling some of the posterior ring of C1 that lies above the C1 lateral mass screw entry point to allow adequate room for the polyaxial head of the C1 screw. The pilot hole is drilled with the hand-held drill in a 5 to 10 degree medial trajectory along a plane parallel to the plane of the C1 posterior arch. We recommend checking the pilot hole with a blunt 1 mm probe and then tapping the hole. A 3.5 mm-diameter polyaxial screw, whose length typically measures 18 to 30 mm, is placed. *(Reprinted with permission from Jandial R, McCormick P, Black PM. Core Techniques in Operative Neurosurgery. Elsevier; 2011.)*

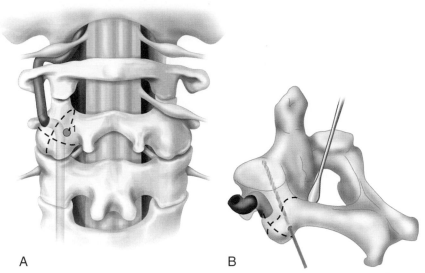

FIGURE 44-4   (A) A no. 4 Penfield dissector is likewise used to feel the medial border of the C2 pars interarticularis. The atlantoaxial membrane is detached using a blunt dissector to expose the upper surface of the C2 pedicle. The inferior articular process of C2 is divided into quadrants. The C2 pedicle screw starting point lies in the superomedial quadrant of the inferior articular process of C2 (approximately 1.75 mm caudal to the lateral mass–pars interarticularis transition zone). **(B)** The pilot hole is again prepared with a high-speed bit, and the pilot hole is drilled in a trajectory oriented 20 degrees medial and 20 degrees cephalad, using lateral fluoroscopic guidance. The hole is checked with a probe and tapped. A 3.5 mm screw is placed. Typical screw lengths are 30 to 35 mm. *(Reprinted with permission from Jandial R, McCormick P, Black PM.* Core Techniques in Operative Neurosurgery. *Elsevier; 2011.)*

sublaminar wiring techniques may be used. Regardless, the cortical bone overlying the C1, C2, and C3 region is decorticated. Autograft and/or allograft are placed over the decorticated segments to achieve bony fusion. Posterior fusions may also require decompressive laminectomy in patients with neurologic injury.

Complication Avoidance and Management

- CT imaging is crucial before instrumentation to assess the location of the vertebral arteries.
- Combined anterior and posterior approaches may provide additional stability in cases of significant displacement and/or angulation.
- Imaging of the entire cervical spine, including the cervico-thoracic junction, should be obtained given the relatively high frequency of adjacent bony injuries.

KEY PAPERS

Ebraheim NA, Fow J, Xu R, et al. The location of the pedicle and pars interarticularis in the axis. *Spine.* 2001;26(4):E34-E37.

Effendi B, Roy D, Cornish B, et al. Fractures of the ring of the axis. A classification based on the analysis of 131 cases. *J Bone Joint Surg Br.* 2013;63:319-327.

Levine AM, Edwards CC. The management of traumatic spondylolisthesis of the axis. *J Bone Joint Surg Am.* 1985;67(2):217-226.

Case 45

Thoracolumbar Burst Fractures

Brandon C. Gabel, MD ● Erik I. Curtis, MD ● Joseph D. Ciacci, MD

Presentation

The patient is a 30-year-old male who fell from height. He complained of mid and low back pain as well as numbness along his right anterolateral thigh.

- PMH: unremarkable
- Exam:
  - 5/5 strength throughout lower extremities, no focal weakness
  - Decreased sensation to light touch on anterolateral right thigh
  - Reflexes 2/4 at patellas and ankles bilaterally
  - Perianal sensation intact
  - Rectal tone intact with good volition

Differential Diagnosis

Thoracolumbar burst fractures most commonly occur in the setting of trauma. Patients with the following diseases may be at an increased risk for burst fractures with minor trauma:

- Neoplastic infiltration
- Osteomyelitis
- Degenerative changes
- Osteoporosis

Initial Imaging

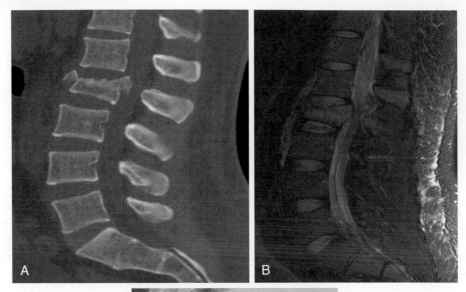

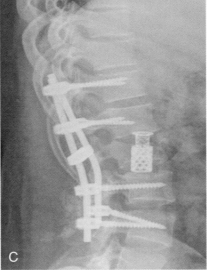

FIGURE 45-1

Imaging Description and Differential

This imaging is consistent with a traumatic L2 burst fracture after a fall from height. Figure 45-1A shows a CT scan with L2 burst fracture. Figure 45-1B is a STIR MRI of the same fracture. Figure 45-1C shows postoperative reconstruction with anterior cage placement and pedicle screw instrumentation.

Further Workup

- Laboratory workup
  - Routine labs
- Imaging
  - MRI of the thoracolumbar spine to assess for ligamentous injury
  - CT imaging to assess bony anatomy, and to aid in potential operative planning
  - Flexion/extension films may be useful in select cases, or at follow-up.

Pathophysiology

Most burst fractures occur at the thoracolumbar junction and are generally considered unstable injuries. These fractures are the result of axial loading forces with a variable degree of flexion force vector. They are one of the most common traumatic injuries seen in the spine, and occur predominately after motor vehicle accidents or falls from significant height. Burst fractures may occur more easily in pathologic conditions of the spine, such as in patients with metastatic disease or in those with osteoporosis. The axial loading forces result in failure of the anterior and middle columns of the spine. The vertebral body "splays" out, and frequently the posterior wall of the vertebral body extrudes into the spinal canal. On anteroposterior bony imaging, the pedicles will often appear more widely separated, compared with adjacent uninjured levels. Neurologic injury depends on the level fractured and the degree of canal compromise. Fractures near the conus medullaris may have the odd combination of bowel and bladder incontinence with normal lower extremity strength (i.e., conus medullaris syndrome). Mid to low lumbar burst fractures with significant retropulsion may cause cauda equina syndrome. Radicular symptoms secondary to nerve root impingement from hematoma or a traumatic disc may also be present and should be distinguished from more severe injury patterns.

Treatment Options

Treatment options depend on the level of injury, degree of canal compromise, neurologic status, and deformity. Treatment options include conservative management with bracing and/or surgical reconstruction with anterior, posterior, lateral, or staged approaches. Decompression may be included if indicated. The most common surgical treatment remains posterior pedicle screw instrumentation and fusion with reduction of the fracture and correction of deformity. Some fractures may require anterior column reconstruction with corpectomy and cage placement to achieve anterior decompression and to provide anterior and middle column support.

- Conservative management is a consideration for patients without neurologic injury and in those with mildly comminuted fractures without significant deformity:
  - External immobilization (i.e., thoracolumbar orthosis)
- Surgical management is indicated for those with significant kyphotic deformity, ligamentous injury, and/or neurologic compromise:
  - Posterior approaches
    - Pedicle screw placement with reduction and correction of deformity
    - Posterolateral fusion with allo/autograft
    - Decompression of neural elements as indicated
    - Corpectomy with cage placement, via a posterior approach, may be considered as indicated
  - Lateral approach
    - Lateral lumbar approach with decompression and reconstruction
      - Corpectomy with cage placement can be performed
      - Consider supplementing construct with posterior instrumentation
  - Anterior or anterolateral approach with corpectomy and reconstruction
    - Allows anterior decompression and reconstruction
    - Consider supplementing construct with posterior instrumentation

Surgical Technique

For posterior approaches the patient is positioned prone on a Jackson table. A Jackson table helps facilitate normal anatomic alignment. The thoracolumbar spine is then prepped and draped in sterile fashion. A lateral fluoroscopic film is taken and the appropriate level is located. An incision is then centered in the midline and extended to include the proposed levels to be fused. The lamina, facet joints, and transverse processes are exposed with electrocautery. Pedicle screws are placed at the levels above and below the fractured vertebrae. Reduction screws, along with decompression and/or osteotomies, may be necessary to achieve reduction of the fracture, aid in correction of deformity, and allow for decompression of the neural elements. If a corpectomy is planned, discectomies are performed above and below the fractured body. Rongeurs, curettes, and high-speed drill are used to complete the corpectomy and decompress the neural elements. The anterior and middle columns are reconstructed using an expandable interbody device combined with auto and/or allograft. The postero-lateral bony surfaces are decorticated. Bone graft is placed over the decorticated areas to augment bony fusion (Figures 45-2, 45-3, and 45-4).

For lateral approaches the patient is placed in the decubitus position. Lateral fluoroscopy is used to locate the fractured level. An incision is made in the flank overlying the fractured fragment. At the L1 and T12 levels it is usually necessary to remove a portion of rib to gain access to the spine. After blunt finger dissection, serial dilators are placed through the psoas muscle; a self-retaining retractor is then introduced. For mid to low lumbar injuries, neuromonitoring potentials should be used to ensure there is no compression of the femoral nerve, which lies adjacent to the psoas muscle. Discectomies and/or corpectomy are performed as indicated. After adequate decompression an interbody device is placed. If supplementation with posterior instrumentation is planned, the patient is turned into the prone position on a Jackson table.

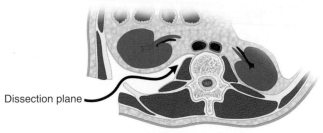

Dissection plane

FIGURE 45-2   Axial view of retroperitoneal dissection. The peritoneum and its contents are swept anteriorly by blunt dissection. The kidney and ureter are retracted anteriorly as well. A self-retaining retractor system, such as the Omni-Tract, aids in maintaining the exposure. *(Reprinted with permission from Jandial R, McCormick P, Black PM.* Core Techniques in Operative Neurosurgery. *Elsevier; 2011.)*

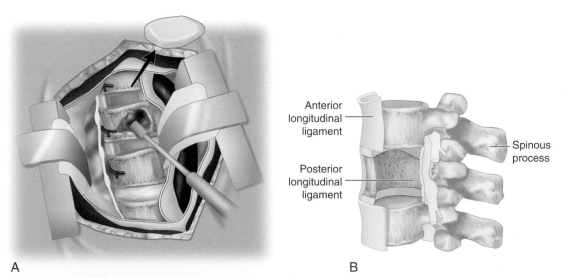

Anterior longitudinal ligament

Posterior longitudinal ligament

Spinous process

A   B

FIGURE 45-3   Corpectomy. Remove the vertebra between the removed disks. Rongeurs and a drill, with cutting burs, may be used **(A)** Cancellous bone can bleed profusely, in contrast to cortical bone. Hemostasis can be maintained by timely resection of cancellous bone out to cortical bone, Gelfoam, or bone wax. Unless contraindicated (e.g., owing to tumor or infection), leave the anterior and contralateral bony cortex intact, and save any resected bone for later grafting. An intact anterior longitudinal ligament and anterior and contralateral cortex help protect great vessels. Decompress the spinal canal carefully to avoid tearing the dura mater, and repair any dural tears primarily if possible. **(B)** *(Reprinted with permission from Jandial R, McCormick P, Black PM.* Core Techniques in Operative Neurosurgery. *Elsevier; 2011.)*

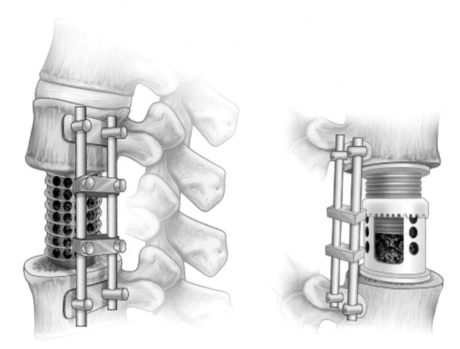

FIGURE 45-4 Instrumentation. Anterior reconstruction generally includes an interbody cage, autograft, or allograft for anterior and middle column support, along with a plate or rods affixed to the adjacent vertebral bodies to limit motion at the fusion site. The specific technique for instrumentation varies by manufacturer. General considerations are listed subsequently. Refer to the manufacturer's guidelines for details of each device. Constructs designed by various manufacturers are illustrated. *(Reprinted with permission from Jandial R, McCormick P, Black PM.* Core Techniques in Operative Neurosurgery. *Elsevier; 2011.)*

Complication Avoidance and Management

- Preoperative imaging with CT is essential to assess bony anatomy before instrumented fusions.
- Patients managed nonoperatively should be followed closely in the clinic with lateral films to ensure no progressive deformity develops.
- Intraoperative neuromonitoring may alert the surgeon to changes in neurologic status. Stimulation of pedicle screws aids in accurate placement.
- Significant blood loss, especially with concomitant corpectomy, should be expected and communicated to the anesthesia team before incision.
- Intraoperative fluoroscopy and/or navigation to assist in placement of instruments.

KEY PAPERS

Dai LY, Jiang SD, Wang XY, et al. A review of the management of thoracolumbar burst fractures. *Surg Neuro.* 2007;67:221-231.

McCormack T, Karaikovic E, Gianes RW. The load sharing classification of spine fractures. *Spine.* 1994; 19:1741-1744.

Wood KB, Li W, Lebl DS, et al. Management of thoracolumbar spine fractures. *Spine J.* 2014;14:145-164.

Case 46

Chance Fractures

Brandon C. Gabel, MD ● Joseph D. Ciacci, MD

Presentation

The patient is a 50-year-old male who fell from a ladder.

- PMH/PSH: tonsillectomy and an umbilical hernia repair
- Examination:
  - 5/5 strength in all muscle groups
  - Sensation intact to light touch throughout
  - Normal reflexes
  - Pain with palpation of high lumbar and low thoracic spine

Differential Diagnosis

Chance fractures may occur in the setting of:

- Trauma (most commonly)
- Osteomyelitis
- Degenerative changes seen in diffuse idiopathic skeletal hyperostosis and ankylosing spondylitis
- Osteoporosis and metabolic bone diseases

Initial Imaging

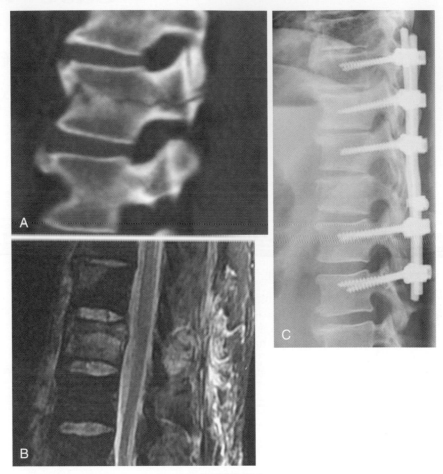

FIGURE 46-1

Imaging Description and Differential

Initial imaging with plain films revealed a subtle fracture through the pedicle of L1. Further imaging with parasagittal CT showed fractures through the bilateral pedicles with extension into the vertebral body (Figure 46-1A). MRI imaging showed STIR signal in the L1 vertebral body, and an increased signal in the posterior ligamentous complex (Figure 46-1B). These images, in the setting of trauma, support a diagnosis of an L1 flexion-distraction injury (aka a "chance" fracture). Postoperative radiograph (Figure 46-1C) shows pedicle screw stabilization from T10 to L3.

Further Workup

- Laboratory workup
  - Routine labs
- Imaging
  - MRI with STIR protocol to assess for posterior ligamentous injury, hematoma, and traumatic disc herniation
  - CT images to assess bony anatomy and to help with potential preoperative planning
  - AP, lateral, and flexion-extension films can be used to assess for biomechanical stability in neurologically intact patients without evidence of ligamentous injury (or if MRI is unavailable).

Pathophysiology

Flexion-distraction injuries, also known as "chance" fractures, or "seat-belt" type injuries, occur in the setting of combined flexion and distraction forces on the spine. They most commonly occur at the thoracolumbar junction. At a minimum, they involve the middle and posterior columns, but may also involve the anterior column; this multicolumn involvement makes them unstable injuries. Chance fractures may be further categorized as "bony," "ligamentous," or both. Ligamentous "fractures" occur in the absence of bony abnormalities, and the only imaging finding may be splaying of the spinous processes on plain films or CT. Therefore a high index of suspicion should be present in a patient with significant back pain and splaying of the spinous processes on bony imaging. The posterior ligamentous complex (i.e., supraspinous ligaments, interspinous ligaments, ligamentum flavum, and facet capsules) is frequently disrupted as a result of the flexion-distraction forces required to create these injuries. Bony findings usually include a fracture line that extends from the posterior elements, through the pedicles, and into the involved body. Flexion-distraction injuries are also seen commonly in patients with diffuse idiopathic skeletal hyperostosis (DISH) after seemingly minor trauma. Most patients with chance fractures are neurologically intact other than pain at the site of injury.

Treatment Options

Treatment options vary and depend strongly on neurologic status, degree of ligamentous injury, and the mechanism of injury. A common, and relatively straightforward, grading system created by Vaccaro et al is frequently used to help guide treatment. In this grading system, flexion-distraction injuries obtain the most number of points and frequently (although not always) require operative intervention to stabilize. In poor operative candidates, or patients with no ligamentous or neurologic injury, a trial of bracing may be appropriate, but close follow-up should be provided. The main worry with conservatively managed patients is the development of posttraumatic kyphosis at the level of the injury.

- Rigid hyperextension braces (i.e., Jewett brace) can be used in patients with bony chance fractures without evidence of significant ligamentous injury, and in those who are poor operative candidates.
- Surgical correction is indicated in most flexion-distraction injuries.
  - Posterior fusion to reconstruct the posterior tension band is the most common surgical treatment:
    - With pedicle screws and auto/allograft
    - Noninstrumented with auto/allograft (in patients who may not tolerate pedicle screw placement)

Surgical Technique

The patient is positioned prone on a Jackson table. The lamina, facets, and transverse processes of the levels being fused are exposed. Typically, although not always, two levels above and below the fracture are selected for fusion; shorter fusions may be considered in select cases. The fractured level is usually skipped. After placement of pedicle screws and rod instrumentation, the adjacent bony structures are decorticated using a high-speed drill. The involved level(s) may need to be decompressed as indicated by the patient's neurologic exam. Reduction screws may be necessary to correct significant kyphotic deformities. A mixture of auto and/or allograft is then placed over the decorticated bone. The wound is closed in layers. The patient is placed in a custom-fitted hyperextension brace postoperatively.

Complication Avoidance and Management

- Preoperative CT imaging should be studied carefully to ensure the pedicles at the adjacent levels are of sufficient size to tolerate screw placement. If they are not, the fusion should be extended to include levels that will support screw placement.

- Reduction screws may be necessary to reduce significant kyphotic deformities.
- Patients managed with hyperextension bracing should be followed closely with repeat X-rays. If a worsening kyphotic deformity develops, then surgical intervention should be offered.

KEY PAPERS

Lee HM, Kim HS, Kim DJ, et al. Reliability of magnetic resonance imaging in detecting posterior ligament complex injury in thoracolumbar spinal fractures. *Spine.* 2000;v.25(16):2079-2084.

Vaccaro AR, Zeiller SC, Hulbert RJ, et al. The thoracolumbar injury severity score. *J Spinal Disord Tech.* 2005;18:209-215.

Weinstein JN, Rydevik BL, Rauschning W. Anatomic and technical considerations of pedicle screw fixation. *Clin Orthop Relat Res.* 1992;(284):34-46.

White AA, Panjabi MM. *Clinical Biomechanics of the Spine.* Philadelphia: Lippincott; 1990.

Case 47

Jumped Cervical Facets

Brandon C. Gabel, MD ● Joseph D. Ciacci, MD

Presentation

The patient is a 40-year-old female with a history of autoimmune labyrinthitis. She suffered a ground-level fall secondary to vertigo. She awoke the following morning with neck pain and paresthesias in her left index finger.

- PMH: autoimmune labyrinthitis, seizure disorder, and hypertension
- Exam:
  - Nystagmus with lateral gaze bilaterally
  - Decreased sensation in left hand to light touch
  - Pain limited left deltoid examination, but otherwise 5/5 strength
  - DTRs were 3+ throughout, without clonus or Hoffmann's reflexes

Differential Diagnosis

Jumped cervical facets are due to traumatic flexion-distraction-rotational injuries involving the cervical spine.

Initial Imaging

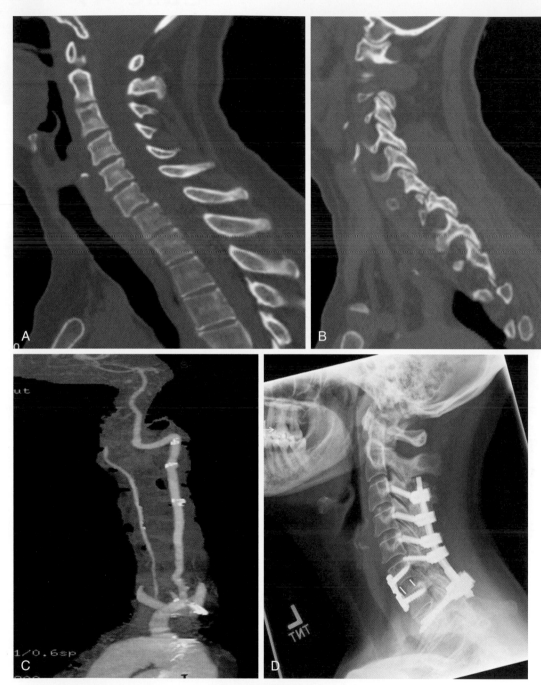

FIGURE 47-1

Imaging Description and Differential

Midline sagittal CT (Figure 47-1A) illustrates a mild anterolisthesis of C6 on C7, which is consistent with a unilateral jumped or perched facet joint. Off-midline sagittal CT (Figure 47-1B) shows the injured facet; notice the perching of the C6 inferior articulating process on the C7 superior articulating process. Also of note is the fracture line extending through the lateral mass. The CT angiogram (Figure 47-1C) shows no evidence of vertebral artery injury at the level of the fracture. These findings are consistent with a diagnosis of traumatic C6-C7 lateral mass fracture with a coexistent perched facet. Postoperative imaging (Figure 47-1D) shows good reduction of the fracture with anteroposterior reconstruction.

Further Workup

- Laboratory workup
  - Routine labs
- Imaging
  - MRI to assess ligamentous injury
  - CT imaging to assess for bony anatomy and to aid in potential operative planning
  - CT or MR angiogram to assess the vertebral arteries

Pathophysiology

Jumped cervical facets occur in the setting of severe distraction, flexion, and usually rotational forces. A unilateral jumped or perched facet occurs under conditions of flexion with a rotational component away from the injured side; bilateral jumped facets occur under conditions of flexion and distractive forces. Regardless of whether the facet is unilaterally or bilaterally jumped, these are always considered unstable injuries given the degree of osteoligamentous disruption needed to create these injuries.

Unilateral jumped facets typically cause a 25% subluxation of the superior vertebral body over the inferior vertebral body on bony imaging. Bilaterally jumped facets usually cause a 50% subluxation. Radiculopathy on the side of the jumped facet is the most common clinical finding in a unilateral jumped facet. Patients with bilateral jumped facets have a high likelihood of spinal cord injury. Most jumped facets occur in the subaxial cervical spine; but, it is important to note that facet dislocations can occur at the C7-T1 junction, which is why visualization of this level on plain film or CT is of paramount importance.

A less severe form of cervical spine subluxation is known as the perched facet, in which the inferior portion of the inferior articulating facet perches on top of the superior portion of the superior articulating facet, without actually locking into place.

Treatment Options

Treatment options usually involve a combination of cervical traction followed by open surgical fusion. Traction is usually done in the awake patient under light sedation with Gardner-Wells tongs. Significant weight may need to be added in order to reduce the jumped facet(s). Occasionally reduction may not be possible with Gardner-Wells tongs and open surgical reduction may be necessary. The patient's neurologic function should be monitored throughout the procedure.

Open surgical fusion usually follows reduction with traction. Controversy exists over ideal operative approach and is decided on a case-by-case basis; a combination of anterior only, posterior only, or combined anterior-posterior approaches are frequently used. Traumatic disc herniations, seen on preoperative MRI, require anterior approaches to address. Patients with traumatic discs and unreducible locked facets (i.e., unable to reduce using Gardner-Wells traction) may require a "front-back-front" approach, in which the disc is removed, the patient is turned prone and fused from behind, and the front is then reapproached with placement of an interbody spacer in the previously removed disc space. This approach prevents worsening central canal stenosis from a herniated disc when the facets are relocated from the posterior approach. It also helps mobilize the spine during the posterior approach.

Surgical Technique

For anterior cervical discectomy/corpectomy, the patient is positioned supine. Additionally, the patient may be placed in traction to aid with alignment. Intraoperative fluoroscopy is used to ensure good alignment before skin incision. Intraoperative neuromonitoring should be used to assess neurologic function while under anesthesia. A combination of blunt and sharp dissection is carried down to the prevertebral fascia. An intraoperative film is taken to ensure the appropriate level(s) is/are exposed. A discectomy is then performed. At this point the incision may be closed and the patient turned prone if a front-back-front approach is used. Otherwise, if there has been reduction in the locked facets with traction, an interbody device, autograft, and/or allograft may be placed in the disc space. Depending on the type of interbody device used, a plate may be secured to the adjacent vertebral bodies to prevent graft extrusion and aid in fusion.

For posterior instrumented fusions, the patient is placed in a Mayfield head holder and turned prone on chest rolls. The patient is placed in slight reverse Trendelenburg with the knees flexed. Before skin incision, lateral fluoroscopy is used to ensure adequate alignment. The fractured level, and several segments above and below the injury, are exposed. The jumped facets will be apparent after exposure. Meticulous removal of the superior facet (i.e., the caudal portion of bone in the operative field) involved in the jump will allow the dislocated facet(s) to reduce. Lateral mass screws are placed above and below the fractured segment and a rod is locked into place (Figures 47-2, 47-3, and 47-4). The cortical bone of the lateral masses is decorticated. Autograft and/or allograft are placed over the decorticated bone to aid in bony fusion.

Complication Avoidance and Management

- Before the placement of traction, craniocervical junction instability should be ruled out. Atlantooccipital dislocation is a firm contraindication to cervical traction.
- Combined anterior and posterior approaches may provide additional stability in cases of significant displacement and/or angulation. They may also be necessary to allow reduction of the jumped or perched facet in some cases.

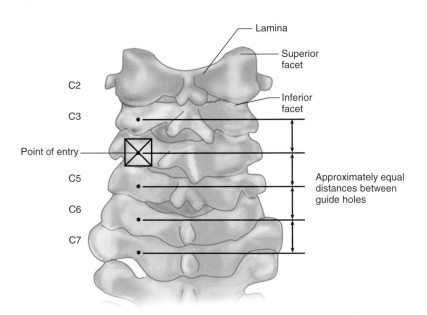

FIGURE 47-2 The appropriate starting point can be determined by creating an imaginary "X" over the lateral mass. The superior and inferior boundaries are the facet joints, and the medial and lateral boundaries of the lateral mass serve as the other boundaries. The ideal starting point is 1 mm medial to the middle of the imaginary "X." *(Reprinted with permission from Jandial R, McCormick P, Black PM. Core Techniques in Operative Neurosurgery. Elsevier; 2011.)*

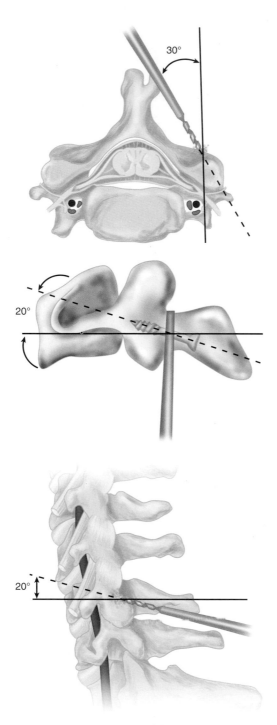

FIGURE 47-3   An up-and-out technique is used for hand drill trajectory. A medial-to-lateral trajectory at 30 degrees avoids injury to the vertebral artery, and a cephalad-caudal trajectory at 20 degrees avoids injury to the nerve root. *(Reprinted with permission from Jandial R, McCormick P, Black PM. Core Techniques in Operative Neurosurgery. Elsevier; 2011.)*

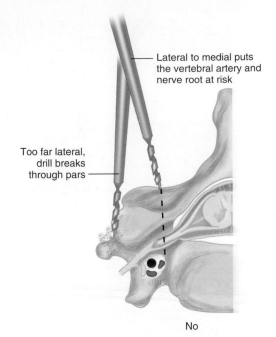

Lateral to medial puts
the vertebral artery and
nerve root at risk

Too far lateral,
drill breaks
through pars

No

FIGURE 47-4   A medial trajectory risks injury to the vertebral artery. Failing to aim the cephalad places the nerve root at risk. Starting too farlateral risks fracture of the lateral mass. *(Reprinted with permission from Jandial R, McCormick P, Black PM. Core Techniques in Operative Neurosurgery. Elsevier; 2011.)*

- Imaging of the entire cervical spine, including the cervicothoracic junction, should be obtained given the relatively high frequency of adjacent bony injuries.
- Preoperative MRI imaging, if available, can help determine the length of fusion required if posterior approaches are used. Longer fusions may be necessary if there is significant posterior ligamentous injury.

KEY PAPERS

Rabb CH, Lopez J, Beauchamp K, et al. Unilateral cervical facet fractures with subluxation: injury patterns and treatment. *J Spinal Disord Tech.* 2007;20(6):416-422.
Shapiro SA. Management of unilateral locked facet of the cervical spine. *Neurosurgery.* 1993;33:832-837.

Section IV
Spinal Neurosurgery

Case 48

Atlanto-Axial Dislocation

Gurpreet S. Gandhoke, MD ● Adam S. Kanter, MD

Presentation

A 31-year-old male plumber presents with sudden onset quadriparesis lasting 5 minutes after hyperextending his neck while at work. The patient reports a similar episode of transient limb weakness after cervical chiropractic manipulation 6 months prior. Upon further questioning, he reports increasing frequency of urination. Positive findings on examination include guarded cervical motion, increased tone in all four extremities, and 3+ hyperreflexia in bilateral biceps, triceps, knee, and ankles.

Differential Diagnosis

- Congenital
  - Atlanto-axial dislocation (AAD)
  - Os odontoideum
- Trauma
  - Odontoid fracture
- Tumor
  - Foramen magnum meningioma or schwannoma
  - Clival malignancy with extension to the craniovertebral junction
- Infection
  - Grisel syndrome
- Inflammation
  - Rheumatoid pannus

Initial Imaging

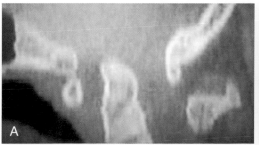 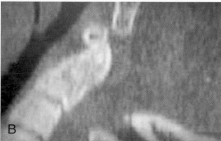

FIGURE 48-1 *(Reprinted with permission from Jain VK. Atlantoaxial dislocation. Neurology India. 2012;60(1):9-17.)*

Imaging Description

CT scan of the craniovertebral junction in flexion (A) and extension (B) demonstrating a reducible atlanto-axial dislocation, with the dens completely reducing in extension.

Further Workup

- MRI cervical spine: helps define relationship of cervico-medullary junction, dens, and posterior arches of C1 and C2 in relation to neural and vascular structures.
- Dynamic flexion/extension X-ray of the cervical spine provides a preoperative anatomic roadmap to compare with intraoperative anatomy and imaging.
- Routine blood work to ensure that the patient is not anemic, protein calorie malnourished, or actively infected (includes CBC, BMP, and PT/INR/PTT)

Pathophysiology

- The C1-C2 facet joints form the most mobile segment of the spine and are thus prone to developing instability. Dislocation at this level predisposes the cervico medullary junction to compression from a mobile dens, causing injuries ranging from transient quadriparesis to respiratory difficulties and sudden death.
- The surfaces of the normal atlanto-axial facet joints are relatively flat and parallel. The movement in these joints includes angular, rotational, linear, and translational motions. However, anterior movement of the axis vertebra is restricted by the anterior arch of C1 when the odontoid is normal. Posterior movement is restricted by the cruciate ligament; largely by the transverse ligament. Rotatory movement is restricted by the alar ligaments.
- It is possible that inadequate extension of C2 to C1 as a result of pain, or a muscle spasm, minimizing C2 mobility, even with adequate extension.
- Atlanto-axial dislocation can be evaluated by measuring the basion-dens interval (BDI) (Figure 48-2).
- Atlanto-axial dislocations are classified into four varieties depending on their direction and plane of dislocation (i.e., anteroposterior, rotatory, central, and mixed dislocations) (Figure 48-3).

Treatment Options

- Posterior fusion is the treatment of choice for reducible AAD.
- If irreducible, an odontoidectomy, followed by a posterior fusion, may be required.
- If the anatomy at the occipito-atlanto-axial region is normal on X-ray, the dislocation should be reducible by cervical traction, or during surgery by mobilizing the joints.
- Approaches
  - Anterior
    - Transoral decompression of odontoid
  - Posterior
    - Bone grafts
      - Bone grafts between occiput-C1 lamina and C2 lamina
      - C1-C2 rib graft; interlaminar
      - C1-C2 interspinous; interlaminar wedge graft (modified Gallie)
    - Instrumentation
      - Semi-rigid occipital loop and sublaminar cables
      - C1-C2 transarticular screws
      - C1 lateral mass to C2 translaminar screws and rods
      - C1 lateral mass to C2 pars screws w/ rods
      - Occipital plate, C1 lateral mass screws, C2 pars screws and rods

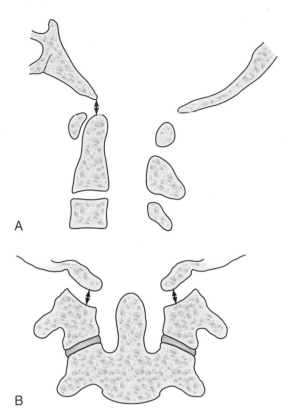

A

B

FIGURE 48-2 Drawings illustrate cervical radiographic techniques for the diagnosis of atlanto-occipital dislocation (AOD). **(A)** Basion-dens interval (BDI) is abnormal in the presence of a displacement between the basion and the dens exceeding 10 mm in adults or more than 12 mm in the pediatric population. **(B)** A distance of more than 2 mm in adults, or 5 mm in pediatric patients, between the occipital condyle and the superior articular facet of the atlas is considered an abnormal condylar gap. *(Redrawn with permission from Barrow Neurological Institute. Reprinted with permission from Ellenbogen RG, Abdulrauf SI, Sekhar LN.* Principles of Neurological Surgery. *3rd ed. Elsevier; 2012.)*

Type 1   Type 2   Type 3

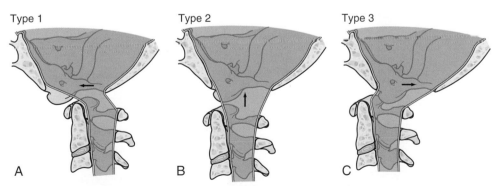

A   B   C

FIGURE 48-3 Classification system for atlanto-occipital dislocation (AOD). **(A)** Type 1 or anterior dislocation of the occiput with respect to the atlas. **(B)** Type 2 or vertical displacement. **(C)** Type 3 or posterior displacement. *(Redrawn with permission from Barrow Neurological Institute. Reprinted with permission from Ellenbogen RG, Abdulrauf SI, Sekhar LN.* Principles of Neurological Surgery. *3rd ed. Elsevier; 2012.)*

Surgical Technique
Occipito-Cervical Fusion

- Fiberoptic intubation is performed and baseline somatosensory-evoked potentials (SSEPs) and motor-evoked potentials (MEPs), while still supine, are obtained.
- Patient is turned prone on chest rolls with cervical alignment maintained in a Mayfield head clamp to maintain neutral occipito-cervical position.
- If autograft is required, the harvest site is included in the prepped area.
- The midline incision extends from the inion to the lowest level to be fused.
- During subperiosteal dissection, a cuff of fascia is left at the inion for subsequent closure, ensuring that the occipital plate is covered by enough soft tissue to prevent hardware erosion.
- The decompression is performed as indicated and the bone saved for use as autograft.
- Occipital fixation can be performed using wiring, in/out buttons, plate, or occipital condyle screw fixation.
- The midline keel is usually between 10 and 14 mm thick and a screw of 4.5 mm can be placed to anchor the occipital plate. Drill in increments of 2 mm, after an initial depth of 8 mm, to avoid injury to the posterior fossa structures. The paramedian bone in this region is not as thick as the midline keel.
- The cervical instrumentation can then be placed and incorporated into the occipital plate using rods bent to the required shape.

Pearls

- Use a flexible endotracheal tube stylet as a template before bending a rod or Steinmann pin.
- If the C2 anatomy is unfavorable for the placement of either pars or pedicle screws, pass the sublaminar cables under the C2 lamina, place lateral mass screws at C3, and wire C2 to the rod from C3 to the occiput (Figure 48-4).

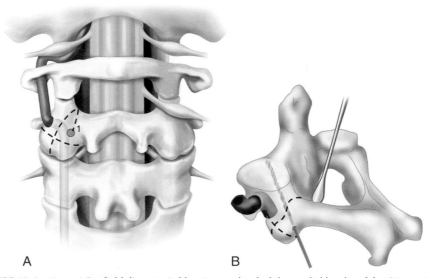

A   B

FIGURE 48-4 A no. 4 Penfield dissector is likewise used to feel the medial border of the C2 pars interarticularis. The atlanto-axial membrane is detached using a blunt dissector to expose the upper surface of the C2 pedicle. The inferior articular process of C2 is divided into quadrants. The C2 pedicle screw starting point lies in the superomedial quadrant of the inferior articular process of C2 (approximately 1.75 mm caudal to the lateral mass-pars interarticularis transition zone). The pilot hole is again prepared with a high-speed bit, and the pilot hole is drilled in a trajectory oriented 20 degrees medial and 20 degrees cephalad with lateral fluoroscopic guidance. The hole is checked with a probe and tapped. A 3.5 mm screw is placed. Typical screw lengths are 30 to 35 mm. *(Reprinted with permission from Jandial R, McCormick P, Black PM. Core Techniques in Operative Neurosurgery. Elsevier; 2011.)*

- Preoperatively review the depth of the midline suboccipital keel, thickness of the paramedian cranium, and the course of the vertebral artery to minimize injury during surgery.
- Verify a neutral occipito-cervical relationship before locking in the construct.

Complication Avoidance and Management

Complication	Management
Inability to intubate	Preoperative evaluation; fiber optic intubation
Worsening in neurologic status, or intraoperative SSEP change	Patient should be in dynamic traction; preoperative assessment of best position; awake positioning
Gross instability at CVJ	Stabilize C1 to C2 with towel clamp during sharp muscle dissection
Excessive bleeding with C1 lateral mass exposure	Subperiosteal dissection behind the C1 posterior arch with progressive bipolar coagulation of the venous plexus; last resort is C2 ganglionectomy to visualize the dorsal rostral C1 lateral mass
Bleeding from vertebral artery in foramen	Place screw and leave in situ; do not place screw on other side; need angiogram
Bleeding from occipital screw placement	Preoperative measurement of occipital keel; position of transverse sinus to gauge depth of screws and avoid sinus; place hemostatic agent (oxidized cellulose) and flat-head screw
CSF egress from occipital screws	Pack with hemostatic agent and place screw; if from spinal dural tear, identify and close leak
Wire cutting through the arch of atlas during sublaminar wiring	Rule out bifid C1 arch, hypoplasia on preoperative images
Hypoglossal nerve injury and pharyngeal penetration	Careful preoperative assessment of C1 screw length; must obtain postop CT scan; if screw is too long, it will need to be withdrawn
Loss of alignment, screw fracture, or pullout	Redo procedure; if no instrumentation performed, place in traction and halo vest
Swallowing or breathing issues	Too flexed position of fusion; will need fusion reposition to improve airway; avoid distraction in flexed position

KEY PAPERS

Behari S, Bhargava V, Nayak S, et al. Congenital reducible atlantoaxial dislocation: classification and surgical considerations. *Acta Neurochir (Wien)*. 2002;144(11):1165-1177.

Bharucha EP, Dastur HM. Craniovertebral anomalies (a report on 40 cases). *Brain*. 1964;87:469-480.

Dastur DK, Wadia NH, Desai AD, et al. Medullospinal compression due to atlanto-axial dislocation and sudden haematomyelia during decompression. Pathology, pathogenesis and clinical correlations. *Brain*. 1965; 88(5):897-924.

Jain VK. Atlantoaxial dislocation. *Neurol India*. 2012;60(1):9-17.

Menezes AH. Craniocervical fusions in children. *J Neurosurgery Pediatr*. 2012;9(6):573-585.

Tulsi RS. Some specific anatomical features of the atlas and axis: dens, epitransverse process and articular facets. *Aust N Z J Surg*. 1978;48(5):570-574.

White AA 3rd, Panjabi MM. The clinical biomechanics of the occipitoatlantoaxial complex. *Orthop Clin North Am*. 1978;9(4):867-878.

Case 49

Basilar Invagination – Rheumatoid Pannus

Zachary J. Tempel, MD ● Robert A. Miller, MD ● Adam S. Kanter, MD

Presentation

A 68-year-old female with known rheumatoid arthritis, controlled with corticosteroids, presents with several months of progressive neck pain and upper extremity weakness. She reports difficulty with fine motor tasks and episodic electrical shock-like pain associated with neck flexion. She reports occasional swallowing difficulty. Other notable history includes osteoporosis and hypertension. Examination reveals a thin woman, head mildly extended. Strength exam reveals 4-/5 in bilateral upper extremities, 4+/5 in the lower extremities, a positive Lhermitte's sign, asymmetric palate elevation, 3+ reflexes throughout, positive Hoffman's, and clonus bilaterally.

Differential Diagnosis

- Degenerative
  - Cervical spondylotic myelopathy
  - Compression fracture
  - Atlanto-axial instability
- Traumatic
  - Odontoid fracture
- Neoplastic
  - Metastasis
  - Cervical spine tumor (astrocytoma or plasmacytoma)
  - CPA tumor (acoustic neuroma or meningioma)
  - Brainstem glioma
  - Chordoma/chondrosarcoma
- Vascular
  - Cavernous malformation
  - Vertebrobasilar insufficiency
- Infectious
  - Discitis +/− osteomyelitis
  - Epidural abscess

Initial Imaging

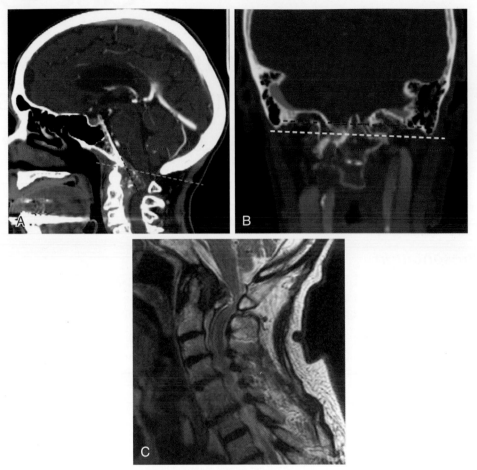

FIGURE 49-1

Imaging Description and Differential

- Sagittal CT (Figure 49-1A), coronal CT (Figure 49-1B), and sagittal MRI (Figure 49-1C) of the cervical spine reveal cranial settling with a large calcified mass posterior to the dens resulting in severe central canal stenosis.
- McRae's line (green): line from the basion to the opisthion; the dens should not cross this line.
- Wackenheim's clivus-canal line (blue): extension of a line drawn along the slope of the clivus; the dens should not cross this line.
- Fischgold's digastric line (red): line connecting the digastric notches; a distance between this line and the middle of the AA joint <10 mm suggests BI.
- Fischgold's bimastoid line (yellow): line connecting the mastoid tips; tip of the dens is 2 mm above this line on average, and the AA joint should not traverse this line.

Further Workup

- Laboratory
  - CBC, BMP, and PT/PTT/INR
  - ESR, CRP, and prealbumin
  - Rheumatoid factor

- Imaging
  - CT chest/abdomen/pelvis
  - MRI brain/cervical spine
  - Dynamic radiographs to evaluate for instability
- Consultants
  - Rheumatology
  - Otolaryngology (swallow evaluation)

Pathophysiology

Rheumatoid spondylitis is subdivided into three categories: atlanto-axial instability with rheumatoid pannus, basilar invagination (superior migration of the odontoid), and subaxial subluxation. RA is an autoimmune condition in which synovial cells produce rheumatoid factor; this initiates an inflammatory cascade with immune complex deposition and leukocyte infiltration in the joint. Fibroblast proliferation creates granulation tissue (rheumatoid pannus), which erodes the surrounding bone and connective tissue (specifically the cruciate ligament) through proteolytic enzyme activity. The end result is ligamentous laxity, atlanto-axial instability, and basilar invagination. The hypermobility that occurs within the occipito-atlanto-axial complex produces further inflammation and arthropathy. Up to 80% of patients with RA develop radiographic evidence of cervical spine involvement.

Treatment Options

- Medical
  - Immunotherapy/DMARDs (TNF inhibitors and monoclonal antibodies)
  - NSAIDs
  - Corticosteroids
- Mechanical
  - Cervical orthosis: does not alter the disease course; mainly protective
- Interventional
  - Nerve blocks: useful for patients with isolated occipital neuralgia
- Surgical
  - <u>Anterior odontoidectomy</u>: traditionally performed through the transoral route with high morbidity. Specific complications include infection and velopalatal insufficiency. Endoscopically assisted expanded endonasal approach (EEA) enables access to the anterior C1 and C2 complex, with lower morbidity, and is ideal for severe anterior compression.
  - <u>Posterior decompression/fusion:</u> allows for rigid fixation of the occipito-atlanto-axial complex. If minimal osseous destruction, a C1 and C2 fusion alone may suffice. Significant osseous destruction warrants a larger construct from the occiput to the subaxial cervical spine. For mild/moderate anterior compression, posterior fixation alone often leads to pannus regression and stabilization.
  - <u>Traction:</u> Gardner-Wells tongs may be an effective means of reducing basilar invagination and indirectly decompressing the cervicomedullary junction. If successful reduction is accomplished, a posterior-only approach is often sufficient.

Surgical Technique
EEA

Positioning is supine, with a Mayfield head holder applied and the head translated anteriorly, slightly flexed and rotated 15 degrees toward the surgeon.

Standard EEA exposure with removal of the middle turbinate, bilateral sphenoidotomies, and detachment of the posterior nasal septum from the rostrum. Boundaries: floor of the sphenoid rostrally, eustachian tubes laterally, soft palate caudally.

The nasopharyngeal mucosa is incised. The soft tissues are dissected laterally from the clivus down to the anterior ring of C1, and then removed with a high-speed drill.

The pannus and odontoid are resected with an ultrasonic aspirator or high speed drill. Reconstruction is accomplished with fibrin glue (Figures 49-2, 49-3, 49-4, and 49-5).

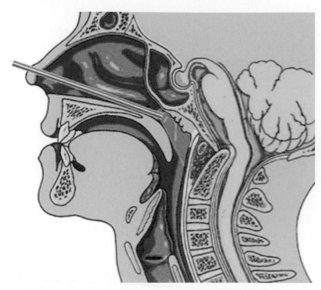

FIGURE 49-2 Expanded endonasal approach to the odontoid. *(Reprinted with permission from Kassam AB, Snyderman C, Gardner P, et al. The expanded endonasal approach: a fully endoscopic transnasal approach and resection of the odontoid process: technical case report.* Neurosurgery. *2005;57(suppl 1):E213, discussion E213.)*

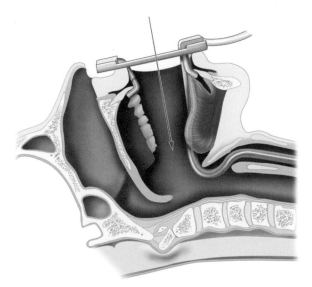

FIGURE 49-3 A Spetzler-Sonntag retractor is placed. It is important to ensure that the tongue and endotracheal tube are behind the retractor. *(Reprinted with permission from Jandial R, McCormick P, Black PM.* Core Techniques in Operative Neurosurgery. *Elsevier; 2011.)*

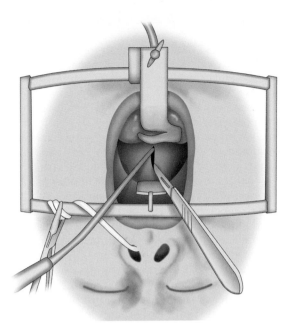

FIGURE 49-4   A linear incision is made in the pharyngeal fascia above the odontoid. *(Reprinted with permission from Jandial R, McCormick P, Black PM.* Core Techniques in Operative Neurosurgery. *Elsevier; 2011.)*

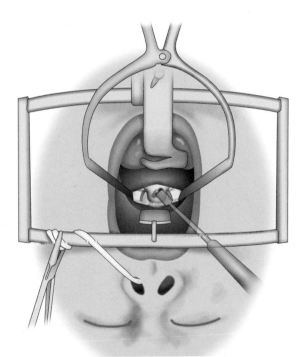

FIGURE 49-5   The C1 ring is removed with a high speed burr. *(Reprinted with permission from Jandial R, McCormick P, Black PM.* Core Techniques in Operative Neurosurgery. *Elsevier; 2011.)*

Posterior Approach

Positioning is prone in a Mayfield head holder with the head in a military tuck position.

The occiput and posterior elements are exposed. The caudal extent of the fusion construct is dependent on several factors: lateral mass anatomy, degree of kyphotic deformity, and bone quality.

C1 and C2 laminectomies may be performed. If C1 screws are placed, the sulcus arteriosus is located on the posterior arch and the vertebral artery is identified. The inferior edge of the C1 lamina is removed laterally, exposing the lateral mass and C2 DRG. The C2 DRG is mobilized inferiorly or sacrificed. The medial wall of the lateral mass and the medial aspect of the transverse foramen are palpated to visualize screw trajectory. The starting point is the center of the lateral mass. Under fluoroscopic guidance, a low-speed drill is aimed 15 degrees medially and cranially toward the anterior tubercle. The screw is placed bicortically and several millimeters proud to properly align with the C2 screw.

C2 screws are placed in the pars interarticularis or the pedicle. The starting point of a pars screw is 3 mm rostral and lateral to the inferior/medial inferior articular process. The trajectory is directed cranially toward the anterior ring of C1 and 20 degrees to 30 degrees medially. The entry point for the pedicle screw is approximately 2 mm superior and lateral to the pars screw with less craniocaudal and more medial angulation (red).

For subaxial screws, the lateral mass is bisected horizontally and vertically, creating four quadrants. The starting point is 1 mm medial and inferior to the midpoint (modified Magerl's technique). The starting point is marked with a high-speed drill. A low-speed drill is used to create a pilot hole aimed to the superolateral corner of the lateral mass.

Occipital plating is performed last because it can be altered to facilitate alignment with the cervical screws. The plate/screw construct is affixed inferior to the inion and superior nuchal line. Bicortical purchase is optimal (Figures 49-6, 49-7, 49-8 and 49-9).

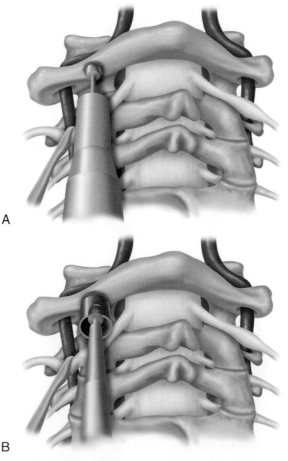

A

B

FIGURE 49-6   (A) Removal of the inferior edge of the C1 lamina to expose the lateral mass, (B) retraction of the C2 DRG and insertion of the C1 lateral mass screw.

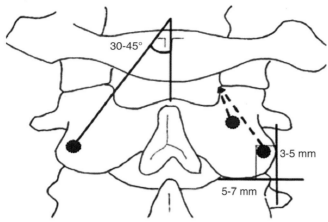

FIGURE 49-7   Various starting points and trajectories for C2 pedicle screws. *(Reprinted with permission from Lee KH, Kang DH, Chul HL, et al. Inferolateral entry point for C2 pedicle screw fixation in high cervical lesions.* J Korean Neurosurg Soc. *2011;50(4):341-347.)*

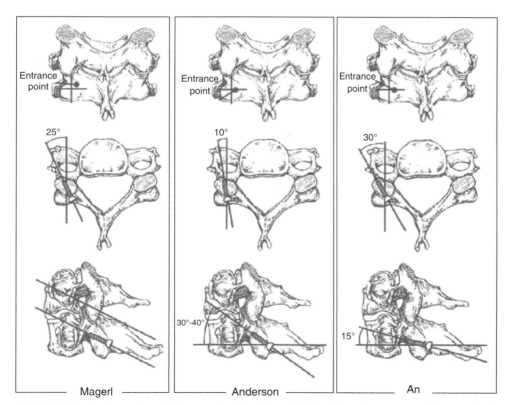

FIGURE 49-8   Starting point and trajectory for subaxial cervical spine lateral mass screws. *(Reprinted with permission from Xu R, Haman SP, Ebraheim NA, et al: The anatomic relation of lateral mass screws to the spinal nerves. A comparison of the Magerl, Anderson, and An techniques.* Spine (Phila Pa 1976). *1999;24(19):2057-2061.)*

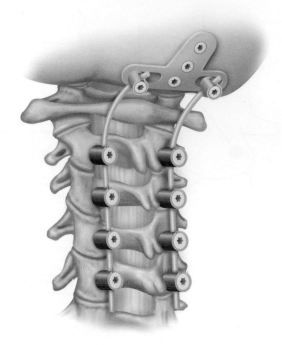

FIGURE 49-9 Occipital plating system with rod connectors to the cervical spine instrumentation.

Complication Avoidance and Management

- Expanded endonasal approach
  - Lateral cautery dissection at the level of the eustachian tubes must be performed carefully to avoid injury to the retropharyngeal carotid arteries.
  - To avoid CSF leak, the odontoid is cored out ventrally, then dissected from the transverse and apical ligaments.
- Posterior approach
  - The head must be optimally positioned for horizontal gaze and bipedal locomotion.
  - Electrocautery is avoided during lateral dissection along the atlas to prevent vertebral artery injury.
  - If vertebral artery injury occurs during placement of the C2 screw, the screw is left in place and the injured vessel is packed off. The wound is closed expeditiously without contralateral instrumentation and immediate postoperative angiography is performed to treat the injury, followed by a stroke protocol MRI.

KEY PAPERS

Harms J, Melcher RP. Posterior C1-C2 fusion with polyaxial screw and rod fixation. *Spine (Phila Pa 1976)*. 2001;26(22):2467-2471.

Kassam AB, Snyderman C, Gardner P, et al. The expanded endonasal approach: a fully endoscopic transnasal approach and resection of the odontoid process: technical case report. *Neurosurgery*. 2005;57(suppl 1):E213, discussion E213.

Lee KH, Kang DH, Chul HL, et al. Inferolateral entry point for C2 pedicle screw fixation in high cervical lesions. *J Korean Neurosurg Soc*. 2011;50(4):341-347.

Mummaneni PV, Haid RW. Atlantoaxial fixation: overview of all techniques. *Neurol India*. 2005;53(4):408-415.

Perrini P, Benedetto N, Di Lorenzo N. Transoral approach to the extradural non-neoplastic lesions of the craniovertebral junction. *Acta Neurochir (Wien)*. 2014;156(6):1231-1236.

Case 50

Cervical Spondylotic Myelopathy

Christian B. Ricks, MD ● Nathan T. Zwagerman, MD ●
Adam S. Kanter, MD

Presentation

A 76-year-old female with history significant for diabetes, hypertension, and arthritis presents with gait unsteadiness that has led to several falls over the past 12 months. She further reports tingling in the bilateral upper extremities, with numbness of her third through fifth digits, hand weakness when picking up objects, and decreased dexterity. She now utilizes a walker for ambulation. Examination reveals an overweight female with depressed affect, full 5/5 strength throughout with bilateral Hoffman's signs, blunted diffuse sensorium and reflexes, and an unsteady gait necessitating assistance for ambulation.

Differential Diagnosis

- Degenerative
  - Herniated cervical disc
  - Opacification of the posterior longitudinal ligament
  - Cervical spondylotic myelopathy
- Neoplastic
  - Tumor of spinal cord, canal, or vertebra
  - Pathologic fracture
- Infectious
  - Epidural abscess
- Other
  - Amyotrophic lateral sclerosis
  - MS
  - Hereditary spastic paraplegia

Initial Imaging

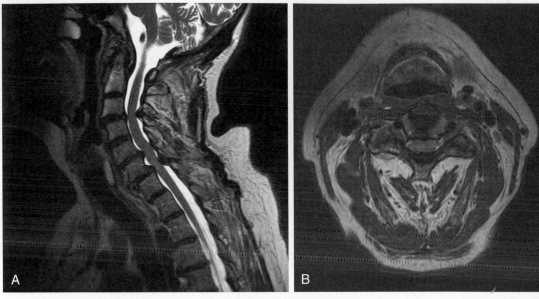

FIGURE 50-1

Imaging Description and Differential

- Sagittal and axial cervical T2-weighted MR images reveal multilevel cervical stenosis at C3-C4, C5-C6, and C6-C7 with T2 cord signal changes, and flattening of the cord with loss of CSF signal at the three levels.

Further Workup

- Laboratory
  - Full set of labs, INR, PTT, type, and screen
  - Preoperative ECG and CXR
- Imaging
  - Cervical plain films with dynamic views to evaluate alignment/stability
  - CT if concern for ossified ligament and considering anterior approach
- Further testing
  - EMG may be beneficial to evaluate other causes or myelopathy, such as peripheral neuropathy or ALS.

Pathophysiology

Myelopathy is due to compression of the cervical cord caused by osteophytes, hypertrophied ligamentum flavum, cervical subluxations, and herniated discs often superimposed upon congenital canal stenosis. Spondylosis can cause repetitive cord trauma from routine movements, or ischemic injury from venous stasis and arterial compromise. Degeneration of the posterior and lateral columns leads to the sensory changes and upper motor neuron findings typical upon presentation, which can become permanent over time.

Treatment Options

- Nonoperative
  - NSAIDs, lifestyle modification to reduce high-risk activities, or rigid cervical bracing may all help reduce further spinal cord compression, particularly in poor surgical candidates.
  - 50% of those treated conservatively will continue to demonstrate disease progression.

- Surgical
  - Anterior cervical discectomy or corpectomy: useful for predominantly anterior compression of three or fewer levels
  - Laminectomy: with or without lateral mass fusion. Useful for posterior compression, greater than three level involvement, severe OPLL, and when anterior approach will not provide >12 mm AP canal diameter. Even with preservation of facet joints, laminectomy without lateral mass fusion risks osteophyte progression and progressive kyphotic deformity.
  - Laminoplasty: includes "French door" (midline enlargement) or "open door" (unilateral) techniques. Does not address neck pain.

Surgical Technique
Posterior Approaches

Neurophysiologic monitoring is performed at baseline and an arterial line for a goal mean arterial pressure >90 mmHg is placed before prone positioning. Moderate neck flexion aids in opening overlapping posterior lamina.

A midline incision is performed with exposure to the spinous processes. Intraoperative imaging is used to confirm levels. The lamina and lateral masses of desired levels are exposed (extent of lateral dissection is dependent on need for fusion); the entire lateral mass is exposed if instrumentation is to be placed.

The laminectomy is performed by burring troughs along the lateral borders of the lamina, followed by removal of the interspinous ligaments and precise lifting of the lamina/ligamentum flavum in an en bloc fashion.

Careful perusal of the foramina can be performed with a Woodson to ensure adequate nerve root decompression. A Kerrison rongeur or drill can be used to open any persistently stenotic neuroforamina.

Once fully decompressed, hemostasis is obtained and a multilayered wound closure performed (Figure 50-2).

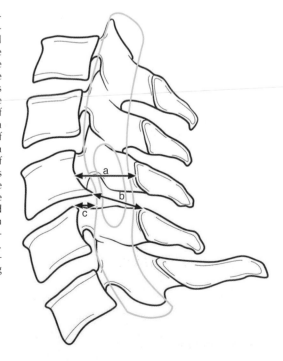

FIGURE 50-2   Illustration depicting the radiographic criteria used in the assessment of cervical stenosis and myelopathy. **(A)** The midsagittal diameter of the spinal canal is measured as the distance from the middle of the dorsal surface of the vertebral body to the nearest point on the spinolaminar line. Patients in whom the osseous canal measures 13 mm are considered to be developmentally stenotic. **(B)** A distance of <12 mm from the posteroinferior corner of a vertebral body to the anterosuperior edge of the lamina of the immediately caudal vertebra with the neck in extension is suggestive of dynamic stenosis. **(C)** Olisthesis of >3.5 mm is a measure of excessive translation between the vertebral bodies. The signal changes within the substance of the spinal cord, noted on T1- and T2-weighted magnetic resonance imaging in some patients, are represented diagrammatically. *(Reprinted with permission from Rao RD, Gourab K, David KS. Operative treatment of cervical spondylotic myelopathy. J Bone Joint Surg Am. 2006;88:1619-1640.)*

Complication Avoidance and Management

- C5 palsies are common due to its short neck and sensitivity to traction injuries; special care should be taken when drilling or retracting at this level.
- Care should be taken when elevating the lamina at both the rostral and caudal ends simultaneously to minimize levering either end into the cord as the other end is raised.
- Poor wound healing from increased tension after laminoplasty can be reduced by selective debulking of prominent spinous processes.
- Hyperlordosis can cause posterior migration of the cervical cord in posterior decompressions, leading to neurologic decline.

KEY PAPERS

Bohlman HH, Emery SE. The pathophysiology of cervical spondylosis and myelopathy. *Spine*. 1988;13(7): 843-846.

Cusick JF. Pathophysiology and treatment of cervical spondylotic myelopathy. *Clin Neurosurg*. 1991;37: 661-681.

Matz PG, Anderson PA, Holly LT, et al. The natural history of cervical spondylotic myelopathy. *J Neurosurg Spine*. 2009;11(2):104-111.

Mitsunaga LK, Klineberg EO, Gupta MC. Laminoplasty techniques for the treatment of multilevel cervical stenosis. *Adv Orthop*. 2012;2012:307916.

Sweet WH, Schmidek HH. *Operative Neurosurgical Techniques; Indications, Methods, and Results*. New York: Grune & Stratton; 1982.

Case 51

Cauda Equina Syndrome

Gurpreet S. Gandhoke, MD ● Adam S. Kanter, MD

Presentation

A 30-year-old male presents 1 day after lifting a heavy box at home that led to excruciating left leg pain, foot drop, perineal tingling, and an inability to void for the past 12 hours. Positive exam findings include weak left knee extension 3/5, left ankle dorsiflexion 2/5, left plantar flexion 4-/5, and left EHL 1/5. He has sensory loss to pin prick in the perineal region, loss of ankle reflexes bilaterally, and a post void residual of 450 mL.

Differential Diagnosis

- Disc herniation/extrusion with cauda equina compression
- Pathological compression fracture
- Spinal stenosis
- Diskitis-osteomyelitis
- Epidural abscess
- Intradural tumor with acute intratumoral hemorrhage
- Epidural hematoma

Initial Imaging

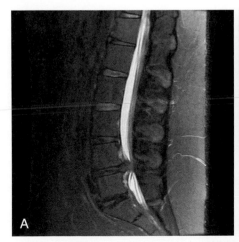 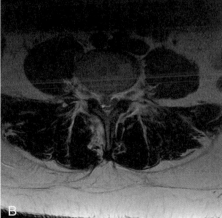

FIGURE 51-1

Imaging Description and Differential

- Sagittal and axial MR images demonstrate a broad-based L4-L5 disc bulge resulting in effacement of the spinal canal; the cauda equina is not visualized at the level of the compression.

Clinical Presentation of Cauda Equina Syndrome (CES)

- Two distinct clinical types of CES have been described: acute and insidious. Acute CES is characterized by the sudden onset of severe low back pain, sciatica, urinary retention, motor weakness of the lower extremities, and perineal anesthesia; typically the result of acute central disk herniation. Insidious CES is characterized by recurrent episodes of low back pain occurring over weeks to years, with the gradual onset of sciatica, sensorimotor loss, and bowel and bladder dysfunction; typically occurs in the setting of long-standing spinal stenosis.
- Genitourinary dysfunction is a hallmark element in CES. Early bladder dysfunction can be subtle and involve difficulty initiating the urinary stream, which may progress to urinary retention and eventually overflow incontinence.
- Dense sensory loss involving the perineum, buttocks, and posteromedial thighs with saddle anesthesia is a relatively late sign of CES and may indicate limited potential for recovery to normal bladder function.

Further Workup

The importance of a thorough clinical examination remains paramount to quickly detecting CES, as prolonged delay in diagnosis and treatment can lead to irreversible consequences.

- CES patients typically have preserved sensation to pressure and light touch, so if discrimination is not made between pinprick and light touch sensation, then the diagnosis can be missed. Sensation to pinprick in the perianal region (S2-S4 dermatomes), perineum, and posterior thigh must be assessed.
- Decreased rectal tone is often an early finding in patients with CES. A rectal examination must be performed on all patients with potential CES to assess the tone and voluntary contracture of the external anal sphincter.
- Both the anal wink test and bulbocavernosus reflex must be evaluated.
- Measurement of postvoid residual volume provides an accurate assessment of urinary retention.
- X-rays, including flexion/extension views, should be quickly obtained to rule out instability for pre-op planning. If instability is present, fusion must be considered.
- CBC/chem 7/coags/T&S performed pre-op; urgent surgery warranted.

Pathophysiology

- The lack of the epi- and perineurium in the nerve roots of the cauda equina (compared with the peripheral nerves) leaves these nerve roots particularly susceptible to mechanical compression.
- Ischemic injury from severe compression to an already hypovascular region heightens the predisposition of the cauda equina to compression.
- Mechanical compression further impairs nutrition of the neural tissue by reducing both blood flow and diffusion from the surrounding CSF.
- The compression of the cauda equina may be compared to a compartment syndrome wherein intraneural edema, caused by the compression, induces a cycle of reducing perfusion to the nerve, which in return begets further edema.

Treatment Options

CES is a surgical emergency and warrants early decompression of the nerve roots to prevent progression of neurological deficits and to maximize potential for recovery. Traditional practice involves surgical decompression preferably within 24 hours. A meta-analysis found a statistically significant improvement in neurologic outcome if patients were operated within 48 hours of the onset of symptoms.

Intraoperative imaging is performed to confirm the surgical level by placing a radiopaque instrument on the spinous processes at the level of interest.

Subperiosteal muscle dissection is performed to the spinolaminar line with lateral dissection proceeding to the medial edge of the facet complex.

A wide laminectomy is performed with high-speed drill, followed by careful removal of the underlying ligament; often tented dorsally due to ventral mass compression. Once the dorsal decompression is complete, the thecal sac is gently reflected medially to perform a discectomy, if ventral compression secondary to disc herniation is the etiologic source.

If hypertrophied facets or lateral ligaments significantly contribute to canal narrowing, partial facetectomies may be required. In most cases a 50% facetectomy on one side, or 25% facetectomy bilaterally, can be accomplished without need for stabilization or fusion.

Complication and Avoidance Management

TABLE 51-1

COMPLICATION AND AVOIDANCE MANAGEMENT

Complication	Avoidance and Management
Persistent bowel and bladder dysfunction	Early intervention with decompression of the cauda equina increases the chance of regaining bladder control (<48 hours).
Recurrence/persistence of symptoms	Inadequate removal of bony, nuclear, and ligamentous compressive elements may allow persistent symptomatology. It is imperative to ensure complete neural decompression, particularly if ventral disc herniation is the culprit.
CSF leak	The severity of the compression of the dural sac with tenting of the dura above and below the level of the compression predisposes to a durotomy. When such occurs, it is crucial to locate the dural injury and close the defect in a water-tight fashion. This can be performed with Nurolon suture, and when necessary a muscle graft and dural sealant. In the case of a ventral defect, or if the defect cannot be closed primarily, a thorough layered musculofascial closure is paramount in preventing external leakage. In such instances, a lumbar drain may be placed to shunt CSF at the level of the back for 4–5 days.

KEY PAPERS

Ahn UM, Ahn NU, Buchowski JM, et al. Cauda equina syndrome secondary to lumbar disc herniation: a meta-analysis of surgical outcomes. *Spine.* 2000;25(12):1515-1522.

Parke WW, Gammell K, Rothman RH. Arterial vascularization of the cauda equina. *J Bone Joint Surg Am.* 1981;63(1):53-62.

Case 52

Foot Drop and Far Lateral Disc Herniation

Christian B. Ricks, MD ● Adam S. Kanter, MD

Presentation

A 55-year-old male presents with progressive left lower extremity radicular pain that began acutely, 1 month prior, after lifting a heavy briefcase. Antiinflammatories were initially successful for pain diminution, but over the past week the pain has become refractory and he is now having difficulty clearing the ground with his left foot. He has scrapes on his knees consistent with recent falls.

Exam reveals an overweight male in obvious discomfort; left lateral bending exacerbates his symptoms, he has a positive left straight leg raise at 10 degrees, 4-/5 left dorsiflexion, 3/5 left EHL, and diminished sensorium along left L5 dermatome.

Differential Diagnosis

- Degenerative
  - Left L4-L5 posterocentral disc herniation
  - Left L5-S1 far lateral disc herniation
  - Lateral recess stenosis
  - Spondylolisthesis
- Neoplastic
  - Schwannoma or neurofibroma involving the left L5 nerve root
  - Retroperitoneal tumor
- Infectious
  - Epidural or psoas abscess
- Other
  - Diabetic neuropathy

Initial Imaging

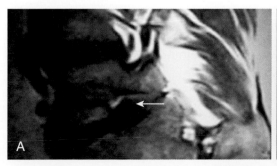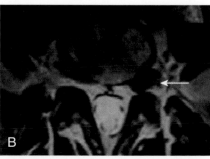

FIGURE 52-1

Imaging Description and Differential

T2-weighted sagittal and axial MR images demonstrate a left-sided disc bulge at the L5-S1 level compressing the exiting L5 nerve root.

Further Workup

- Laboratory
  - Preoperative labs including INR, PTT, type, and screen
  - Preoperative EKG and CXR
- Imaging
  - Plain film dynamic radiographs (flexion and extension) to rule out instability at the L5-S1 level and to delineate bony anatomy for surgical planning
- Further testing
  - EMG may be beneficial to evaluate other causes of radiculopathy if imaging is inconclusive.

Pathophysiology

Intervertebral discs that undergo degenerative changes when combined with increased mechanical stress can overwhelm the posterolateral annulus where the supportive PLL is absent. In most cases this causes paramedian breaches, but foraminal or extraforaminal herniations do occur in 7%–12% of cases. The exiting nerve root is compressed, causing radicular pain, weakness, and/or sensory changes. Pain may be exacerbated by direct compression on the dorsal root ganglion, which may also impede full or timely recovery. The most common level is L4-L5 (60%), followed by L3-L4 (24%), L2-L3 (8%), L5-S1 (7%), and L1-L2 (1%). Whereas a straight leg test is only positive in a minority of patients, most will have reproducible pain with lateral bending toward the pathology.

Treatment Options

- Nonoperative
  - Activity modification to limit strenuous movements, physical therapy, analgesics, and spinal manipulation
  - A period of conservative treatment is indicated except with progressive neurological deficit, profound weakness, or severe refractory pain.
- Percutaneous
  - Epidural injections are generally minimally effective for long term radicular symptom relief, but transforaminal injections may provide transient relief and help confirm diagnosis.
  - Chemonucleolysis-chymopapain injected intradiscally is less effective than discectomy for pain control, and most patients eventually undergo surgery.
  - Intradiscal spinal procedures including nucleoplasty, laser disc decompression, intradiscal endothermal therapy, and percutaneous endoscopic lumbar discectomy rely on removal of material from the center of the disc to reduce the herniated portion. May be useful for contained herniation with intact anulus fibrosus, but not recommended in the presence of neurological deficits.
- Surgical
  - Midline hemilaminectomy – removal of ipsilateral medial facet with foraminotomy allows for disc and bone decompression to address concomitant stenosis or spondyloarthrosis; can lead to instability, necessitating fusion
  - Posterolateral approach – paramedian incision preserves facet, but does not enable medial access; lumbo-sacral herniations require drilling of the sacral ala for access to extra-foraminal herniations.
  - Extreme lateral transpsoas approach – minimally invasive lateral corridor enables removal of laterally extruded fragments, but may require significant nerve root retraction for more posterior access and can only be performed at L4-L5 and above.

- Transpars approach – superior laminotomy for lateral pars resection; preserves facet complex, but aggressive drilling may lead to instability
- Lumbar fusion – PLIF, TLIF, and ALIF are generally reserved for cases of spinal deformity, instability, or chronic axial pain in addition to radicular symptoms.

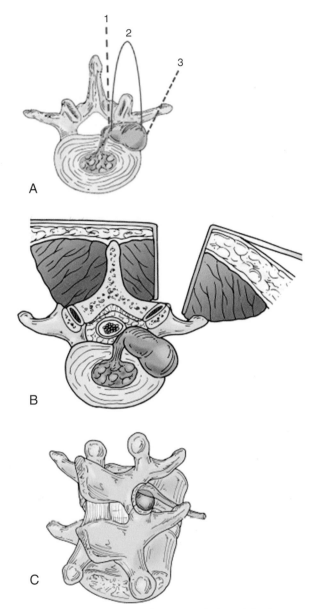

FIGURE 52-2   Trajectories achieved by a variety of exposures for lateral disc herniation. **(A)** *1*, midline; *2*, interlaminar and extralaminar approach; *3*, paramedian muscle splitting. **(B)** Paramedian muscle splitting approach achieves an optimal angle of exposure to discs situated beyond the pedicle. **(C)** For most approaches to a lateral disc hernia, a modest lateral facetectomy is performed, thus providing direct access to the hernia. *(Reprinted with permission from Benzel EC, Francis TB.* Spine Surgery: Techniques, Complication Avoidance, and Management. *3rd ed. Elsevier; 2012.)*

Surgical Technique
Posterolateral Approach

- A 3 cm vertical incision is made approximately 4 cm lateral to midline on the symptomatic side.

- Longitudinal fascia opening is performed, followed by blunt separation of the multifidus and longissimus muscles, to identify the superior and inferior transverse processes.
- A probe is inserted for radiographic level localization, followed by retraction and utilization of the operating microscope.
- The intertransversarius ligament is divided to reveal the nerve root and disc, and the radicular artery and vein.
- The herniated disc material is removed; the lateral facet can be resected if further medial exposure is necessitated.
- If herniation is at L5-S1, a portion of the sacral ala must be drilled to enable safe access to the disc space.

Complication Avoidance and Management

- Total medial facetectomy can precipitate instability, and should be avoided if possible.
- The DRG is sensitive to manipulation and thermal injury from electrocautery. Bipolar should be used over monopolar when working in proximity to the nerve root.
- The disc herniation may translocate the nerve by axillary impingement, so careful blunt dissection should be performed during anatomic identification.
- EMG stimulation may be utilized to assist with nerve localization.

KEY PAPERS

Abdullah AF, Wolber PG, Warfield JR, et al. Surgical management of extreme lateral lumbar disc herniations: review of 138 cases. *Neurosurgery.* 1988;22(4):648-653.

Epstein NE. Evaluation of varied surgical approaches used in the management of 170 far-lateral lumbar disc herniations: indications and results. *J Neurosurg.* 1995;83(4):648-656.

Madhok R, Kanter AS. Extreme-lateral, minimally invasive, transpsoas approach for the treatment of far-lateral lumbar disc herniation. *J Neurosurg Spine.* 2010;12(4):347-350.

Marquardt G, Bruder M, Theuss S, et al. Ultra-long-term outcome of surgically treated far-lateral, extraforaminal lumbar disc herniations: a single-center series. *Eur Spine J.* 2012;21(4):660-665.

Pirris SM, Dhall S, Mummaneni PV, et al. Minimally invasive approach to extraforaminal disc herniations at the lumbosacral junction using an operating microscope: case series and review of the literature. *Neurosurg Focus.* 2008;25(2):E10.

Case 53

Thoracic Disc Herniation

Zachary J. Tempel, MD ● Adam S. Kanter, MD

Presentation

A 59-year-old female with a history of subarachnoid hemorrhage, s/p MCA aneurysm clipping 30 years prior, presents with 3 months of severe mid-low back pain radiating under the left chest wall below the ribs. She reports tingling in her left leg and progressive unsteadiness while ambulating; her left leg feels as though it "gives out" on her. She denies bowel/bladder incontinence. Her symptoms remain refractory to antiinflammatory medications and chiropractic therapy. Exam reveals normal strength throughout, but vague sensory changes to pinprick on the left flank. She has 3+ reflexes in bilateral lower extremities, a positive left Babinski, clonus, and Hoffmann's negative.

Differential Diagnosis

- Degenerative
  - Thoracic disc herniation (TDH)
  - Compression/burst fracture
  - Spondylotic myelopathy
- Neoplastic
  - Metastasis
  - Extradural tumor (aneurysmal bone cyst or plasmacytoma)
  - Intradural-extramedullary tumor (meningioma or neurofibroma)
  - Intramedullary tumor (ependymoma or astrocytoma)
- Vascular
  - AVM
- Infectious (DM, IV drug use, or immunodeficiency)
  - Discitis +/− osteomyelitis
  - Epidural abscess
- Other
  - Multiple sclerosis
  - Transverse myelitis

Initial Imaging

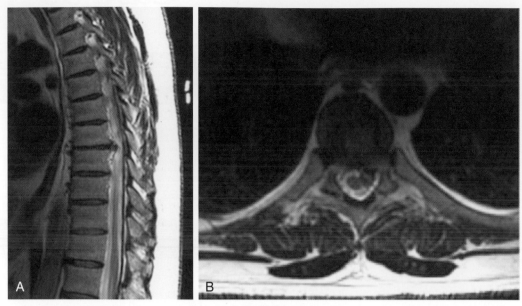

FIGURE 53-1

Imaging Description

Sagittal and axial CT myelogram of the thoracolumbar spine demonstrates a focal disc herniation at T10-T11, eccentric to the left, with loss of CSF signal anterolaterally.

Further Workup

- Laboratory
  - CBC, BMP, and PT/INR/PTT
- Imaging
  - CT reveals calcifications/osteophytes (MRI cannot be performed due to unknown material of aneurysm clip).
- Other tests
  - EMG/NCS (exclude other diagnoses if vague/equivocal signs/symptoms)
- Consultants
  - Internal medicine: preoperative evaluation, particularly pulmonary status (transthoracic approach consideration)

Pathophysiology

The vast majority of TDHs result from degenerative processes. Articulation of the ribs with the sternum anteriorly, and vertebral bodies and transverse processes posteriorly, stabilize the upper thoracic spine. Most herniations occur below T7, the last level of individually fused ribs. The prevalence of asymptomatic TDH ranges from 10% to 37%. Symptomatic TDH is rare and accounts for approximately 0.5% of all symptomatic disc herniations. The ratio of canal-to-cord diameter is lowest in the thoracic spine, increasing the potential for mass lesions to become symptomatic. The dentate ligaments and natural kyphosis tether the spinal cord anteriorly, rendering it more susceptible to compression from disc herniation.

Each rib articulates with the superior posterior part of the same level vertebra, and with the inferior part of the above vertebra, except at T1, T11, and T12 where it meets only

VERTEBRAL LIGAMENTS
THORACIC

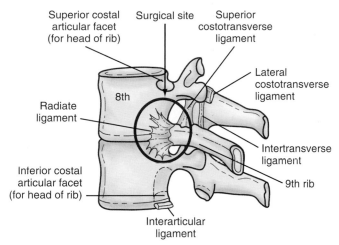

FIGURE 53-2   Diagram illustrating the surgical site and its relationship to the surrounding ligaments from an anterior approach. *(Reprinted with permission from Winn HR.* Youmans Neurological Surgery. *6th ed. Elsevier; 2011.)*

the same level vertebra. Accordingly, access to disc space often requires resection of a rib head (Figure 53-2).

Treatment Options

- Medical
  - Back pain: NSAIDs, oral corticosteroids, muscle relaxants
  - Radicular or neuropathic pain: gabapentin, pregabalin, antidepressants
- Mechanical
  - Physical therapy: activity modification, muscle strengthening, optimizing posture and mechanics to limit axial loading on the disc space
  - Electrical stimulation (TENS) unit
  - Chiropractic manipulation is contraindicated
- Interventional
  - Thoracic epidural steroid injections: may be useful in a subset of neurologically normal patients with radicular pain refractory to medications
- Surgical
  - Transpedicular approach +/− laminectomy: less extensive posterior approach allows access to lateral canal and disc space; limited access medially. Unilateral approaches typically do not require instrumentation. Optimal for soft, paracentral TDH. It is not advisable to remove most TDHs via a laminectomy alone.
  - Costotransversectomy: posterolateral approach involving more extensive soft tissue dissection and resection of the proximal rib for better visualization and medial access. Increased postoperative pain and risk of pneumothorax. Used for central/paracentral soft and calcified TDH.
  - Lateral extracavitary: most aggressive posterolateral approach, simultaneously allows ventral access to the anterior and posterior columns. Technically difficult operation with higher morbidity. Used for large central disc/osteophyte complexes or multilevel TDH with osteophytic disease.
  - Transthoracic: anterior approach, direct access to the ventral spine, and requires single-lung ventilation. Highest morbidity, especially in smokers and the elderly; contraindicated in patients with severe respiratory disease. Three distinct approaches: standard thoracotomy, endoscopic thoracoscopy, and MIS direct lateral. Used for intradural herniations and large central disc/osteophyte complexes (Figure 53-3).

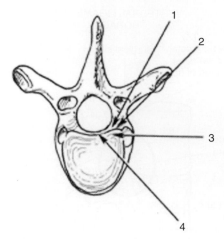

FIGURE 53-3   Schematic demonstrating the trajectory and access of the transpedicular (1), costotransver-sectomy (2), lateral extracavitary (3), and transthoracic (4) approaches. *(Reprinted with permission from Stillerman CB, et al. The transfacet pedicle-sparing approach for thoracic disc removal: cadaveric morphometric analysis and preliminary clinical experience. J Neurosurg. 1995;83[6].)*

Surgical Technique

Transpedicular Approach

Prone positioning is used with neuromonitoring and fluoroscopy for localization. Locate the lumbosacral junction and count rostrally, utilize live fluoroscopy and ensure that images correlate with preoperative films. Ribs may be used as an adjunct marker. Subperiosteal dissection is performed unilaterally to expose the superior and inferior facets of the index level. (The exposure is performed bilaterally if performing a complete laminectomy or bilateral transpedicular approach.)

The inferior articular process and the inferior lamina of the rostral vertebra are removed with a high-speed drill for pedicle-to-pedicle exposure. The superior half of the inferior pedicle is drilled approximately 1 cm beyond the PLL into the dorsal aspect of the caudal vertebra, then medially, ventral to the dura, then rostral, through the disc space and into the upper vertebral end plate, creating a void ventral to the disc pathology (Figures 53-4 and 53-5).

A low-profile instrument (blunt nerve probe) is used to carefully dissect the dura from the underlying PLL/osteophyte/TDH. A down-biting curette is carefully inserted into this plane atop the pathology and directed ventrally and laterally to persuade the disc material into the cavity, away from the cord. The disc material is removed with an angled rongeur forceps (Figure 53-6).

If ligamentous hypertrophy or osteophytes are contributory factors, posterior decompression can be performed after addressing the ventral pathology to avoid dorsal herniation and kinking of the cord ventrally. Neurophysiologic monitoring remains essential throughout the procedure.

If the index level is at the thoracolumbar junction, or multiple sequential levels are involved, or bilateral pediculectomy is required, internal fixation may be necessary.

Complication Avoidance and Management

- CT imaging is integral for preoperative planning. Failure to adequately assess the location and consistency of the TDH may lead to selection of an inappropriate surgical approach. Accurate localization prior to incision is crucial to verify the correct operative level in the thoracic spine and should be performed using the same method as was performed pre-operatively. After initial dissection, the level should again be verified prior to any bony removal.

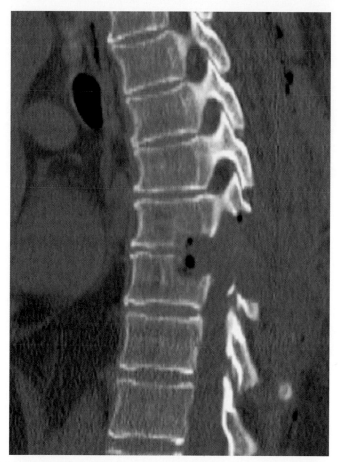

FIGURE 53-4   Sagittal CT scan demonstrating the cavity created ventral to the disc pathology.

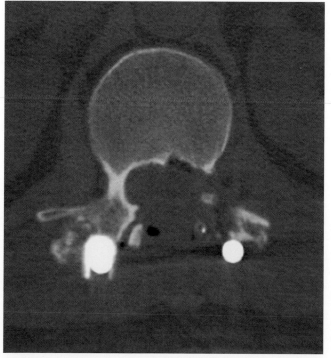

FIGURE 53-5   Axial CT scan demonstrating removal of the left pedicle.

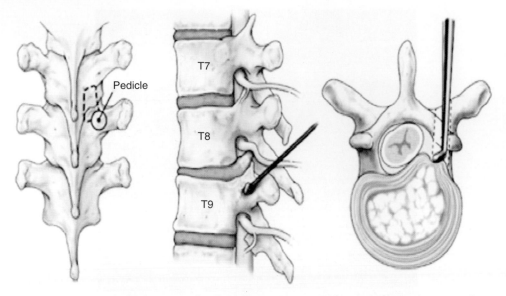

FIGURE 53-6 Transpedicular approach, a back-down curette is used to persuade the disc material ventrally. *(Reprinted with permission from Bilsky MH. Transpedicular approach for thoracic disc herniations. Neurosurg Focus. 2000;9.)*

- While drilling the pedicle, care should be taken to identify its medial edge to avoid incidental breach and durotomy. Prior to manipulating the TDH, it is critical to create a large enough ventral cavity to accept the disc material. Extreme caution must be used when persuading the disc material into the cavity to avoid rocking the curette into the cord. Early removal of the lamina may lead to posterior stretching and translation of the cord, manifesting as neurophysiologic signal loss and injury. It is therefore recommended that ventral decompression be performed prior to posterior decompression when feasible.
- Perfusion of the thoracic spine is tenuous. Anesthetic vigilance is required to maintain elevated MAPs and maximize volume status. Appropriate selection of anesthetic agents is important (e.g., propofol compromises blood flow to the cord and ketamine is often utilized to optimize perfusion).

KEY PAPERS

Arts MP, Bartel RH. Anterior or posterior approach of thoracic disc herniation? A comparative cohort of mini-transthoracic versus transpedicular discectomies. *Spine J.* 2014;14(8):1654-1662.

Bilskey MH. Transpedicular approach for thoracic disc herniations. *Neurosurg Focus.* 2000;9(4):E3.

Oppenlander ME, Clark JC, Kalyvas J, et al. Surgical management and clinical outcomes of multiple-level symptomatic herniated thoracic discs. *J Neurosurg Spine.* 2013;19(6):774-783.

Case 54

Spinal Epidural Abscess

Christian B. Ricks, MD ● Adam S. Kanter, MD

Presentation

A 77-year-old male presents with left lower extremity cellulitis and edema. Blood cultures reveal streptococcus bacteremia, and antibiotics are administered per culture sensitivities. Two weeks later, the patient again has complaints of progressive back pain and right lower extremity weakness. Past medical history further includes diabetes mellitus and congestive heart failure. Examination reveals a confused elder with nonspecific low back pain. Other positive findings include 2/5 RLE weakness, 4+/5 LLE weakness, diminished LE sensorium, reflexes, and rectal tone. Gait cannot be assessed.

Differential Diagnosis

- Degenerative
  - Herniated lumbar disc
  - Severe stenosis (CES)
  - Vertebral body fracture
- Neoplastic
  - Spinal cord tumor/metastasis
  - Pathologic fracture
- Infectious
  - Epidural abscess
- Other
  - Epidural hematoma
  - Transverse myelitis

Initial Imaging

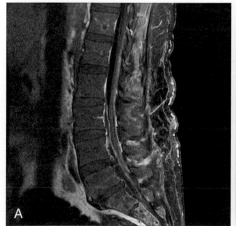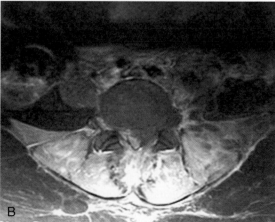

FIGURE 54-1

Imaging Description and Differential

- Mid-sagittal and axial lumbar T1-weighted MRI with gad contrast reveals enhancing epidural collection from L3-S1 with mass effect on the thecal sac and exiting nerve roots.

Further Workup

- Laboratory
  - CBC, BMP, ESR, CRP, repeat blood cultures, UA and culture, type and screen, and PT/INR/PTT
- Imaging
  - MRI of the entire spinal axis, with and without contrast
  - CT abdomen and pelvis with contrast if concern for psoas, paraspinal, or abdominal involvement
  - CT spine if concern for vertebral osteomyelitis
- Consultants
  - Infectious disease

Pathophysiology

Epidural abscesses can occur in the lumbar (48%), thoracic (31%), and cervical (24%) spine. Coexisting chronic disease is common, and risk factors include: diabetes mellitus, IV drug use, renal failure, alcoholism, prior spinal procedures, and trauma. Symptoms typically present with pain followed by weakness; weakness can progress to paraplegia in hours. Symptoms are generally attributed to compression and thrombophlebitis of epidural veins, causing infarction and edema of the spinal cord, although arterial compromise and mechanical compression are also contributing factors. *Staphylococcus aureus* is the most common organism; however, approximately 50% of abscesses go without species identification. Inoculation is typically through hematogenous spread to the vertebra or epidural space, direct extension from adjacent infection, or following spinal procedures.

Treatment Options

- Medical
  - Antibiotics – while some patients may recover with appropriate antibiotic therapy, others may progress to irreversible neurologic injury despite appropriately directed antibiotics.
  - Medical management alone for patients without motor deficits remains controversial.
  - Conservative management can be reserved for those with prohibitive operative risk factors, or complete paralysis for longer than 72 hours, although symptoms present for longer than 36 hours often remain permanent.
- Interventional
  - CT-guided biopsy of epidural collection, psoas abscess, or involved disc
- Surgical
  - Goals are decompression of the neural elements, followed by drainage and debridement of infection, cultures for pathogen identification, and stabilization (if needed) with minimal instrumentation.
  - <u>Laminectomy</u>: for focal compression or multilevel laminotomies with catheter irrigation; works well for dorsal pathology when abscess is liquid purulence
  - <u>Transpedicular, costotransversectomy, or lateral extracavitary</u>: for extensive ventral pathology or compressive phlegmon below the cervical spine
  - <u>Thoracotomy</u> or <u>cervical corpectomy</u>: anterior approaches for ventral compressive nonliquid collections infrequently required

Surgical Technique

The patient is placed prone. A midline incision is performed followed by dissection to the spinous processes. The correct level is confirmed with intraoperative imaging after which the paraspinal musculature is taken down in a subperiosteal fashion to expose the desired lamina.

Midline strip laminectomies of L4 and L5 are performed. The underlying ligament is gently parted to expose any purulent drainage and cultures are taken. The ligament is removed and gentle retraction of the thecal sac is performed to expose the ventral epidural space, which is copiously irrigated.

Rubber catheters are passed both rostral and caudal and ventral and dorsal to the thecal sac. Copious irrigation is flooded throughout the epidural space until the fluid returns clear. Discectomy should be done in the setting of discitis.

Epidural drains are placed and the wound is closed in a layered fashion.

Complication Avoidance and Management

- Antibiotics should be held until cultures are obtained to maximize identification of causative organism.
- Laminectomy without instrumentation is well tolerated; however, removal of junctional bone and its tension band may result in destabilization that necessitates internal fixation. It is reasonable to acutely clear the infection and treat the stability issue at a later date. In instances where a single operation is preferred, titanium hardware can be placed at the index surgery and the infection can still be successfully cleared with long-term antibiotics.
- Extreme care must be taken when removing the lamina and ligament to minimize chance of durotomy, as bacterial meningitis can occur with subarachnoid contamination
- When liquid purulence is found, strip laminectomies can be performed, sparing the facets and minimizing destabilization. When protracted treatment, or a failed attempt with antibiotic therapy occurs, granular fibrosis may result, necessitating a more aggressive laminectomy and neural manipulation to clear the epidural space of debris; extreme care must to taken with blunt instruments to prevent dural tear.

KEY PAPERS

Arko LT, Quach E, Nguyen V, et al. Medical and surgical management of spinal epidural abscess: a systematic review. *Neurosurg Focus.* 2014;37(2):E4.

Curry WT Jr, Hoh BL, Amin-Hanjani S, et al. Spinal epidural abscess: clinical presentation, management, and outcome. *Surg Neurol.* 2005;63(4):364-371, discussion 371.

Hlavin ML, Kaminski HJ, Ross JS, et al. Spinal epidural abscess: a ten-year perspective. *Neurosurgery.* 1990;27(2):177-184.

Kaufman DM, Kaplan JG, Litman N. Infectious agents in spinal epidural abscesses. *Neurology.* 1980;30(8):844-850.

Russell NA, Vaughan R, Morley TP. Spinal epidural infection. *Can J Neurol Sci.* 1979;6(3):325-328.

Case 55

Spinal Metastases

Todd Harshbarger, MD ● Mike Y. Chen, MD, PhD

Presentation

A thin 66-year-old female with a history of chronic lumbar spondylosis and no significant trauma presents with mid thoracic back pain for 10 weeks refractory to conservative measures and progressive difficulty with ambulation.
- PMH: otherwise unremarkable
- Exam: tender to palpation at mid thoracic midline spine
  - Normal UE examination
  - Right LE 4/5 weakness at iliopsoas and quadriceps
  - Sensory level at T7 with decreased pinprick
  - Normal rectal tone

Differential Diagnosis

- Degenerative
  - Thoracic disc herniation
  - Osteoporotic compression fracture
- Neoplastic
  - Metastasis (h/o cancer)
  - Spinal cord tumor
- Vascular
  - AVM (more chronic course often with stepwise progression)
- Infectious
  - Spinal abscess (h/o IVDA and manifestations of infection)
- Other
  - MS
  - Transverse myelopathy (acute onset)
  - Vitamin B_{12} deficiency (h/o alcoholism)
  - Radiation myelopathy

Initial Imaging

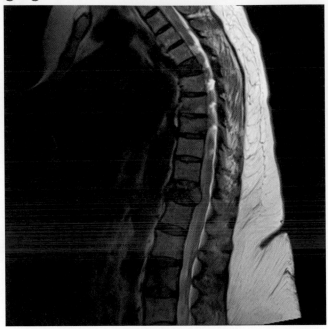

FIGURE 55-1

Imaging Description and Differential

- Thoracic spine MRI shows sagittal and axial images of a T7 enhancing lesion with dural extension. Involvement of the pedicle and posterior elements is suggestive of the metastatic process. No serpiginous vessels suggestive of AVM are seen. No other segments of the spine are involved.
- Differential: spinal metastasis with anterior cord compression; less likely, spinal epidural abscess

Further Workup

- Laboratory
  - Routine labs
  - ESR, CRP
- Imaging
  - CT chest/abdomen/pelvis, mammogram (evaluation of systemic burden)
  - CT for evaluation of bone quality and precise localization
- Consultants
  - Medical oncology

Pathophysiology

Ninety percent of spinal tumors are metastatic in origin. This patient has metastatic involvement of the mid thoracic spine. In the setting of malignancy, circulating tumor cells can lead to colonization of different organs. The bone marrow of the mid thoracic spine receives abundant blood flow and provides a nutrient-rich microenvironment for metastatic cells. With time, the macrometastases lead to erosion of the bone and pathological fracture with potential of epidural extension. With recent improvement in molecular therapies, the prognosis for patients is heterogeneous, with some surviving multiple years in the setting of stage IV cancer.

Treatment Options

- Medical
  - Corticosteroids are indicated for cord compression.
- Biopsy
  - Very rarely performed in the setting of active cancer.
- Radiation
  - Radiation can provide pain palliation and at times reduce the epidural component. However, these benefits require time and do not address pathological fractures that are often present. Renal cancer, melanoma, triple negative breast cancer and NSCLC are relatively radioresistant. Prospective randomized trials indicate that circumferential decompression for cord compression is superior to radiation alone. Thus, in the setting of symptomatic cord compression, radiation by itself is typically reserved for poor surgical candidates or extremely radiosensitive lesions.
- Interventional
  - Vertebroplasty with posterior vertebral wall disruption is contraindicated, as is balloon expansion with kyphoplasty. These modalities can be effective with metastases that result in compression fractures. Vertebroplasty can also be augmented with ablation.
  - Preoperative embolization of hypervascular tumors can dramatically reduce blood loss.
- Surgical
  - <u>Laminectomy</u>: thoracic laminectomy may provide some benefit by removing the posterior elements, but prospective studies have shown poor outcomes in the setting of anterior cord compression. Separation surgery – wide laminectomies +/–instrumentation with removal of tumor immediately adjacent to the cord – followed by XRT (often SRS) is appealing when the vertebral body is mostly intact.
  - <u>Transthoracic corpectomy</u>: anterior corpectomy with mini thoracotomy usually supplemented with posterior decompression and instrumentation. This is the standard approach.
  - <u>Posterior corpectomy and fusion</u>: circumferential decompression and reconstruction via a lateral extracavitary approach has become less challenging due to advancements in instrumentation. In general, corpectomies provide significant benefits when there is a severe fracture or deformity.

Surgical Technique

Posterior modified lateral extracavitary approach: Prone positioning, neuromonitoring, and fluoroscopy for marking incision are performed. Bilateral transverse processes two levels above and below tumor segment are dissected. For costotransversectomy, the rib head at the tumor segment and the rib head one level below should be exposed on the right (Figure 55-2A).

Laminectomies are performed at the level of the vertebrectomy and at the level above. The superior and inferior facets of the vertebrectomy level are drilled away. The inferior facet of the level above and the superior facet of the level below are also removed without damaging the attached pedicles. By removing these structures, the relevant disc spaces, pedicles, and nerve roots are fully exposed. In the thoracic spine the nerve roots can be tied off (Figure 55-2B).

For the costotransversectomy, approximately 2 cm of the rib distal to the transverse processes of the level of the vertebrectomy and the rib at the level below are exposed. The transverse processes at those levels are then removed. At approximately 1.5 cm, distal to the lateral tip of the resected transverse processes, a plane is developed between the pleura and the rib. The proximal ribs could then be removed in a piecemeal fashion. Of note, a Cobb elevator is often useful to dissect the tissue away from the rib head and lateral vertebral body. The removal of the rib heads exposes the lateral aspect of the disc space above and below (Figure 55-2C).

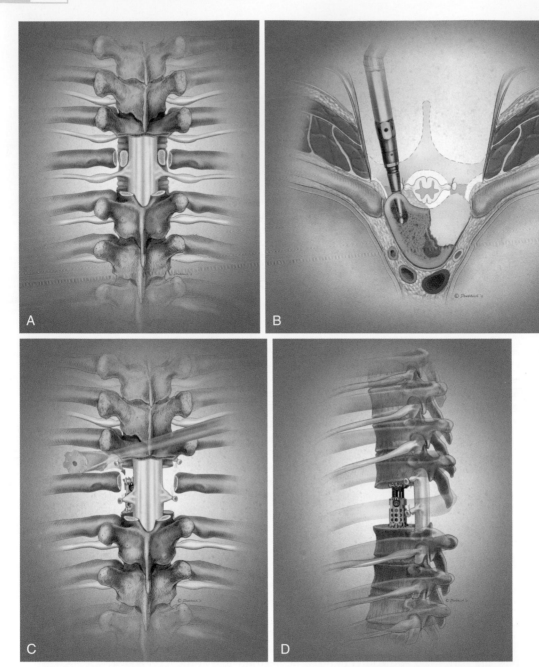

FIGURE 55-2 **(A)** Midline incision with laminectomy and facetectomy exposing the spinal cord from the pedicle above to the pedicle below of the affected level. **(B)** Removal of pedicle and use of transpedicular corridor to perform corpectomy and removal of discs above and below. **(C)** After tying of thoracic root, delivery of expandable cage. **(D)** Expansion of cage to span the inferior end plate of the vertebral segment above the superior end plate and vertebral segment below. *(Copyright Jim Dowdalls)*

The pedicles are then removed bilaterally and a vertebrectomy or corpectomy is performed using the extracavitary approach on the right. A transpedicular approach is employed on the contralateral side, which allows complete vertebral segment removal (Figure 55-2D).

The placement of the expandable cage should then be straightforward; an angled holder for the cage is extremely helpful to place the cage in the midline. Posterior fixation 2-3 levels above and below is then employed.

Complication Avoidance and Management

- Transthoracic corpectomy
  - During this approach it is key to position the patient in true lateral with fluoroscopy at the beginning of the case. During the resection of the vertebral segment, care should be taken to identify the pedicle and foramen to avoid incidental durotomy. Preoperative embolization, when available, can help reduce blood loss, particularly in the case of renal cell cancer.
- Posterior corpectomy and fusion
  - During this approach it is preferable to perform costotransversectomy or transpedicular decompression on the right to avoid inadvertent aortic injury. Prior to resection of vertebral body, vertical control and alignment should be maintained with temporary rod fixation. If insertion of titanium cage is difficult, polymethylmethacrylate (PMMA) with pins can be used. Polyetheretherketone (PEEK) cages allow for better visualization of neural elements on follow-up MRI. Meticulous multi-layer closure is required as there is a high incidence of wound healing complications.

KEY PAPERS

Patchell RA, Tibbs PA, Regine WF, et al. Direct decompressive surgical resection in the treatment of spinal cord compression caused by metastatic cancer: a randomized trial. *Lancet.* 2005;366:643-648.

Complication Avoidance and Management

Case 56

Spinal Intradural Extramedullary Mass

Hazem Mashaly, MD ● Zachary J. Tempel, MD ●
Adam S. Kanter, MD

Presentation

A 55-year-old male presents with lower thoracic/upper lumbar back pain, with a sense of "heaviness and weakness" in his lower extremities, greater on the left than the right, without symptoms of bowel or bladder dysfunction.

- PMH: otherwise unremarkable
- Exam: no tenderness to palpation or muscle spasms of the thoraco-lumbar spine
  - UE examination: normal
  - LL examination: grade 4/5 weakness in the left leg; 5/5 on right.
  - Sensory: decreased pain and temperature sensation in left leg, diminished vibratory sense in right leg
  - 2+ reflexes, no clonus, and negative Hoffman's
  - Normal rectal tone
  - No obvious skin lesions or abnormal pigmentation

Differential Diagnosis

- Degenerative
  - Thoracic disc herniation
  - Thoracic spondylosis
- Neoplastic
  - Extradural spinal cord compression (e.g., primary bone tumor)
  - Intradural intramedullary spinal cord tumor (e.g., astrocytoma, ependymoma)
  - Intradural extramedullary spinal cord tumor (e.g., meningioma, schwannoma)
  - Metastatic spinal cord tumor
- Vascular
  - AVM (typically more indolent course; often with stepwise progression)
- Other
  - MS
  - Transverse myelopathy (acute onset)
  - Vitamin B_{12} deficiency (h/o alcoholism)
  - Syringomyelia

Initial Imaging

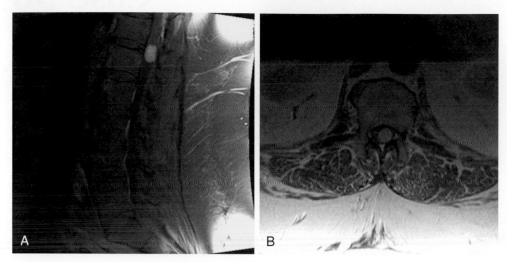

FIGURE 56-1

Imaging Description and Differential

- Thoracic spine MRI with contrast-enhanced sagittal and axial views reveals an intradural extramedullary lesion at T12-L1, compressing the cord from the left side. The mass reveals homogenous enhancement with no dural tail or extension through the intervertebral foramen.
- Differential
- Schwannoma, neurofibroma; less likely meningioma or intramedullary tumor

Further Workup

- Laboratory
  - CBC, PT/PTT/INR, LFT, KFT, electrolytes
  - ESR, CRP
- Imaging
  - CT thoraco-lumbar spine for bony anatomy detail and preoperative planning
  - X-ray thoraco-lumbar spine with dynamic flexion/extension views to evaluate preoperative stability of the thoracolumbar junction

Pathophysiology

Tumors of the spine are anatomically classified by their relationship to the dura mater and spinal cord parenchyma. Intradural tumors can be intramedullary or extramedullary, the latter accounting for approximately 75% of all intradural spinal tumors. Nerve sheath tumors account for nearly 25% of intradural spinal tumors in adults and are typically categorized as schwannomas or neurofibromas. Most are solitary schwannomas, and can occur throughout the spinal canal. The fourth through sixth decades of life represent the peak incidence of occurrence, affecting both men and women equally.

The majority of schwannomas arise from a dorsal nerve root, while ventral root tumors are more commonly neurofibromas. Most nerve sheath tumors are entirely intradural, but 10%–15% extend through the dural root sleeve as a dumbbell tumor with both intradural and extradural components. About 10% of nerve sheath tumors are epidural or paraspinal in location and 1% are intramedullary and arise from the perivascular nerve sheaths that accompany penetrating spinal cord vessels. Although the majority of nerve sheath tumors are benign, 2.5% of intradural nerve sheath tumors are malignant, with at least one half of these occurring in patients with neurofibromatosis.

Treatment Options

Incidentally identified benign nerve sheath tumors can be managed conservatively with serial imaging unless symptoms develop or growth prompts resection.

The optimal treatment for a symptomatic intradural extramedullary tumor is surgical excision. For nerve sheath lesions, this can often be accomplished via standard laminectomy.

Recurrences are rare when gross total removal has been achieved. Most nerve sheath tumors are dorsal or dorsolateral to the spinal cord and well visualized with a midline opening of the dura mater.

Ventrally located tumors may require facetectomy, transthoracic, or far lateral approaches, and may require stabilization if iatrogenic instability ensues.

Surgical Technique

For typical schwannomas, the patient is positioned prone, neuromonitoring is applied consisting of SSEPs, MEPs, and EMGs, and fluoroscopy is utilized for incision localization.

Laminectomies are performed beyond the level of the upper and lower edges of the mass to achieve unobstructed exposure. It is important to remove enough bone to be able to open the dura and adequately visualize the rostral and caudal edges of the mass (limited dural opening can lead to excessive neural element manipulation).

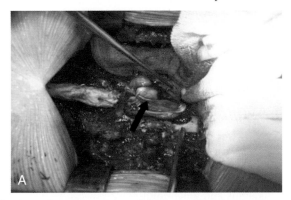

FIGURE 56-2 **(A)** Dural opening and exposure of the tumor. *(Reprinted with permission from Ahn DK, Park HS, Choi J. The surgical treatment for spinal intradural extramedullary tumors.* Clinics in Orthopedic Surgery. *2009;1:165-172.)*

The operative microscope is used to open the dura at its midline, and the leaflets are tethered laterally with suture. There is often an arachnoid membrane tightly applied to the tumor surface. This layer is sharply incised and dissected off the tumor capsule, which is then cauterized to diminish vascularity and shrink tumor volume.

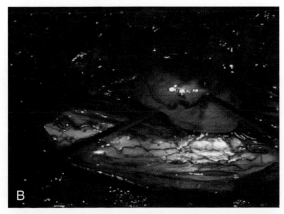

FIGURE 56-2 **(B)** Dissection of the schwannoma from the spinal cord. *(Reprinted with permission from Jandial R, McCormick P, and Black PM.* Core Techniques in Operative Neurosurgery. *Elsevier; 2011.)*

Tumor removal requires identification and division of the proximal and distal nerve root attachments; these are often immediately apparent with large tumors. Stimulate to determine if the root can be sacrificed. Internal decompression with a laser or ultrasonic aspirator can be used in such cases. Ventrally located tumors maybe adherent to the anterior spinal artery.

Sacrifice of the nerve rootlets of origin may be required. It is often possible to preserve the corresponding intradural nerve root as the fenestrated arachnoid sheaths allow anatomic separation of the dorsal and ventral nerve roots just distal to the dorsal root ganglion.

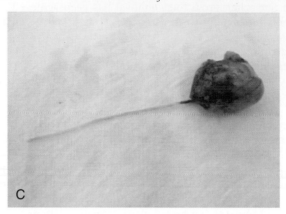

FIGURE 56-2 **(C)** Nerve rootlet that is connected to a schwannoma. *(Reprinted with permission from Ahn DK, Park HS, Choi J. The surgical treatment for spinal intradural extramedullary tumors.* Clinics in Orthopedic Surgery. *2009;1:165-172.)*

Once the tumor has been removed, hemostasis is obtained and a watertight dural closure is performed, and dural sealant is used to fortify the suture line. Multilayered musculofascial closure is performed to the skin.

Complication Avoidance and Management

- Meticulous hemostasis is key in spinal cord tumor surgery; particularly prior to dural opening, as epidural venous bleeding often increases after its opening due to the decrease in mural pressure. It is also critically important to minimize bleeding into the intradural space and to clear any such blood prior to dural closure; this will minimize postoperative meningismus and arachnoiditis.
- Inadequate bony removal that limits dural opening and visualization of the rostral and caudal aspects of the intradural mass can lead to unnecessary retraction and manipulation of neural structures. Intraoperative ultrasonography can be used prior to dural opening to confirm adequate bony removal.
- The use of an ultrasonic aspirator is often essential during microsurgical resection of intradural nerve sheath tumors. These instruments allow for resection of the tumor with minimal retraction on the spinal cord.
- MEPs are essential for monitoring during spinal cord surgery. Muscle MEPs are reported in an all-or-none fashion; their loss is typically associated with a postoperative motor deficit.
- Preservation of the facet joints during exposure and laminectomy reduces the incidence of postoperative kyphosis and instability, particularly at junctional levels of the spine. Osteoplastic laminoplasty may also reduce the incidence of postoperative deformity in children and young adults.
- Instrumented fixation should be performed when facet joint disruption is required for safe tumor resection; this will prevent postoperative deformity development and the need for additional surgery.

KEY PAPERS

Mehta V, Bettegowda C, Kretzer RM, et al. Intradural nerve sheath tumors. In: Jandial R, McCormick P, Black P, eds. *Core Techniques in Operative Neurosurgery*. Philadelphia: Elsevier Inc; 2011:661-665.

Parsa AT, Lee J, Parney IF, et al. Spinal cord and intradural-extraparenchymal spinal tumors: current best care practices and strategies. *J Neurooncol*. 2004;69:291-318.

Case 57

Intradural Intramedullary Mass

Hazem Mashaly, MD ● Zachary J. Tempel, MD ●
Adam S. Kanter, MD

Presentation

A 41-year-old male presents with nonradiating diffuse midline cervicothoracic pain that
has progressed over a 6-month period. He recently developed numbness and weakness in
the bilateral distal upper extremities, primarily his hands. He further reports several episodes of urinary incontinence and a sense of incomplete evacuation with bowel
movements.

- PMH: otherwise unremarkable
- Exam: no tenderness or muscle spasm to palpation of the cervicothoracic spine
  - UE exam: grade 4/5 weakness in hand grip bilaterally, 4+/5 wrist flexors/extensors,
    and diffuse sensory dysesthesias
  - LL exam: grade 4+/5 weakness diffusely in both lower limbs, decreased pain and
    temperature sensation with sensory level at T4
  - Reflexes 3+ in lower limbs, 2 beats of clonus, positive Hoffmann's sign bilaterally
  - Normal rectal tone

Differential Diagnosis

- Degenerative
  - Cervical disc herniation
  - Cervical spondylosis
- Neoplastic
  - Intradural intramedullary spinal cord tumor (e.g., astrocytoma, ependymoma)
  - Intradural extramedullary spinal cord tumor (e.g., meningioma)
  - Extradural spinal cord compression (e.g., primary bone tumor, epidural
    lymphoma)
  - Metastatic spinal cord tumor
- Vascular
  - Spinal AVM
  - Spinal dural AVF (congestion leads to increased signal in cord)
- Infectious
  - Spinal epidural abscess (fever and toxic manifestations)
- Other
  - MS (relapsing and remitting course)
  - Transverse myelopathy (acute onset)
  - Devics
  - ADEM
  - Vitamin B_{12} deficiency (h/o alcoholism)

Initial Imaging

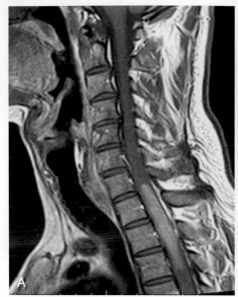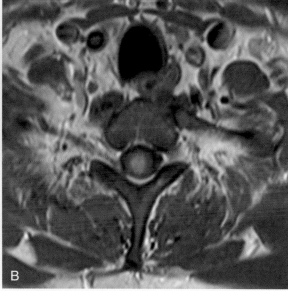

FIGURE 57-1

Imaging Description and Differential

- Figure 57-1 shows cervical/upper thoracic contrast enhanced sagittal (A) and axial (B) MRI of an intradural intramedullary oblong lesion extending from the inferior border of C7 to T3 expanding the spinal cord. The lesion reveals homogenous enhancement with no dural tail.
- Differential: ependymoma; less likely astrocytoma or extramedullary tumor

Further Workup

- Laboratory
  - Routine lab: CBC, PT/PTT/INR, LFT, KFT, and electrolytes
  - CSF: if canal is not obstructed by expanded cord and there is suspicion of infection or inflammation
- Imaging
  - CT cervicothoracic spine for better evaluation of bony anatomy
  - X-ray cervical spine with flexion/extension to evaluate for dynamic instability
  - MRI brain to exclude intracranial ependymoma or demyelinating disease
  - MRI pan-spine to rule out further disease
  - CT chest/abdomen and pelvis to rule out metastasis or tumors associated with Von-Hippel Lindau (VHL)

Pathophysiology

- Primary spinal cord tumors account for 5% to 10% of adult spinal tumors and 4.5% of primary central nervous system tumors. They are classified by their anatomic sub-location: intradural intramedullary, intradural extramedullary, or extradural. Intradural intramedullary spinal cord tumors constitute 20% to 30% of all primary spinal cord tumors.
- Approximately 90% of intramedullary tumors are either ependymomas (~60%) or astrocytomas (~30%). The remaining 10% include hemangioblastomas (especially in VHL, often have associated syrinx), cavernomas, and metastases. Ependymoma is the most common intradural intramedullary tumor type in adults, and peak incidence is in the fourth decade, with males being more commonly affected than females.

- The most common symptoms are nonspecific axial pain, followed by slowly progressive neurologic decline; urogenital and anorectal dysfunction occur early. Rare cases of acute neurologic compromise from tumor hemorrhage have been reported.
- Myxopapillary ependymoma (WHO grade 1) is a distinct type, predominantly extra-medullary, and located in the lumbar cistern.
- Cellular ependymomas arise from the ependymal lining of the central canal and are classified as WHO grade 2 tumors. Anaplastic ependymomas are rare and are WHO grade 3 tumors.
- Histologically, ependymoma cells are characterized by round to oval nuclei containing finely dispersed chromatin with perivascular and ependymal rosettes. The most common location of ependymomas is the cervical spine, followed by the cervicothoracic and thoracic spine.

Treatment Options

- Microsurgery
  - The most important factor influencing surgical objective is the nature of the tumor and spinal cord interface.
  - Benign tumors, such as ependymomas and hemangioblastomas, although unencapsulated, are noninfiltrative lesions that typically exhibit a distinct tumor–spinal cord interface; gross total removal is the treatment of choice.
  - Astrocytomas rarely exhibit a definitive dissection plane; gross total resection may be achieved in some cases, but the extent of removal is uncertain and poorly defined in most cases. Biopsy rather than resection of spinal GBMs maybe prudent.
- Radiotherapy
  - Radiotherapy is the mainstay treatment in high-grade glioma cases; it can also be administered for recurrent or residual tumors with evidence of progression when surgical resection is not possible.
  - Side effects include: spinal cord edema, radiation myelopathy, spinal kyphosis or subluxation, and delayed radiation necrosis.
- Chemotherapy
  - High-grade astrocytomas are treated with concomitant radiation and chemotherapy and postradiotherapy temozolomide.

Surgical Technique

- The patient is placed prone on the operating table. A Mayfield is used for cervical and upper thoracic lesions above the T6 level. Neuromonitoring is utilized including MEPs and EMGs; SSEPs are not uncommonly lost following midline myelotomy and are of minimal use in surgical resection of intramedullary spinal cord tumors. Fluoroscopy is used for localization. Ultrasonography is useful for tumor localization and assurance of adequate bony exposure.
- A midline skin incision is made followed by subperiosteal bony dissection, and a standard laminectomy is performed. This should extend to at least one segment above and one segment below the solid tumor component, with preservation of the facet joints where possible. Meticulous hemostasis is necessary before dural opening.
- The dura is opened at the midline under magnification of the operating microscope. Dural traction sutures are placed (Figure 57-2A).
- The arachnoid is opened separately; the spinal cord is inspected for any surface abnormality. The tumor area of the spinal cord usually appears enlarged, swollen, tense, and more or less vascularized.
- Exposure of most intramedullary neoplasms is typically performed via dorsal midline myelotomy. Some authors prefer to part the dorsal columns using microscissors and microdissectors. Eccentrically located tumors may be exposed by paramedian myelotomy that extends longitudinally from both ends of any visible tumor (Figure 57-2B).
- The use of pial sutures improves surgical exposure and reduces the severity of repeated trauma during dissection.

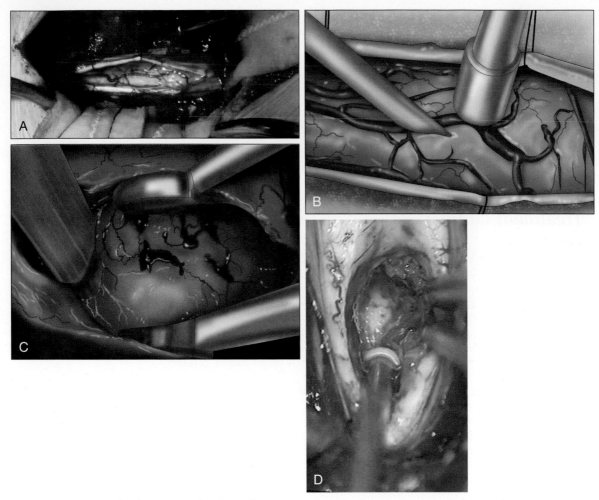

FIGURE 57-2   **(A)** The dura is incised in the midline using a no. 15 blade scalpel and Metzenbaum scissors. An attempt should be made to keep the arachnoid membrane intact at the time of initial dural opening. Dural tenting sutures are placed bilaterally to minimize the flow of blood products into the subarachnoid space and to aid in operative exposure. **(B)** The microscope is brought into the field, and the arachnoid membrane is incised. Dorsal midline myelotomy is performed through the posterior median sulcus using a microknife or contact neodymium:yttrium-aluminum-garnet (Nd:YAG) laser. **(C)** Because intramedullary lesions typically lie several millimeters below the posterior surface of the cord, dissection is carried through the midline myelotomy until pathologic tissue is encountered. Biopsy specimens are obtained and sent for preliminary pathologic examination. Any polar cysts that are accessible should also be drained to allow relaxation of the spinal cord. The tumor is debulked internally using an ultrasonic aspirator starting in the middle of the lesion; resection at the superior and inferior portions of the tumor is typically delayed because of the proximity to the normal spinal cord parenchyma. Microsuction or a contact laser can also be used to resect the residual tumor from the margins, with the extent of resection guided by MEP readings. Plated bayonets are used to aid in exposure of the resection cavity and can be used to develop the tumor–spinal cord interface in cases of intramedullary ependymomas. *(Reprinted with permission from Jandial R, McCormick P, and Black PM. Core Techniques in Operative Neurosurgery. Elsevier; 2011.)* **(D)** The tumor is progressively resected by dissection of the tumor–spinal cord interface and debulking with an ultrasonic aspirator. *(Reprinted with permission from Quiñones-Hinojosa A. Schmidek and Sweet Operative Neurosurgical Techniques. 6th ed. Elsevier; 2012.)*

- The technique of tumor removal depends on the presence of a clean plane of the spinal cord and its size. Development of the tumor–spinal cord interface is preferred for circumscribed tumors with a well-defined plane (e.g., ependymoma) (Figure 57-2C). It is of paramount importance that in the absence of a plane of dissection in an infiltrating tumor, surgical resection is limited to areas of absolute gross pathology to avoid injury to adjacent neural tissues.
- Larger tumors require internal decompression to allow better visualization and mobilization of the lateral and ventral tumor margins. Intratumoral resection is performed from inside to outside (Figure 57-2D). Hemangioblastomas should be removed en bloc and

not be debulked. Like AVMs, arterial supply should be deprived pior to venous drainage.

- Hemostasis followed by a meticulous dural closure is performed to prevent CSF leakage.

Complication Avoidance and Management

- Muscle MEPs and epidural D-wave MEPs should be used in combination during surgical resection of intramedullary tumors. As long as D-wave amplitude remains >50%, any postoperative motor deficits are likely to be transient.
- Care should be taken to avoid facet disruption during exposure to reduce the risk of postsurgical kyphosis, especially in young patients with lesions in the cervical and cervicothoracic spine.
- During surgery, if there is significant change in MEP, options include medications to increase the mean arterial pressure, the use of warm saline or papaverine-soaked cotton in the resection cavity, tumor removal at a different site, or cessation of the operative procedure.
- Neurologic deficits are common after surgery for intramedullary lesions; most deficits are transient and correlate with the patient's preoperative baseline level of functioning. Dysesthesias and proprioceptive difficulties commonly occur secondary to the midline myelotomy. These deficits generally improve over the first 3 months after surgery with the aid of physical therapy.

KEY PAPERS

Aghayev K, Vrionis F, Chamberlain MC. Adult intradural primary spinal cord tumors. *J Natl Compr Canc Netw*. 2011;9(4):434-447.

Bowers DC, Weprin BE. Intramedullary spinal cord tumors. *Curr Treat Options Neurol*. 2003;5(3):207-212.

Bruneau M, Brotchi J. Surgical management of intramedullary spinal cord tumors in adults. In: Gokaslan ZL, Belzberg AJ, eds. *Schmidek and Sweet Operative Neurosurgical Techniques Indications, Methods, and Results*. 6th ed. Philadelphia: Elsevier Inc; 2012.

Kretzer RM, Bettegowda C, Jallo GI. Intramedullary glioma. In: Jandial R, McCormick P, Black P, eds. *Core Techniques in Operative Neurosurgery*. Philadelphia: Elsevier Inc; 2011:673-679.

McCormick PC, Anson JA. Intramedullary spinal cord lesions. In: Benzel EC, Francis TB, eds. *Spine Surgery Techniques, Complication Avoidance and Management*. 3rd ed. Philadelphia: Elsevier Inc; 2012:983-990.

Case 58

Cervical Ossified Posterior Longitudinal Ligament

Hazem Mashaly, MD ● Adam S. Kanter, MD

Presentation

A 79-year-old male presents with progressive weakness in his upper and lower extremities, although most pronounced in the hands. He further reports numbness, tingling, and the inability to perform fine motor tasks. He additionally has been having increasing difficulty with gait and balance function. His symptoms have been progressively worsening over the last 12 months. He denies any recent trauma.

- PMH: HTN, type 2 DM
- Exam:
  - Reduced range in cervical motion, and electric shocks extending down his spine during passive neck flexion
  - Wasting of intrinsic hand muscles bilaterally
  - Increased tone in bilateral lower extremities
  - Quadriparesis grade 4-/5, affecting extensors more than flexors in upper extremities; most evident in the hands, and affects flexors greater than extensors in lower extremities
  - Reflexes: brisk hyperreflexia in upper and lower extremities
  - Severe gait ataxia

Differential Diagnosis

- Degenerative
  - Cervical spondylotic myelopathy
  - Cervical stenosis: OPLL
- Neoplastic
  - Metastasis
  - Spinal cord tumor
- Vascular
  - Vertebrobasilar insufficiency
- Cervical instability
  - C1-C2 subluxation
- Other
  - Amyotrophic lateral sclerosis
  - Syringomyelia
  - Vitamin B_{12} deficiency
  - Chiari malformation

Initial Imaging

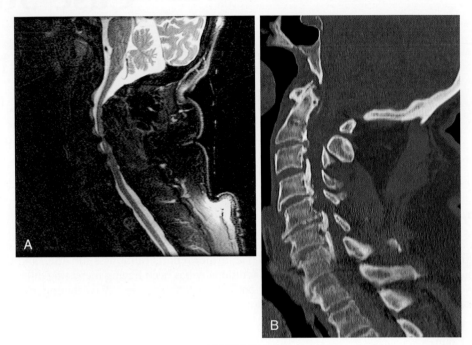

FIGURE 58-1

Imaging Description and Differential

- Sagittal MRI of cervical spine reveals severe cervical spinal cord compression from both anterior and posterior pathology, extending from C3 to C7; note the compression is not limited to the disc space.
- Sagittal CT scan reveals cervical OPLL of mixed type; note the double layer sign most evident behind the caudal C3 vertebral body is possibly indicative of dural penetrance.

Further Workup

- Laboratory
  - CBC, BMP, PT/INR/PTT
- Imaging
  - X-ray cervical spine with dynamic views
  - CTA: to map vertebral artery course if considering multilevel corpectomy

Pathophysiology

- OPLL most commonly occurs in males (2 : 1) in their mid-50s; it contributes to 25% of cervical myelopathy cases in North America and has higher percentages in the Asian population.
- Originates as early hypertrophy of the PLL with accompanying punctate ossification centers (early OPLL). These foci coalesce and become loci of frank ossification in the PLL.
- The increased prevalence of OPLL in East Asians, particularly among blood relatives, suggests a genetic predisposition.
- OPLL enlarges an average of 0.4 mm per year in its anterior-posterior dimension, and longitudinal expansion occurs at a rate of 0.67 mm per year.

- Two major mechanisms contribute to neural injury in patients with OPLL: direct mechanical compression and indirect ischemic injury.
- There are four types of OPLL: the segmental variant (39%), located behind the vertebral bodies, does not cross the intervening disc spaces; the continuous type (27%) extends from vertebra to vertebra, traversing the disc spaces; the mixed form (29%) simultaneously includes both continuous and segmental elements with "skip" areas; and the localized form (5%) is localized to the disc spaces.

Treatment Options

- Conservative
  - Observation is appropriate in patients without signs or symptoms of myelopathy, and in those deemed high-risk surgical candidates.
  - Nonsurgical management includes immobilization with a neck brace, steroidal or nonsteroidal antiinflammatory medications, activity modification, and physical therapy.
- Surgical
  - Surgical approach is selected based upon the degree of myelopathy, number of involved segments, sagittal balance of cervical spine, and surgeon preference/experience.
  - Significant controversy exists in regards to anterior versus posterior surgical approach for managing cervical OPLL. Anterior surgery offers direct OPLL removal typically through multilevel corpectomy and fusion, whereas posterior procedures allow for indirect dorsal decompression of multilevel pathology via laminectomy (+/– fusion) or laminoplasty.
  - Laminectomy (+/– fusion): laminectomy may sufficiently decompress the cervical spinal canal in patients with OPLL if the cervical spine is stable and the lordotic curvature remains adequately preserved. In some patients, stabilization may be performed to diminish the evolution of instability, whereas in others, instability may already be present.
  - Multilevel anterior corpectomy and fusion (ACF): improved outcomes have been reported in some series for OPLL patients undergoing multilevel anterior corpectomy and fusion procedures.
  - Combined anterior and posterior approach: for specific cases with localized severe anterior compression accompanied by cervical canal stenosis, the combined anterior and posterior approach can be used.
  - Laminoplasty: simultaneously offers dorsal decompression and augments stability without the need for traditional fusion.

Surgical Technique

Positioning

Laminectomy

- Laminectomies alone can be performed, but posterior cord herniation is possible especially if the OPLL causes a bulky anterior mass in the canal
- Neuromonitoring, including SSEPs, are established pre- and post-prone positioning; lamina and spinous processes are removed with a high-speed drill; ligamentum flavum is removed, and any necessary foraminotomies are performed.
- The decompression typically includes C3-C7, or at minimum one segment above and below the radiographically compressed levels.
- Because of the risk of post-laminectomy kyphosis, lateral resection should not incorporate more than the medial 25% of the facets on either side (Figure 58-2).

Laminectomy with Fusion

- In some patients, prophylactic stabilization may be performed to avoid the evolution of instability, whereas in others, instability may already be present.
- Following neural decompression, lateral mass screws (typically 14 mm) are placed by drilling approximately 1 mm infero-medial to the intersection of the rostro-caudal and

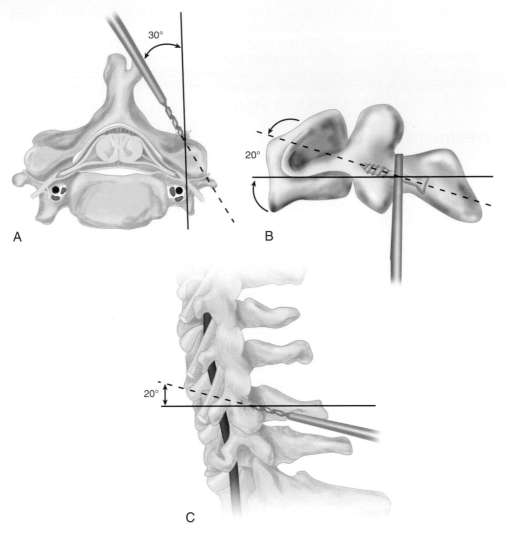

FIGURE 58-2 An up-and-out technique is used for hand drill trajectory. **(A)** Medial-to-lateral trajectory at 30 degrees avoids injury to the vertebral artery, **(B,C)** and a cephalad-caudal trajectory at 20 degrees avoids injury to the nerve root. *(Reprinted with permission from Jandial R, McCormick P, and Black PM. Core Techniques in Operative Neurosurgery.* Elsevier; 2011.)

medio-lateral midline, and aiming the trajectory to the supero-lateral edge of the lateral mass (Figure 58-3 and 58-4). The intervening joints are than decorticated with the drill, and rods are placed and secured under minimal compression force. Morselized bone graft is placed into the dorsolateral joints for arthrodesis (Figure 58-5).

Anterior Corpectomy and Fusion (ACF)

- The corpectomy is performed by drilling a longitudinal groove approximately 15 mm wide through the index vertebrae. Exceeding 15 mm in width increases the risk of vascular injury and decreases the bony surface area to aide in arthrodesis.
- The OPLL is carefully dissected free of the ossified dura and either resected or thinned; microscopic magnification is mandatory to assist in distinguishing the PLL from ossified dura that must be left intact.
- Arthrodesis is then performed using structural bone graft or interbody cages, with the use of anterior cervical plating to solidify the construct (Figure 58-6A and B).

Laminoplasty

- Laminoplasty has classically been associated with a lower risk of postoperative kyphotic deformity compared with standard laminectomy.

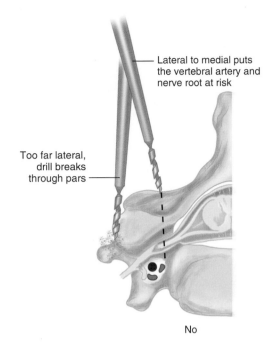

Lateral to medial puts
the vertebral artery and
nerve root at risk

Too far lateral,
drill breaks
through pars

No

FIGURE 58-3   An up-and-out technique is used for hand drill trajectory. A medial-to-lateral trajectory at 30 degrees avoids injury to the vertebral artery, and a cephalad-caudal trajectory at 20 degrees avoids injury to the nerve root. *(Reprinted with permission from Jandial R, McCormick P, and Black PM.* Core Techniques in Operative Neurosurgery. *Elsevier; 2011.)*

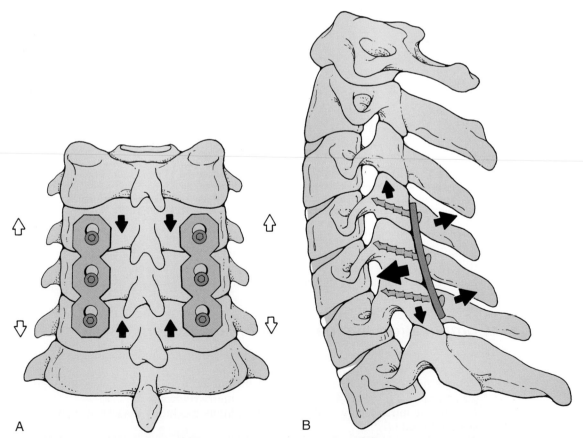

A   B

FIGURE 58-4   Coronal **(A)**-58.3 and lateral **(B)**-58.4 views of a lateral mass fixation construct. *(Reprinted with permission from Benzel EC.* Spine Surgery: Techniques, Complication Avoidance and Management, *3rd ed. Elsevier; 2012.)*

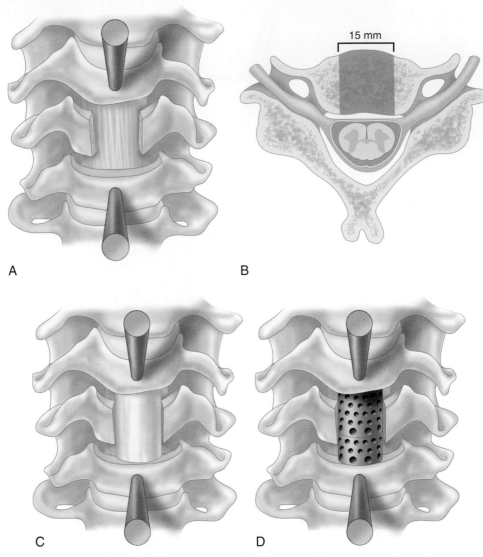

FIGURE 58-5   **(A)** The width of the corpectomy should not exceed 15 mm to avoid vascular injury and allow the lateral walls to help with bony fusion. The corpectomy can be completed with a high-speed drill and various rongeur forceps. **(B)** Bone graft or interbody cage is placed in the corpectomy defect. *(Reprinted with permission from Jandial R, McCormick P, and Black PM.* Core Techniques in Operative Neurosurgery. *Elsevier; 2011.)*

- Laminoplasty requires drilling a partial trough on one side, and a complete trough on the other, enabling a hinge-like opening of the spinal canal, followed by placement of bone or metal implant stabilizers that are secured into place to maintain canal expansion and cervical rigidity.

Complication Avoidance and Management

- Awake fiber-optic intubation and positioning are performed under continuous SSEP and intermittent MEP monitoring.
- Complications of anterior cervical surgery include a 2% to 10% incidence of quadriplegia and up to a 17% incidence of nerve root injury (typically the C5 root).
- Continuous intraoperative SSEP monitoring limits morbidity associated with cervical surgery for OPLL.
- The incidence of a CSF leak after anterior cervical OPLL resection is between 6.7% and 31.8%. If CT signs of dural penetrance are observed prior to surgery, then intraoperative

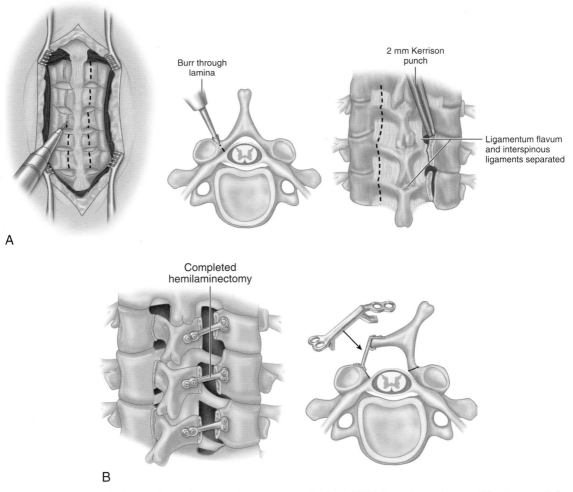

FIGURE 58-6 **(A)** At the lamina-lateral mass junction, a 3 mm cutting burr drill bit is used to make a small laminotomy hole at the lowest level. Then a footed drill bit is used to open all levels on one side, moving in an upward direction. It is also acceptable to complete the opening in this fashion or with a 2 mm Kerrison punch. **(B)** A trough at the lamina-lateral mass junction, on the contralateral side, is drilled using a 3 mm burr. Care is taken not to breach the anterior cortical bone. A fixation plate is screwed in position connecting the lateral mass, graft, and lamina. *(Reprinted with permission from Jandial R, McCormick P, and Black PM.* Core Techniques in Operative Neurosurgery. *Elsevier; 2011.)*

fistulas may be anticipated, allowing the surgeon to plan for a complex dural/wound repair. Head elevation and lumbar drains may be employed postoperatively to minimize pseudomeningocele formation.

- Posterior surgery is often contraindicated in the presence of significant kyphosis, as removal of the posterior elements may leave the cord tethered over ventral disease.

KEY PAPERS

Cardoso MJ, Koski TR, Ganju A, et al. Approach-related complications after decompression for cervical ossification of the posterior longitudinal ligament. *Neurosurg Focus.* 2011;30(3):E12.

Nancy E. Epstein, Kazuo Yonenobu. Ossification of the posterior longitudinal ligament. In: Benzel EC, Francis TB, eds. *Spine Surgery Techniques, Complication Avoidance and Management.* 3rd ed. Philadelphia: Elsevier Inc; 2012:859-870.

Case 59

Ankylosing Spondylitis

Michael M. McDowell, MD ● Zachary J. Tempel, MD ●
Adam S. Kanter, MD

Presentation

An 84-year-old male with a known history of ankylosing spondylitis presents to the emergency room 8 days following a ground-level fall with progressive cervicothoracic axial pain and limited range of motion. He reports experiencing tingling in both hands after the fall, but these symptoms resolved within a couple of days. He denies numbness, weakness, or bowel/bladder dysfunction.

- Exam:
  - 5/5 strength throughout
  - 2+ reflexes in bilateral lower extremities
  - Sensation intact to light tough and pinprick
  - No clonus or Hoffmann's; down-going toes

Differential Diagnosis

- Degenerative
  - Acute disc herniation
  - Compression fracture
  - Facet or laminar fracture
  - Cervical spondylotic myelopathy
  - Central cord syndrome
- Vascular
  - Epidural hematoma
- Infectious (history of immunosuppressant therapy)
  - Discitis +/- osteomyelitis
  - Epidural abscess

Initial Imaging

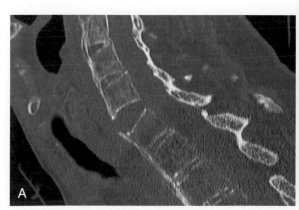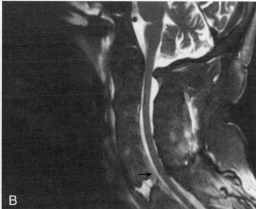

FIGURE 59-1

Imaging Description

Sagittal CT of the spine demonstrates C6-C7 fracture with disruption of the prevertebral ankylosis and "fish-mouthing" of the intervertebral disk space (Figure 59-1A). MRI demonstrates associated prevertebral hematoma (arrow) and disruption of the disc space. (Figure 59-1B).

Further Workup

- Laboratory
  - ESR, CRP, prealbumin, vitamin D, ionized calcium, vitamin D
- Imaging
  - Complete trauma workup, as indicated by mechanism and exam
  - CT head, chest, abdomen, pelvis
- Consultants
  - Internal medicine: preoperative evaluation

Pathophysiology

AS is a challenging disease that predisposes patients to major bony injuries from low-energy kinetic trauma (e.g., mechanical falls) due to a combination of predisposition toward osteoporosis and a loss of dynamic force redistribution as individual vertebral elements are fused into a single long bone. When fractures occur, they frequently involve the intervertebral disc space (usually spared from ossification in AS), resulting in a high risk of subsequent instability and neurological dysfunction.

AS is the third most common type of arthritis in the United States, affecting 0.5% of the population, and classically involves patients with major histocompatibility complex class 1 HLA-B27 variant. The primary theories of pathogenesis suggest that HLA-B27 may be predisposed to molecular mimicry of bacterial antigens when bound by certain selfpeptides, or alternatively, may directly stimulate autoreactive cytotoxic T-cells through misfolding and inappropriate dimerization within the endoplasmic reticulum.

Clinically, patients complain of morning back stiffness and often have kyphoscoliosis. AS can results in bowstring myelopathy, cauda equina (from dural ectasia), C1-2 instability (these segments are spared) and chalkstick fractures.

Treatment Options

- Medical
  - Back pain: NSAIDs (most effective), short courses of opioids, muscle relaxants
  - Progression of disease: disease-modifying antirheumatic drugs, such as sulfasalazine (not effective in axial spine), with small amounts of evidence available for methotrexate
  - Corticosteroid injections into peripheral joints; TNF-α antagonists appear to have more profound effects on disease activity within the spine;
- Mechanical
  - Cervical collar for prolonged duration in patients without unstable fractures
  - Chiropractic manipulation is not recommended given the fragility of the spine, with the cervical spine being contraindicated due to the risk of vertebral dissection.
- Surgical
  - Pedicle screw fixation +/- traction: in patients with kyphotic or hyperlordotic deformity from the fracture; reduction via light traction (<5 pounds) can be attempted, followed by intraoperative reduction when needed; given the diminished purchase available due to AS, constructs frequently require extensive posterior instrumentation several levels above and below the injury.
  - Anterior segmental fixation: rarely acceptable as a stand-alone approach for fixation in ankylosing spondylitis fractures; bone quality is important due to the low number of feasible levels; can be combined with pedicle screw fixation (PSF) in patients with

persistent deformity, circumferential fractures, or who are at high risk of construct pullout.

- Wedge osteotomy with pedicle screw fusion: most aggressive approach and ideal in patients with severe sagittal deformity; unlikely to be corrected with the above-mentioned techniques; preferentially performed for injuries at, or below, C7 to avoid the vertebral artery should complications occur intraoperatively; technically a difficult operation with high morbidity; numerous variations have been described, including those utilizing subsequent PSF to avoid immobilization postoperatively.
- Nonoperative intervention: the high risk of morbidity in the surgical treatment of AS has led some to elect for hard collar or halo fixation, especially in those without deficit or frank deformity; however, progressive neurological injury has been found in over half of conservatively managed patients, with other complications including fracture nonunion, skin ulceration, aspiration risk, and pulmonary impairments.

Surgical Technique
Pedicle Screw Fixation

Prone positioning with neuromonitoring and fluoroscopy for localization. Place the patient in Mayfield pin fixation. Subperiosteal dissection is performed bilaterally to expose the entire spinous process and lamina out to and including the lateral masses of the cervical spine and the medial edge of the transverse processes of the thoracic spine. (Figure 59-2).

Bony landmarks and ligamentous structures are examined for evidence of fracture or disruption, respectively. Screws are inserted into the lateral masses of the cervical vertebrae and pedicles of thoracic vertebrae, with the angulation based on anatomic landmarks for each level. In this vignette, C4, C5, and C6 were utilized bilaterally, C7 was not instrumented due to deep angulation. Bilateral pedicle screws were inserted into T1, T2, and T3.

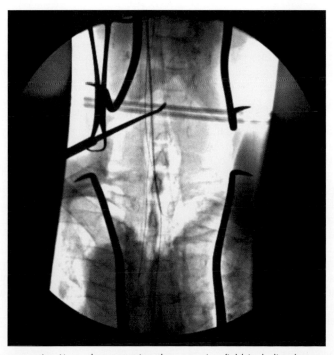

FIGURE 59-2 Intraoperative X-ray demonstrating the operative field including low cervical and high thoracic vertebrae.

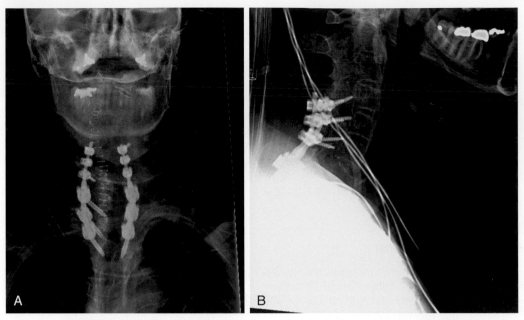

FIGURE 59-3   AP and lateral X-ray demonstrating the fusion construct from C4-T3.

After thorough decortication with a high-speed drill, morselized bone allograft is placed to induce arthrodesis. The wound is copiously irrigated and closed in layers following hemostasis.

Neurophysiologic monitoring is essential in these cases due to the highly unstable nature of the fracture. Postoperative CT and X-rays may be obtained to evaluate reduction and instrumentation (Figure 59-3).

Complication Avoidance and Management

- A CT scan is required for preoperative planning; a complete evaluation of the spine for additional injuries is crucial in identifying the appropriate correction to restore spinal alignment and balance, and prevent inadequate reduction or construct length, particularly if other fractures, even if chronic, become apparent at adjacent levels to the index injury.
- Detailed knowledge of the anatomy of the spine is crucial, particularly adjacent landmarks due to the fact that central spinal anatomy may be disfigured in AS; extrapolation based on the remaining cues, combined with judicious use of fluoroscopy, permits safe instrumentation placement.
- A thorough understanding of spinal biomechanics is required to maximize long-term efficacy of surgical stabilization; anterior procedures that could typically suffice to treat similar fractures in patients without AS provide inadequate strength to support the longer torque arms created by the underlying pathology.
- Transcranial electrical motor–evoked potential (TES-MEP) monitoring is an alternative or adjuvant to somatosensory-evoked potential monitoring; TES-MEP potentials above 20% of reference value in all muscle groups are a strong predictor of motor preservation postoperatively; care must be taken by the anesthesia team to avoid agents that may compromise neurophysiologic monitoring
- Be wary of epidural hematomas in AS patients.

ACKNOWLEDGEMENTS

We would like to thank Ahsan Nabiha for her artistic contribution.

KEY PAPERS

Apple DF Jr, Anson C. Spinal cord injury occurring in patients with ankylosing spondylitis: a multicenter study. *Orthopedics*. 1995;18:1005-1011.

Bronson WD, Walker SE, Hillman LS, et al. Bone mineral density and biochemical markers of bone metabolism in ankylosing spondylitis. *J Rheumatol*. 1998;25:929-935.

Broom MJ, Raycroft JF. Complications of fractures of the cervical spine in ankylosing spondylitis. *Spine (Phila Pa 1976)*. 1988;13:763-766.

Chin KR, Ahn J. Controlled cervical extension osteotomy for ankylosing spondylitis utilizing the Jackson operating table: technical note. *Spine (Phila Pa 1976)*. 2007;32:1926-1929.

Einsiedel T, Schmelz A, Arand M, et al. Injuries of the cervical spine in patients with ankylosing spondylitis: experience at two trauma centers. *J Neurosurg Spine*. 2006;5:33-45.

Kanter AS, Wang MY, Mummaneni PV. A treatment algorithm for the management of cervical spine fractures and deformity in patients with ankylosing spondylitis. *Neurosurg Focus*. 2008;24:E11.

Langeloo DD, Journee HL, Pavlov PW, et al. Cervical osteotomy in ankylosing spondylitis: evaluation of new developments. *Eur Spine J*. 2006;15:493-500.

Simmons ED, DiStefano RJ, Zheng Y, et al. Thirty-six years experience of cervical extension osteotomy in ankylosing spondylitis: techniques and outcomes. *Spine (Phila Pa 1976)*. 2006;31:3006-3012.

Yilmaz N, Pence S, Kepekci Y, et al. Association of immune function with bone mineral density and biochemical markers of bone turnover in patients with ankylosing spondylitis. *Int J Clin Pract*. 2003;57:681-685.

Case 60

Spinal Chordoma

Michael M. McDowell, MD ● Zachary J. Tempel, MD ●
Adam S. Kanter, MD

Presentation

A 62-year-old female smoker presents with 3 weeks of mild low back pain, urinary incontinence, and numbness/tingling in the saddle region. She denies weakness and bowel incontinence. Her symptoms persist despite treatment of an otherwise asymptomatic UTI.

- Normal strength throughout
- 2+ reflexes in bilateral lower extremities
- Decreased perianal sensation
- Normal rectal tone
- Negative Babinski and Hoffmann's

Differential Diagnosis

- Degenerative
  - Degenerative scoliosis
  - Compression fracture
  - Disk herniation
  - Cauda equina syndrome
- Neoplastic
  - Metastasis
  - Extradural tumor (chordoma, aneurysmal bone cyst, plasmacytoma)
  - Intradural-extramedullary tumor (meningioma, neurofibroma)
  - Intramedullary tumor (ependymoma, astrocytoma)
- Vascular
  - AVM
  - Cavernous malformation
- Infectious (DM, IV drug use, immunodeficiency)
  - Discitis +/- osteomyelitis
  - Epidural abscess

Initial Imaging

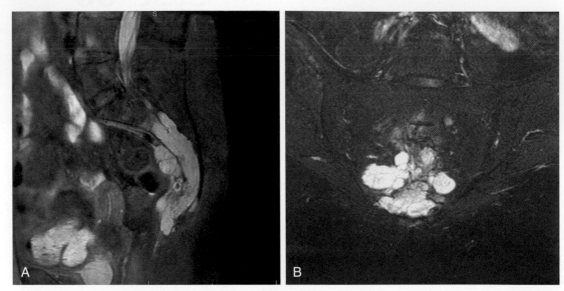

FIGURE 60-1

Imaging Description

Sagittal T2 MRI demonstrating an abnormal hyperintense mass in the distal spinal canal, sacrum, and adjacent soft tissues (Figure 60-1A). The mass is further emphasized on the coronal T2 MRI demonstrating anterior extension to the sacrum and into the adjacent soft tissues (Figure 60-1B).

Further Workup

- Laboratory
  - CBC, BMP, PT/INR/PTT
  - ESR, CRP, prealbumin
- Procedural radiology
  - Biopsy to confirm diagnosis of chordoma. When chordoma is suspected, great care must be taken to prevent seeding. For this reason transrectal biopsies are contraindicated. Ideally, biopsy tracts are marked to facilitate their resection if chordoma is confirmed.
- Imaging
  - CT of lumbar spine, abdomen, and pelvis to evaluate bony involvement for presurgery planning. Systemic metastasis is frequent.
  - Contrasted pelvic MRI to evaluate for other potential malignant etiology seeding the spine, and for preoperative planning
  - Contrasted MRI of the neuraxis to rule out metastases to other CNS regions

Consultants

- Internal medicine: preoperative evaluation

Pathophysiology

Chordomas are a malignant neoplasm resulting from embryonal remnants of the fetal notochord. The fourth most common malignant tumor of the bone, it comprises approximately 1%–4% of primary bone tumors. There is a 2:1 male to female preponderance. Chordomas manifest most commonly in the sacrum (50%), the spheno-occipital area (35%), the cervical region (10%), and rarely in the thoracic vertebrae (5%).

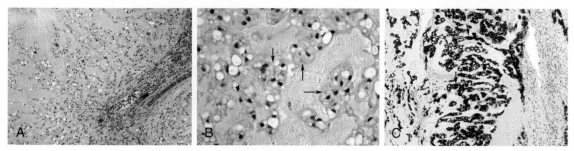

FIGURE 60-2 Key histopathological features of chordomas.

Given the large volume of the sacrum and adjacent cavities, patients often remain asymptomatic until substantial tumor growth within the pelvis has occurred. Symptoms can include urinary incontinence, bowel dysfunction, and weakness, but most patients present with lumbar and/or buttocks pain.

Disease recurrence and local metastasis are aided by this tumor's tendency to form a pseudocapsule with satellite lesions, which may be released by surgical manipulation. The key histopathological feature of these tumors is the presence of physaliferous cells (Figure 60-2).

Treatment Options

* Medical
  * Back pain: NSAIDs, oral corticosteroids, and muscle relaxants
  * Radicular or neuropathic pain: gabapentin, pregabalin, and antidepressants
  * Chemotherapy is rarely indicated as stand-alone therapy in chordomas; dedifferentiated tumors may have a higher rate of response; identification and targeting of stem cell-like components of chondromas may prove useful in future studies.
* Mechanical
  * Physical therapy: activity modification, muscle strengthening, optimizing posture, and mechanics to limit sacral loading
* Radiation therapy
  * Chordomas tend to require high-dose radiation treatment for disease control, resulting in tissue injury to the spinal cord and other adjacent tissues; adjuvant therapy is indicated in some patients with positive resection margins, inoperable tumors, or large tumor burden. Proton beam is a particularly effective.
* Surgical
  * Posterior approach sacrectomy: less invasive, single-stage approach that does not require assistance of a general surgeon; ideal for smaller tumors that are predominantly posterior in extension and caudal; preserves more function, but may result in a higher rate of local recurrence in cases where encapsulated components are not completely resected; lack of visualization and translation of visceral organs may increase the risk of injury during osteotomy
  * Combined anterior-posterior approach sacrectomy: more invasive, two-stage approach that is best performed with assistance by a general surgeon for laparotomy and protection of visceral organs via dissection and movement outside of the planned resection trajectory; sacrifice of sacral nerve roots may be necessary, requiring fecal diversion via ostomy; risks are higher because of the additional surgical procedure, but increases ability to obtain negative resection margins; ideal for large or rostral tumors

Surgical Technique
Anterior-Posterior Sacrectomy

Supine positioning with neuromonitoring (appendix Y) and fluoroscopy for localization. The anterior approach exposure is performed with the assistance of a general surgeon. Once completed, intraoperative imaging is used to confirm sacral levels (Figure 60-3). The

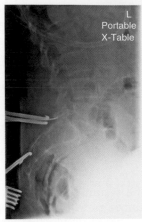

FIGURE 60-3   Intraoperative x-ray localizing the posterior aspect of S1.

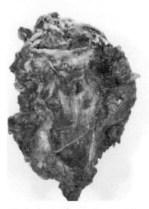

FIGURE 60-4   Pathological specimen status postsacrectomy.

high-speed drill is used to perform osteotomies to achieve a partial corpectomy and allow for removal of the remaining bony structures posteriorly (in this vignette S1 and S2). Hemostasis is achieved and the wound is closed with general surgery's assistance.

The patient is transferred to a prone position and the appropriate level confirmed. Subperiosteal dissection is performed (L5 to the coccyx in this vignette). Laminectomies are performed with care taken to expose the end of the thecal sac, and the lateral margin of the sacrum is identified and dissected, further into the soft tissues depending on tumor spread. The coccyx is dissected free of soft tissue attachments, and the bowel is identified to ensure its preservation.

The sacral nerves are identified and followed to the osteotomy site. Release of entangled sacral nerves is performed. The osteotomies continue posteriorly until sacroiliac joint sparing sacrectomy has been achieved and the specimen removed as one (Figures 60-4 and 60-5). Tumor outside of the sacral boundaries is resected until 1–2 inches of normal tissue is observed.

Complication Avoidance and Management

- Obtaining negative tumor margins is an important prognostic indicator in preventing recurrence and maximizing long-term survival; intraoperative rupture of the capsule greatly increases the risk of recurrence and reduces long-term survival; review of pelvic anatomy and preoperative imaging is crucial to planning negative resection margins.

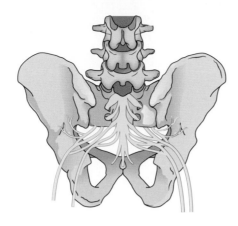

FIGURE 60-5   Artistic depiction of sacrectomy.

- The sacroiliac joints form a barrier that reduces tumor spread; resection of the joints allows for greater dissemination intraoperatively into adjacent viscera and musculature; when necessary, partial or total resection of the sacroiliac joints should be preceded by consideration of the need for instrumentation to prevent instability.
- Care must be taken to identify uninvolved visceral or neurological structures; however, tissues in which chordoma has grossly invaded must be resected aggressively to prevent local recurrence.

ACKNOWLEDGEMENTS

We would like to thank Alexandra Nikas for her artistic contribution.

KEY PAPERS

Bergh P, Kindblom LG, Gunterberg B, et al. Prognostic factors in chordoma of the sacrum and mobile spine: a study of 39 patients. *Cancer*. 2000;88:2122-2134.

Casali PG, Stacchiotti S, Sangalli C, et al. Chordoma. *Curr Opin Oncol*. 2007;19:367-370.

Chugh R, Tawbi H, Lucas DR, et al. Chordoma: the nonsarcoma primary bone tumor. *Oncologist*. 2007;12:1344-1350.

Fleming GF, Heimann PS, Stephens JK, et al. Dedifferentiated chordoma. Response to aggressive chemotherapy in two cases. *Cancer*. 1993;72:714-718.

Fuchs B, Dickey ID, Yaszemski MJ, et al. Operative management of sacral chordoma. *J Bone Joint Surg Am*. 2005;87:2211-2216.

Kaiser TE, Pritchard DJ, Unni KK. Clinicopathologic study of sacrococcygeal chordoma. *Cancer*. 1984;53:2574-2578.

Kayani B, Hanna SA, Sewell MD, et al. A review of the surgical management of sacral chordoma. *Eur J Surg Oncol*. 2014;40:1412-1420.

Ozger H, Eralp L, Sungur M, et al. Surgical management of sacral chordoma. *Acta Orthop Belg*. 2010;76:243-253.

Safari M, Khoshnevisan A. An overview of the role of cancer stem cells in spine tumors with a special focus on chordoma. *World J Stem Cells*. 2014;6:53-64.

Tharmabala M, LaBrash D, Kanthan R. Acute cauda equina syndrome secondary to lumbar chordoma: case report and literature review. *Spine J*. 2013;13:e35-e43.

York JE, Kaczaraj A, Abi-Said D, et al. Sacral chordoma: 40-year experience at a major cancer center. *Neurosurgery*. 1999;44:74-79, discussion 79-80.

Section V Pediatric Neurosurgery

Case 61

Pineal Tumor

Bond Nguyen ● Melanie G. Hayden Gephart, MD ●
Alexa Smith, MD ● Michael L. Levy, MD, PhD

Presentation

An 8-year-old girl was referred by her pediatrician for a concern of rapid development. After referral to an endocrinologist, a preliminary diagnosis of precocious puberty was made, and an MRI revealed hydrocephalus and a lesion in the pineal region. She has also been noted to be clumsy at school lately, and mom describes her daughter as "off balance." Initial assessment shows a child who appears older than her stated age. Neurologic examination reveals mild cerebellar dysmetria and difficulty with rapid alternating movements.

Differential Diagnosis

- Hydrocephalus
- Pineal cyst
- Lipoma
- Epidermoid
- Vascular malformation
- Pineal region tumor – including germ cell tumor, glioma, meningioma, metastasis

Initial Imaging

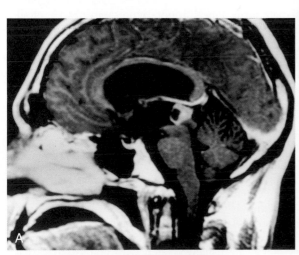
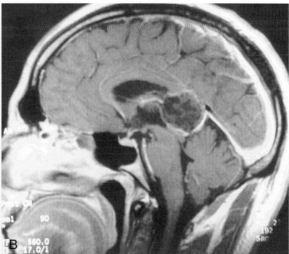

FIGURE 61-1 MRI showing the variability of the deep venous system in relation to pineal region tumors. (**A**) The deep venous system is located superior and dorsal to the tumor. This is the most common configuration and is conducive to an infratentorial-supracerebellar approach. (**B**) The deep venous system is located inferior and ventral to this epidermoid tumor and is conducive to a supratentorial approach. *(Reprinted with permission from Winn HR. Youmans Neurological Surgery. 6th ed. Elsevier; 2011.)*

Imaging Description and Differential
CT

May demonstrate hydrocephalus and calcifications, but will not further assist in differential diagnosis.

MRI

May suggest a germ cell tumor if the mass is iso- or hypointense relative to gray matter on a T1-weighted image and iso- to hyperintense on a T2-weighted image (T2WI). Contrast images of germ cell tumors demonstrate enhancement and sometimes cystic components, which do not enhance. Teratomas may be characterized by heterogeneity on T1 and hyperintensity on a T2WI. Teratomas may also be calcified. Pineal gland tumors, such as pineocytomas and pineoblastomas, can be differentiated on T2WI. Pineoblastomas have an isointense signal on T2WI and demonstrate brain invasion and edema. Pineocytomas have a hyperintense signal on T2WI.

Pineal cysts are round, smoothly demarcated on MRI, and appear similar to CSF with occasional rim enhancement. (Table 61-1)

Further Workup

Measurement of germ cell markers (beta-human chorionic gonadotropin (bhCG) and alpha-fetoprotein) in the CSF and serum should be obtained in all patients. (Table 61-2) Although most pineal region tumors are not marker producing, their presence indicates a malignant germ cell tumor. In the setting of elevated germ cell markers, a tissue diagnosis is not necessary and most centers proceed with chemotherapy and radiation. After therapy, germ cell markers can also be used to assess effectiveness of treatment and followed to monitor potential recurrence. In the absence of positive serum or CSF markers, a tissue sample is required. CSF cytology is useful as pinealblastomas and the germ cell tumors have a propensity to seed the CSF.

Pathophysiology

Pineal region masses include simple cysts, germ cell tumors, and tumors arising from cells in the pineal gland itself: pineoblastomas and pineocytomas. (Figure 61-2) Pineocytoma is a slow-growing, grade 2 tumor. Pineoblastoma is a more aggressive, grade 4, malignant tumor. There is also a grade 3 intermediate form. Pineal tumors represent only 1% of all brain tumors; however, they account for 3%–8% of all intracranial tumors in pediatric cases. Pineal tumors can cause hydrocephalus. Directly related to the function of the pineal gland are endocrine syndromes, which arise from secretion of hormones by germ cell tumors. Pseudoprecocious puberty, initiated by bhCG, can be observed with germ cell tumors in either the pineal or suprasellar region.

Treatment Options

Clearance of the obstructive hydrocephalus from the pineal mass must be performed, commonly before the removal of the pineal tumor. An endoscopic third ventriculostomy and biopsy of the tumor, performed in one operative procedure, is ideal especially as it prevents potential for peritoneal seeding. Benign pineal tumors including mature teratomas can be cured with surgery alone. Radiation is the primary curative treatment for pure germinomas arising intracranially and is beneficial for many malignant germ and parenchymal tumors that are not completely resectable. Pinealblastomas and germ cell tumors-including geminomas with positive cytology- are usually treated with craniospinal XRT which generally follows chemotherapy. Mature teratomas and benign tumors or cysts are not treated with radiation. Malignant tumors (except germinomas) will benefit from total resection followed by chemotherapy and irradiation especially if significant brainstem compression is evident.

TABLE 61-1

MOST FREQUENT TUMORS OF THE PINEAL REGION: TYPICAL CHARACTERISTICS

Tumor Feature	Germinoma	Teratoma	Pinealo-blastoma	Pinealo-cytoma	Glioma	Meningioma
Age	Child	Child	Child	Adult	Child	Adult
Sex predilection	Male	Male	None	None	None	None
Pineal versus parapineal	Pineal	Pineal	Pineal	Pineal	Parapineal (usually)	Parapineal (usually)
Signal intensity (heterogeneous versus homogeneous)	Homogeneous (but often hemorrhagic)	Strikingly heterogeneous	Homogeneous (unless hemorrhagic)	Homogeneous	Homogeneous (usually)	Homogeneous
Hemorrhage	Common	Typical	Common	Common	Rare	Rare
Calcification	Rare	Typical	Common	Common	Uncommon	Common
Brain edema or invasion	Common	Variable	Common	Uncommon	Primarily midbrain neoplasm	Occasional
Tendency to metastasize	Yes	Variable	Yes	No	Variable	No
Enhancement	Dense	Variable	Dense	Dense	Variable	Dense
Prognosis with 10-year survival rate, if available	Good with additional therapy: ~85% to >35%	Variable	Poor	Variable	Variable	Excellent

(Reprinted with permission from Ellenbogen RG, Abdulrauf SI, and Sekhar LN. Principles of Neurological Surgery. 3rd ed. Elsevier, 2012.)

TABLE 61-2

IMMUNOHISTOCHEMICAL PROFILES (TUMOR MARKERS) OF TUMORS OF THE PINEAL REGION

	Alpha Fetoprotein ⊥ (<5 ng/mL)	Human Chorionic Gonadotropin ⊥ (<5 ng/mL)	Human Placental Lactogen HPL	Placental Alkaline Phosphatase	Cytokeratin (CAM 5.2, AE 1/3)	c-kit (CD 117)	OCT 4	Melatonin
Germinoma	−	+ (<770 ng/mL)	−	++	−	+	+	−
Teratoma	+ (<1000 ng/mL)	−	−	−	+	+/−	−	−
Yolk sac tumor	+++	−	−	+/−	+	−	−	−
Embryonal carcinoma	++ (<1000 ng/mL)	++ (<770 ng/mL)	−	+	+	−	+	−
Choriocarcinoma	−	+++ (>2000 ng/mL)	++	+/−	+	−	−	−
Pinealocytoma	−	−	−	−	−	−	−	+
Pinealoblastoma	−	−	−	−	−	−	−	++
Papillary tumor	−	−	−	−	++	−	−	−

Modified, with additional data, from Rosenblum et al: In Louis DN, Ohgaki H, Wiestler OD, Cavenee WK. *WHO Classification of Tumours of the Central Nervous System.* Lyon: International Agency for Research on Cancer (IARC); 2007.
(Reprinted with permission from Ellenbogen RG, Abdulrauf SI and Sekhar LN. Principles of Neurological Surgery. 3rd ed. Elsevier; 2012.)

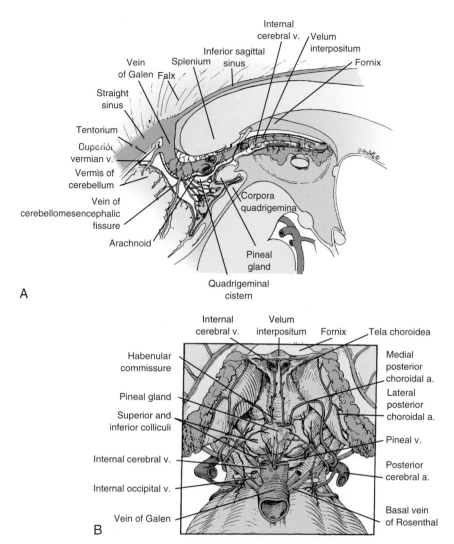

FIGURE 61-2   Sagittal **(A)** and dorsal **(B)** drawings of pineal region anatomy. *(From McComb J, Levy M, Apuzzo M. The posterior intrahemispheric retrocallosal and transcallosal approaches to the third ventricle region. In: Apuzzo M, ed. Surgery of the Third Ventricle. 2nd ed. Baltimore: Williams & Wilkins; 1998:743-777.)*

Surgical Technique

The pineal region can harbor lesions that exhibit a wide range of anatomical extensions. The mass can be below the tentorial apex and midline, extend above and below the tentorium, laterally in either direction, or be mostly encased within the posterior third ventricle. The surgical approach should be tailored to each patient with consideration given to the tumor size, extension, advantages and disadvantages of each approach, and surgeon familiarity.

The infratentorial supracerebellar approach performed in the sitting, prone with neck flexed, or Concorde position provides a good corridor to the pineal region for masses that are midline and below the tentorial apex. Furthermore, the lesion is encountered first when the deep venous system is displaced superiorly and is best for small midline lesions (Figure 61-3). The supratentorial–occipital transtentorial approach is best when the lesion has significant extension below the tentorium or laterally. It can also be used when the torcula is low lying, precluding the infratentorial supracerebellar approach. This approach provides the most extensive view of the pineal region, and tumors extending even to the cerebello-mesencephalic cistern can be accessed. This approach is also performed in the three-quarter prone position to provide gravity retraction to the nondominant hemisphere for assistance with the development of the parafalcine corridor. (Figure 61-4) A posterior transcallosal approach is another option particularly useful if the splenium is invaded by tumor.

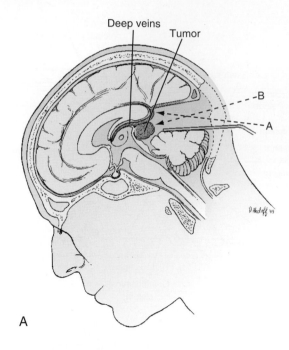

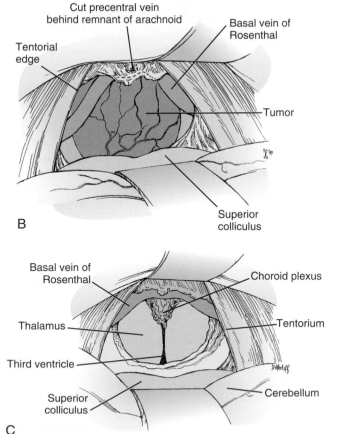

FIGURE 61-3 The infratentorial supracerebellar approach. **(A)** Sagittal diagram showing the initial trajectory, in line with the vein of Galen. After opening the arachnoid over the quadrigeminal plate, the trajectory should be adjusted several degrees downward and in line with the center of the tumor to avoid damage to the deep venous system. **(B)** Diagram of the tumor exposure. **(C)** Diagram of the tumor bed. *(From Bruce J, Stein B. Supracerebellar infratentorial approach. In: Kaye A, Black P, eds.* Operative Neurosurgery. *Vol 1. London: Churchill Livingstone; 2000:815-824.)*

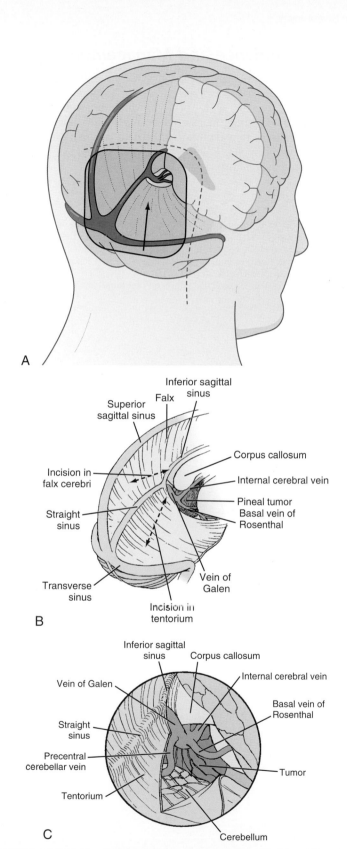

FIGURE 61-4 **(A)** The occipital transtentorial approach, showing the trajectory of the approach, skin incision, and position of craniotomy. *(Modified from Day JD, Koos WT, Matula C, Lang J, eds.* Color Atlas of Microneurosurgical Approaches. *Stuttgart: Thieme; 1997.)* **(B)** Occipital transtentorial approach showing the exposure of the pineal region that can be expanded by dividing the tentorium and the falx. **(C)** Exposure of the tumor after dividing the tentorium. *(From Rosenfeld J. Supratentorial approaches to pineal tumors. In: Kaye A, Black P, eds.* Operative Neurosurgery. *Vol 1. London: Churchill Livingstone; 2000:825-840.)*

Complication Avoidance and Management

- If the infratentorial supracerebellar approach is taken, minimize the risk of venous embolism with meticulous hemostasis and the use of intraoperative Doppler. However, care must be taken to spare the lateral bridging veins or a venous infarct may ensue. Cerebellar relaxation by opening the cisterna magna should always be considered. For the supratentorial–occipital transtentorial approach, a three-quarter prone position allows the nondominant occipital lobe to retract with the aid of gravity, avoiding any postoperative homonymous hemianopsia.

KEY PAPERS

Farnia B, Allen PK, Brown PD, et al. Clinical outcomes and patterns of failure in pineoblastoma: a 30-year, single-institution retrospective review. *World Neurosurg.* 2014;82(6):1232-1241.

Jakacki RI, Burger PC, Kocak M, et al. Outcome and prognostic factors for children with supratentorial primitive neuroectodermal tumors treated with carboplatin during radiotherapy: a report from the children's oncology group. *Pediatr Blood Cancer.* 2015;doi:10.1002/pbc.25405.

Mori Y, Kobayashi T, Hasegawa T, et al. Stereotactic radiosurgery for pineal and related tumors. *Prog Neurol Surg.* 2009;23(1):106-118.

Case 62

Myelomeningocele

Alexa Smith, MD ● Bond Nguyen ● Michael L. Levy, MD, PhD

Presentation

After routine prenatal ultrasound reveals a fetus has an anomaly of the lower back, a fetal MRI is performed. The radiologist concludes with a myelomeningocele and the mother and father are referred for a prenatal consultation and discussion of the MRI results.

Differential Diagnosis

- Myelomeningocele
- Sacral agenesis

Initial Imaging

- Prenatal MRI

Imaging Description and Differential

- Open neural tube defect
- Closed neural tube defect

Further Workup

- Once the baby is delivered via C-section, an ultrasound
- Pediatric specialists to evaluate swallowing, respiration and rule out lethal cardiac or renal anomalies that can be associated with Chiari II.

Pathophysiology

Myelomeningocele is the most severe form of spina bifida. The disorder is caused by failure of the neural tube to close, resulting in a lesion where the spinal cord and meninges are exposed on the back of the newborn. Myelomeningoceles occur in approximately 1 in 4000 births, with probability further reduced by supplementation of folic acid by the mother. Nearly exclusive to the formation of myelomeningocele is the Chiari II structural malformation. The Chiari II malformation is characterized by the extension of cerebellar and brainstem tissue into the spinal canal through the foramen magnum. The severity of the symptoms of myelomeningocele vary from case to case.

Clinical Features

- Partial or complete paralysis of the legs from damage to the spinal cord; partial or complete sensation in the legs may result

- Loss of bladder or bowel control due to spinal cord damage is common.
- Symptoms of raised intracranial pressure or hydrocephalus (headache, nausea, vomiting, increased head circumference)

Treatment Options

Surgery is the only treatment option. There has been debate surrounding prenatal versus postnatal surgical timing, although better outcomes with prenatal surgery have been shown. However, this approach also carries an increased risk for complication.

Surgical Technique

The patient is intubated and sedated by a pediatric anesthesiologist. Because the closure is generally performed within 24 hours of birth, hemostasis is extremely important as blood volume is low. Either a 15 blade scalpel or a Colorado bovie tip is used to perform the initial dissection of the edge of the neural placode from the dural edge. Once the initial layer is dissected, a 5-0 Prolene suture can be used to reapproximate the neural tube in an interrupted fashion. The normal skin edges (Figures 62-1, 62-2, 62-3, and 62-4) can then be further separated from the elements of the placode with the 11 blade and then closed using resorbable suture in an interrupted or running fashion.

Complication Avoidance and Management

- Delay in surgery can lead to further issues of infection; therefore operate as soon as reasonably possible (within 24 hrs) regardless of rupture status. Given that the skin is open, antibiotic prophylaxis is key. Additionally, keep the placode moist and the patient prone prior to surgery. The theory of latex allergy is not a true allergy and concern over future allergy development, given the use of gloves for catheterization of the bladder, etc., is why latex precautions are taken immediately.

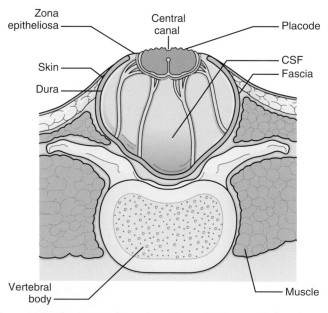

FIGURE 62-1   Cross-sectional anatomy of a myelomeningocele. The neural placode is visible on the back, usually at the center of the sac. It is separated from the full thickness skin by a fringe of pearly tissue, called the "zona epitheliosa." The neural tissue herniates through a defect in the skin, fascia, muscle, and bone. The dorsal dura and zona epitheliosa converge to attach laterally to the placode, forming the roof of the sac. *(Reprinted with permission from Ellenbogen RG, Abdulrauf SI, and Sekhar LN. Principles of Neurological Surgery. 3rd ed. Elsevier; 2012.)*

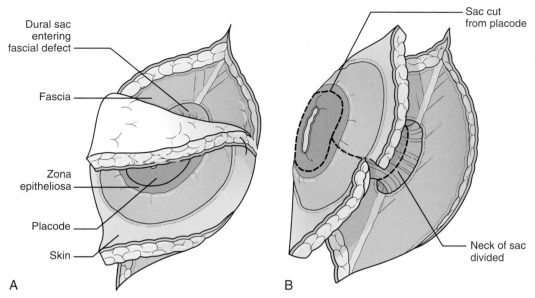

FIGURE 62-2   **(A)** Mobilizing the sac. The skin is undermined medially until the dural sac is seen to enter the fascial defect. **(B)** Excising the fringe of skin surrounding the placode. A radial cut is used to enter the sac and is continued around the placode to excise the skin. A separate circumferential cut amputates the base of the sac. *(Reprinted with permission from Ellenbogen RG, Abdulrauf SI, and Sekhar LN.* Principles of Neurological Surgery. *3rd ed. Elsevier; 2012.)*

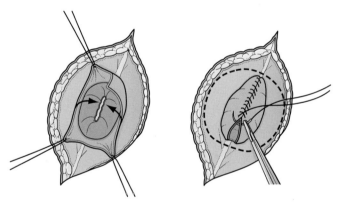

FIGURE 62-3   Mobilizing and closing the dura. The dura is undermined and closed using a continuous 4-0 nonabsorbable suture. *(Reprinted with permission from Ellenbogen RG, Abdulrauf SI, and Sekhar LN.* Principles of Neurological Surgery. *3rd ed. Elsevier; 2012.)*

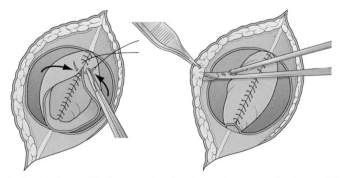

FIGURE 62-4   The fascial closure. The fascia is closed with a continuous stitch. The caudal end of the repair may be incomplete. Skin is mobilized by blunt dissection with scissors or a finger. *(Reprinted with permission from Ellenbogen RG, Abdulrauf SI, and Sekhar LN.* Principles of Neurological Surgery. *3rd ed. Elsevier; 2012.)*

- Monitor for hydrocephalous postoperatively.
- Longterm complications include: syringomyelia, tethering (spasticity, scoliosis and urinary problems) and shunt failure.

KEY PAPERS

Marreiros H, Loff C, Calado E. Who needs surgery for pediatric myelomeningocele? A retrospective study and literature review. *J Spinal Cord Med*. 2015;38(5):626-640.

Meuli M, Moehrlen U. Fetal surgery for myelomeningocele: a critical appraisal. *Eur J Pediatr Surg*. 2013;23(2):103-109. doi:10.1055/s-0033-1343082; [Epub 2013 Apr 9].

Case 63

Cerebellar Medulloblastoma

Michael L. Levy, MD, PhD ● John R. Crawford, MD, PhD ●
Alexa Smith, MD

Presentation

A 4-year-old girl arrived in the emergency room with a history of nausea and emesis for the past 2 months. Her pediatrician had initially thought her nausea and emesis was as a result of aggravated gastroesophageal reflux disease (GERD), which was in her family history. However, over the past 2 weeks, she has had more prominent gait ataxia. She had never complained of headaches.

- PMH: GERD
- Exam:
  - Alert and oriented to self, situation, and location
  - CN II-XII grossly intact
  - No sun-setting of her eyes
  - Strength 5/5 throughout
  - Sensation to light touch normal throughout
  - Coordination revealed bilateral dysmetria with mild ataxia on tandem straight line gait examination

Differential Diagnosis

- Neoplastic
  - Medulloblastoma
  - Ependymoma
  - Astrocytoma (juvenile pilocytic astrocytoma or a high-grade glioma)
  - Atypical teratoid rhabdoid tumor (ATRT)
- Vascular
  - AVM
- Infectious
  - Cerebellar abscess
- Other
  - GERD episode exacerbation

Initial Imaging

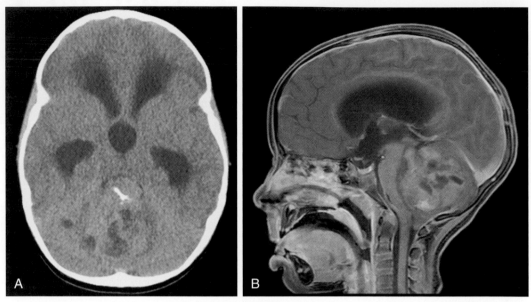

FIGURE 63-1

Imaging Description and Differential

Figure 63-1A shows a large heterogeneous mass in the posterior fossa, centrally located with areas of calcification and a predominantly solid appearance with some cystic areas. This leads to obstructive hydrocephalus with dilation of the lateral and third ventricles, and transependymal flow of CSF. Basal cisterns and the fourth ventricle are effaced.

Figure 63-1B shows a large heterogeneously enhancing T2 hyperintense, T1 hypointense cystic mass with restricted diffusion occupying the entirety of the fourth ventricle, causing obstructive hydrocephalus with transependymal flow and inferior herniation of the cerebellar tonsils. Multiple cerebellar satellite lesions are compatible with metastases. Note the absence of tumor components below the foramen magnum, which would also be consistent with ependymoma.

The MRI features of medulloblastoma are diverse, but generally include DWI positivity and heterogeneous and/or homogeneous enhancement. Medulloblastoma, because of its location, can be associated with obstructive hydrocephalus and in up to 10%–25% of cases can have leptomeningeal dissemination.

Further Workup

- Laboratory
  - Routine laboratory analysis
  - CSF: glucose, protein, and cytology (generally obtained 7 days postoperatively, via lumbar puncture)
- Imaging
  - MRI entire brain and spine, with and without contrast to check for drop metastases
- Consultants
  - PICU – if ventriculostomy needs to be placed, ICU admission is also necessary for frequency of neuro checks, which is every hour in the immediate pre- and postoperative period.
  - Neuro-oncology – to initiate a team-directed approach for care, and to coordinate care pre- and postoperatively for complementary modalities of treatment

TABLE 63-1

CHANG'S STAGING OF MEDULLOBLASTOMA WITH METASTATIC STAGE (M SYSTEM)

T1	Tumor <3 cm in diameter
T2	Tumor ≥3 cm in diameter
T3a	Tumor >3 cm in diameter with extension
T3b	Tumor >3 cm in diameter with unequivocal extension into the brainstem
T4	Tumor >3 cm in diameter with extension past the aqueduct of Sylvius and/or down past the foramen magnum (i.e., beyond the posterior fossa)
M0	No evidence of subarachnoid or hematogenous metastasis
M1	Tumor cells found in cerebrospinal fluid
M2	Intracranial tumor beyond primary site
M3	Gross nodular seeding in spinal subarachnoid space
M4	Metastasis outside the cerebrospinal axis (especially to bone marrow and bone)

Pathophysiology

Medulloblastoma is the most common malignant tumor during childhood. While the incidence of pediatric brain tumors is 4.88 per 100,000 person-years, medulloblastoma is the most common malignant type. Medulloblastoma is derived from cells of the external granular cell layer and can be classified into four molecular subgroups based on gene expression data: wingless (WNT), sonic hedgehog (SHH), group C, and group D.

Medulloblastoma is a WHO grade 4 tumor and is histologically composed of classic, large cell, anaplastic, and nodular desmoplastic features. The nodular desmoplastic are generally SHH-driven tumors and are seen in both younger and older patients in a bimodal age distribution.

Chang's staging of medulloblastoma, with regards to metastatic stage (M system), is summarized in Table 63-1.

Standard-risk medulloblastoma, previously defined as >3 years of age, classic pathology, <1.5 cm^2 of residual, and no dissemination at diagnosis, was associated with survivals of >80%–85% with standard chemotherapy and radiation treatments. However, we now know that the molecular underpinnings of the tumor, as described above, are what determine survival.

The treatment for both newly diagnosed and recurrent medulloblastoma is not uniform and is dependent on patient age, degree of spread, and availability of clinical trials.

Treatment Options

- Medical
  - Decadron preoperatively can improve the patient's nausea and vomiting. It is important to remember GI prophylaxis and glucose checks during administration of steroid.
- Biopsy
  - Not necessary as full surgery indicated and once craniotomy and exposure performed, resection of mass should be attempted given that extent of resection is an important variable in determining subsequent treatment and outcome.
- Adjuvant therapy (radiation and/or chemotherapy)
  - Craniospinal radiation and adjuvant chemotherapy are the therapies of choice for patients older than 5 years. Alternative treatment strategies are currently being used to delay radiation therapy in children younger than 5 years due to the associated neurocognitive effects. Additionally, new approaches are being used to risk stratify patients based on molecular subgroups. Cranial radiation can also be utilized as necessary, after surgical resection, for any metastases or remaining tumor in the resection cavity that is not amenable to further surgery. Both photon and proton beam irradiation therapy are used in the treatment of childhood medulloblastoma.

- Surgical
  - External ventricular drain if indicated
  - Posterior fossa craniotomy for resection of tumor
  - Consideration of "second-look" surgery if >1.5 cm^2 of residual noted on postoperative imaging

Surgical Technique

The head of the bed is rotated 180 degrees away from the anesthesia team. The patient's head is placed in a Mayfield head holder at a weight appropriate for the size/age of the patient. All appropriate pressure points should be padded as the patient is placed in a three-quarter lateral position. It is our preference to place the majority of patients with the right side of the body facing upward. Tumor lateralization into the "gutter" or within the fourth ventricular chamber may modify the need to place the patient left side up. The patient's head is significantly flexed and then angled in 30 to 45 degrees regard to the floor. We attempt to keep the base of the Mayfield pin head holder parallel with the floor so as to facilitate the utilization of Mayfield-based retraction systems. Stereotactic registration should be performed and good accuracy ensured at this time.

Colorado tip monopolar cautery is used in cutting mode to make the initial scalp incision to a depth of approximately 1 mm. The Colorado tip cautery is then used to take the incision down to the underlying bone in coagulation mode. Cerebellar self-retaining retractors are then placed and the operating microscope brought into the field. We performed a C1 laminectomy in this case, utilizing the craniotome to maximize the angle of access into the fourth ventricle. Burr hole placement, followed by the use of rongeur forceps, is also a viable technique. The suboccipital craniotomy should be performed using a craniotome running from the foramen magnum superiorly and ending inferiorly to the inion and likely to the location of the torcula. In our experience, the height of the craniotomy is not as important as maximizing the width at the foramen magnum and above. It should be noted that this approach will open the cisterna magna and maximize one's view of the fourth ventricular chamber and lateral gutters, allowing for visualization up to the aqueduct. This approach additionally minimizes retraction/resection of the cerebellar vermis and minimizes the potential for postoperative mutism.

The dura should be opened sharply with an 11 blade scalpel in a Y configuration. The dural leaflets should be retracted and secured with 4-0 Nurolon. The cerebellar hemispheres should be dissected in the midline. Tumor is usually immediately encountered. Self-retaining retractor blades can then be placed to elevate the inferior edges of the cerebellar hemispheres, and dissection of the tumor using suction and bipolar cautery can be performed. We prefer to use variable action, Fukushima-type suction for these cases. Care should be taken to maintain hemostasis while detaching the small feeding vessels with microscissors from the tumor periphery. Tumor should be biopsied at this point and a specimen sent for frozen and permanent examination by the neuropathologist.

Debulking of the tumor can be performed using surgical microscissors, biopsy forceps, and ultrasonic aspiration. The floor of the fourth ventricle can be encountered at any point during surgery and most often when the majority of the tumor is resected. It is our preference to identify the floor very early in our resection and protect it with cotton surgical paddies. The floor may be smooth or irregular if it has been invaded by tumor. It is rare to find tumor invasion of the floor at the time of initial surgery. In subsequent surgeries, should tumor invasion of the floor be noted, consideration of the anatomy and potential complications should be considered prior to progressing to resection.

Attention should then be turned laterally to the gutters to confirm the absence of any residual tumor. The lateral gutters will frequently harbor residual tumor, even if this is not apparent on preoperative contrast-enhanced imaging studies. Additionally, evaluating tissue planes below the retractor blades should be performed at this time.

Once resection is completed, irrigation of the tumor resection cavity with copious amounts of irrigant is followed by lining the resection cavity with Surgicel fibrillar to maximize hemostasis prior to closing the dura. A dural graft and fibrin glue can be used to augment the duraplasty as needed. The bone flap should be replaced using absorbable or nonabsorbable plates and screws. The paraspinal muscles and galea should be closed in the usual fashion with Vicryl and the skin closed with either a permanent suture or a subcuticular Monocryl suture, followed by skin glue based on the surgeon's preference. The patient's head should be taken out of the Mayfield head holder at this time and a sterile dressing applied.

Complication Avoidance and Management

- Of importance in children, intraoperative blood loss must be controlled and monitored closely with careful attention to hemostasis throughout the procedure. Usually tumor ooze and bleeding will decrease as more tumor is resected. As was previously noted, careful examination of the gutters to avoid residual tumor is also important. Avoiding injury to the floor of the fourth ventricle is also of key importance, as injury of the facial colliculus can result in a permanent injury to either unilateral or bilateral CN VII function. Additionally, such injuries can result in paresis/plegia. Significant injury resulting in aberrant extraocular movement can occur from injury to the MLF or PPRF. Be very aware that manipulation of the tumor causes traction on the floor when invasion is present. Aggressive vermian manipulation and/or resection should be avoided to minimize the incidence of postoperative mutism. Obviously, PICA branches can be in close proximity. Strict attention should be paid to the closure with either a primary watertight closure or a graft and dural fibrin glue, as needed, to minimize postoperative CSF leaks. Additionally, the skin may be closed with an absorbable suture, such as Monocryl or chromic, and covered with Dermabond. However, as previously noted, if CSF leakage is a concern, a permanent suture such as Prolene or nylon should be used. Temporary ventriculostomy placement is often helpful for larger tumors but must be judiciously used so as to prevent upwards herniation.

KEY PAPERS

Crawford JR, MacDonald TJ, Packer RJ. Medulloblastoma in childhood: new biological advances. *Lancet Neurol.* 2007;6:1073-1085.

DeSouza RM, Jones BR, Lowis SP, et al. Pediatric medulloblastoma – update on molecular classification driving targeted therapies. *Front Oncol.* 2014;4:176.

Kool M, Korshunov A, Remke M, et al. Molecular subgroups of medulloblastoma: an international meta-analysis of transcriptome, genetic aberrations, and clinical data of WNT, SHH, Group 3, and Group 4 medulloblastomas. *Acta Neuropathol.* 2012;12:473-484.

Case 64

Brainstem Glioma

Michael L. Levy, MD, PhD ● John R. Crawford, MD, PhD ●
Alexa Smith, MD ● Salman Abbasifard, MD

Presentation

An 8-year-old boy experiences several weeks of difficulty playing. Upon closer history taking, he also complains of difficulty watching TV, with the picture becoming "blurry." His mother has also noticed that his eyes "don't seem together." He has had nausea for the past 3 days and has complained of a severe headache today. His mother brought him to the ER because the pediatrician's office is closed Saturdays. The ER obtained a CT scan showing a mixed density irregular mass in his brainstem.

Differential Diagnosis

- Brainstem glioma, which is a subtype of astrocytoma; histopathology usually reveals fibrillary and pilocytic types of astrocytomas
- Cavernoma
- Metastases (rare)
- Transverse myelitis

Initial Imaging

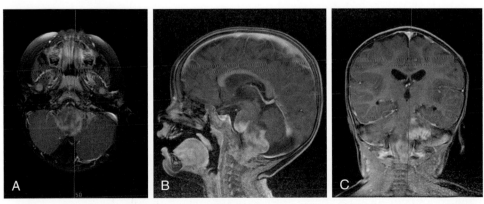

FIGURE 64-1

Imaging Description and Differential

MRI – cysts may be seen with either the high- or low-grade forms; necrosis and hemorrhage within the mass can be noted in later stages and in malignant forms.

MRA or CTA can be useful to rule out a cavernoma, and attention must be paid to determine if the tumor is diffuse or focal. Diffuse intrinsic pontine gliomas spread widely throughout the brainstem. A focal tumor could potentially be low grade and more amenable to a resection as opposed to solely a biopsy.

Further Workup

Biopsy – if an exophytic component is present that is safe to biopsy (usually only in a focal glioma); diffuse intrinsic pontine gliomas are generally not biopsied

CSF – protein may be elevated; be cautious during a lumbar puncture as hydrocephalus is generally present

Pathophysiology

Most of the astrocytomas in this location are grade 3 or 4, and even grade 2 grow rapidly. Molecular analysis may aid in treatment and it is therefore important to obtain tissue if it is safe to do so.

Treatment Options

Given location of tumor, surgery is not usually an option as vital functions, including wakefulness and breathing control, are in this location. Radiation is most effective and the most common initial treatment therapy. This is typically done over a 6-week period. Standard agent chemotherapy or experimental drugs can be used to complement the treatment and attempt to control tumor growth. "Radiosensitizers" are drugs that make tumor cells more sensitive to radiation therapy and can be used. Molecular analysis of the tumor has been used to link the particular profile of a specific patient's tumor to target the specific aberrations found in that tumor. For example, the Pacific Pediatric Neuro-Oncology Consortium opened such a trial in 2013. If a biopsy reveals a grade 1 brainstem glioma, a more aggressive resection in the OR can be attempted and control with radiation therapy for the remainder can be effective.

Surgical Technique

Biopsy may be attempted to confirm diagnosis, obtain tissue for specialized chemotherapy protocols unique to each patient, and assist in making the patient eligible for clinical trials that may be available. The patient can be placed in a prone or three-quarter lateral position. Stereotactic image guidance registration should be performed because the anatomy is severely distorted in these cases. Standard anatomic landmarks cannot be trusted. A small suboccipital craniotomy and C1 laminectomy can be performed in standard fashion. The dura should be opened under the microscope as neovascularization may occur with these tumors. A judicious biopsy should be performed with micro biopsy forceps. We prefer to take biopsies from the junction of the cerebellar peduncle and the lateral and superior most aspect of the adjacent fourth ventricle. In our experience, this approach has minimized complications.

Discussion in advance with the neuro-oncologist and pathologist should determine how much specimen is necessary and the preferred method of it being managed from the operating room en route to the pathology laboratory. As the specimen here is usually not a large amount, a permanent specimen may be preferred over using tissue for a frozen specimen. The need for a diagnosis based upon frozen sections to verify the presence of tumor must be determined based upon the quantity of tissue obtained and the amount required for permanent section.

The dura should be reapproximated in a watertight fashion and supplemented with a graft and fibrin glue if necessary. As these patients frequently have aggressive chemotherapy and radiation protocols, attention to keeping CSF from forming a pseudomeningocele, fistula, or wound dehiscence is extremely important. Fascia and skin should be closed in standard fashion with consideration of nonabsorbable sutures or staples for closure.

The patient should be extubated in the OR, if possible, to determine if any deficits are present that have been aggravated by or are resultant from surgery that would require rapid reintubation. Admission to the ICU overnight should be considered for hourly vitals, neurologic examinations, and further assessment of any changes noted immediately following surgery.

Complication Avoidance and Management

- Counseling regarding the dangers of biopsy should be explained very carefully to the patient's family and that surgical cure is not the goal. At times, if hydrocephalus is the issue, a ventriculoperitoneal shunt or endoscopic third ventriculostomy should be offered to ameliorate symptoms and allow for improved quality of life.

KEY PAPERS

Bouffet E, Hargrave D, Baruchel S. Clinical trials for brainstem glioma patients (BGS): critical review of statistical endpoints and results. *Neuro Oncol*. 2003;5:29.

Grimm SA, Chamberlain MC. Brainstem glioma: a review. *Curr Neurol Neurosci Rep*. 2013;13(5):346.

Hargrave D, Bartels U, Bouffet E. Diffuse brainstem glioma in children: critical review of clinical trials. *Lancet Oncol*. 2006;7(3):241-248.

Sun T, Wan W, Wu Z, et al. Clinical outcomes and natural history of pediatric brainstem tumors: with 33 cases follow-ups. *Neurosurg Rev*. 2013;36(2):311-319, discussion 319-320.

Case 65

Hypothalamic Hamartoma

Michael L. Levy, MD, PhD ● John R. Crawford, MD, PhD ●
Alexa Smith, MD ● Salman Abbasifard, MD

Presentation

A 10-year-old girl is referred for precocious puberty workup. Her mother notices that she has become inappropriate in her laughter and has had difficulty passing her classes. She formerly was a top student and a quiet child. The mother is not sure if she has ever had seizures, but she has an appointment with a pediatric neurologist in 3 months.

Differential Diagnosis

- Optic glioma
- Hypothalamic glioma
- Suprasellar germ cell tumors
- Craniopharyngioma

Initial Imaging

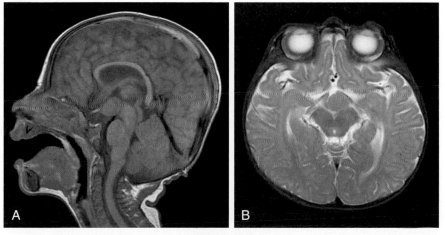

FIGURE 65-1

Precontrast MRI reveals a large isointense suprasellar mass in close proximity to the optic chiasm/nerve. A posterior pituitary bright spot is observed. Axial T2-weighted sequence reveals the hypothalamic location.

Imaging Description and Differential

The neuroradiographic differential includes a low-grade glioma, hypothalamic hamartoma (HH), and germ cell tumor (pure germinoma versus nongerminomatous germ cell tumor).

Further Workup

EEG to confirm the presence of gelastic seizures, which would be typical of HH

Pathophysiology

HHs are a rare, benign tumor type that only affect approximately 1 in 200,000 people. Symptoms can include: seizures, precocious puberty, hormone imbalances, cognitive impairment, and behavioral and emotional problems. Gelastic or laughing seizures usually begin in infancy and may be difficult to distinguish from normal laughter at their onset. Seizure may evolve into complex partial, generalized, or drop seizures. Tantrums, rage attacks, and social isolation may ensue.

Treatment Options

- Surgery – transcallosal approach or orbitozygomatic craniotomies; endoscopic surgery may be possible
- Gamma knife stereotactic radiosurgery may be effective.

Surgical Technique

The patient is placed in the supine position in Mayfield three-point fixation with the head in either the neutral position or slightly rotated to the contralateral side about 20 to 30 degrees. Preferably, a right-sided approach is chosen. Stereotactic registration should be performed and good accuracy ensured. The skin incision is usually semi-arcuate, running from within the hairline, 2–3 cm lateral of the midline, to a point slightly above the anterior border of the ear. It therefore runs parallel to a portion of the coronal suture and ends at the sphenofrontal suture. Scalp incision using Colorado tip monopolar cautery should be created.

The craniotomy should be performed using a craniotome. The flap is centered on the coronal suture and can be oriented slightly more anterior or posterior, depending on the location of pathology. The dura is opened in a horseshoe fashion with its base on the sagittal sinus. Cortical veins draining into the sinus should be protected. The arachnoid is incised, allowing visualization of both cingulate gyri. The paired callosomarginal arteries must be identified, coursing superficial to the cingulate gyrus, and must be protected. The cingulate gyri, which are often adhered, are separated; the very white corpus callosum, overlying the paired pericallosal arteries, is visualized. The midline interhemispheric approach is performed with a small corpus callosotomy just behind the genu. A midline transseptal dissection, an interforniceal approach between the uppermost section of the columns before they converge to form the arches of the fornix, is next. Entering the anterior end of the roof of the third ventricle, remove the hamartoma using the long, curved, microtip of the ultrasonic aspirator. The consistency of the HH is tougher than normal cerebral tissue, slightly brown in color, relatively avascular, and can usually be differentiated from the surrounding normal cerebral tissue. The perforating arteries from the basilar apex demarcate the posterior limit of the dissection and, for some large HH, the optic chiasm demarcates the most anterior extent of the resection. Frameless stereotactic navigation is helpful in choosing the ideal trajectory and defining the margins for resection. Closure is done in a standard fashion with a watertight closure of the dura, followed by replacement of the bone flap. Scalp is closed in a two-layered fashion, and the skin is reapproximated.

Patient's head should be taken out of the Mayfield head holder and a sterile dressing applied.

Complication Avoidance and Management

- Concern regarding seizure control is the goal. The main surgical complications are related to hypothalamic disturbance. Total resection can be difficult because preserving the normal hypothalamus is important. Radiosurgery can be challenging, so close to the optic nerve. It can take 2 to 3 years to control symptoms completely, but seizure activity can decrease in months.

KEY PAPERS

Mittal S, Mittal M, Montes JL, et al. Hypothalamic hamartomas. Part 1. Clinical, neuroimaging, and neurophysiological characteristics. *Neurosurg Focus*. 2013;34(6):E6.

Mittal S, Mittal M, Montes JL, et al. Hypothalamic hamartomas. Part 2. Surgical considerations and outcome. *Neurosurg Focus*. 2013;34(6):E7.

Pati S, Sollman M, Fife TD, et al. Diagnosis and management of epilepsy associated with hypothalamic hamartoma: an evidence-based systematic review. *J Child Neurol*. 2013;28(7):909-916.

Wait SD, Abla AA, Killory BD, et al. Surgical approaches to hypothalamic hamartomas. *Neurosurg Focus*. 2011;30(2):E2.

Case 66

Endoscopic Third Ventriculostomy

Michael L. Levy, MD, PhD ● John R. Crawford, MD, PhD ●
Alexa Smith, MD ● Salman Abbasifard, MD ●
Ali H. A. Muhammad Altameemi, MD

Presentation

The patient is a 4-year-old male with no significant past medical or surgical history who presented to the emergency department with progressive ataxia and eye movement abnormalities. The child reportedly had become progressively ataxic over the past few weeks. Approximately 1 week prior, the child had a mild head injury at which time he was noted to have internal deviation of the left eye, potentially consistent with a sixth nerve palsy. On ophthalmologic exam, the extraocular movement abnormalities were verified and bilateral papilledema was noted. CT of the head documented marked hydrocephalus, possibly as a result of an aqueductal stenosis.

- PMH: otherwise unremarkable
- Review of systems: positive for visual disturbance; negative for nausea and vomiting
- Exam:
  - Alert
  - Head circumference well above the ninety-fifth percentile; it was 38 cm at birth (around the ninetieth percentile)
  - Gait ataxic
  - No other significant findings noted

Differential Diagnosis

- Familial
  - Macrocephaly with normal-sized ventricles
  - No underlying cause
- Pathological macrocephaly
  - Macrocephaly and hydrocephalus
    - Obstructive (e.g., tumor, aqueduct stenosis)
    - Communicating (e.g., perinatal hemorrhage, meningitis)
  - Macrocephaly without hydrocephalus
    - A large space-occupying lesion:
      - Arachnoid cyst
      - Tumor
      - Subdural hematoma, chronic subdural hematoma, and subdural effusion
    - Neurocutaneous syndromes (most commonly neurofibromatosis)
    - Increased volume of brain tissue (megalencephaly)
    - Venous hypertension due to a large arteriovenous malformation; may cause macrocephaly
    - Genetic conditions including autism and PTEN mutations (e.g., Cowden disease, fragile X syndrome, glutaric aciduria type 1, and D-2-hydroxyglutaric aciduria)

- Metabolic causes, including the endocrinopathies of hypoparathyroidism and adrenal insufficiency, megaloencephalic leukoencephalopathy, Alexander's disease, and Canavan's disease
- Overgrowth syndromes, including Soto's syndrome, Weaver's syndrome, Simpson-Golabi-Behmel's syndrome, and macrocephaly-capillary malformation (M-CMTC) syndrome
- Cranial hyperostosis
- Tuberous sclerosis
- Neurocardiofacial – cutaneous syndromes including Noonan's syndrome, Costello's syndrome, and cardiofaciocutaneous syndrome

Initial Imaging

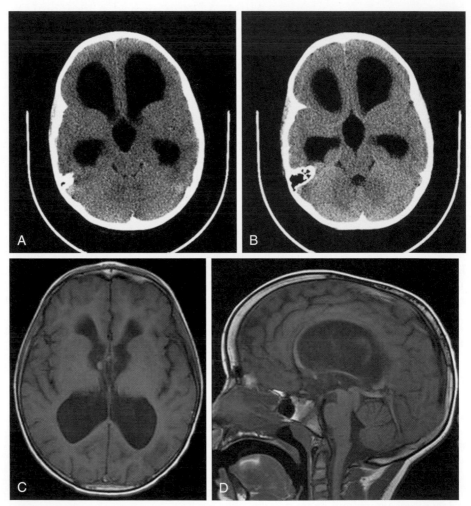

FIGURE 66-1

Imaging Description and Differential

Figure 66-1 A and B depict a CT of the brain without contrast, demonstrating marked dilation of the lateral ventricles; however, the fourth ventricle is small. Therefore this is a noncommunicating hydrocephalus with an obstruction either in the third ventricle or between the third and fourth ventricles. Obstruction in the third ventricle would most commonly be a tumor. Obstruction between the third and fourth ventricles could also be a tumor in the pineal region or aqueduct stenosis. The reformatted CT clearly shows the enlarged third and the small fourth ventricles. The pineal region is seen clearly and appears normal. The cerebral aqueduct is not seen clearly at all, and therefore the diagnosis is aqueduct stenosis. (Images courtesy of Dr. Michael Levy.)

Figure 66-1 C and D show MRI of the brain without contrast in a patient with a known aqueductal stenosis status post ETV with a decrease in size of the lateral and third ventricles. Redemonstration of stably marked third and bilateral or lateral ventriculomegaly. Flow through the reported endoscopic third ventriculostomy is seen. Stable fullness of the dorsal midbrain, tectum, and superior and inferior colliculi; left greater than right, with marked narrowing of the Sylvian aqueduct. This may represent a hamartoma or a low-grade glioma. (Images courtesy of Dr. Michael Levy.)

Further Workup

- Laboratory
  - Routine labs
  - ESR, CRP
- Imaging
  - If there is doubt about the underlying cause of the hydrocephalus, an MRI should be performed to better identify the aqueductal anatomy, the tectum (for potential benign neoplasms), and the presence of transependymal edema. Additionally, a Cine MRI flow study can be performed to assess flow through the aqueduct.
- Consultants
  - Pediatrics
  - Genetics
  - Oncology
  - Ophthalmology

Pathophysiology

Pediatric hydrocephalus represents a mismatch in normal cerebral spinal fluid production and reabsorption. One variant is the presence of choroid plexus hypertrophy, which results in an increased production of CSF and progressive hydrocephalus. In children, the normal CSF formation rate is about 20 mL/hour or 500 mL/day. Any failure to reabsorb 100% of the produced fluid results in a discrepancy and progressive accumulation of CSF. The symptoms in hydrocephalic children can be acute or progressive in nature. In compensated hydrocephalics, symptoms may take years and minimal to no symptoms may be present at the time of diagnosis. In the acute scenario, it is considered to be a neurosurgical emergency, which if left untreated, can rapidly lead to brain herniation and death. Infants can tolerate an increase in CSF volume more than adults because of the nonunion of cranial sutures; the head enlarges, causing macrocephaly, a common symptom of hydrocephalus among infants. Hydrocephalus can be classified as obstructive or communicating; the former results from obstruction of CSF flow within the ventricular system and the latter from obstruction at the arachnoid villi. In obstructive hydrocephalus the ventricles proximal to the obstruction will be dilated, whereas those distal will be relatively small.

Treatment Options

- Surgical
  - Endoscopic third ventriculostomy
  - Shunting

Surgical Technique

- This patient was treated by endoscopic third ventriculostomy: supine position with the head flexed, ranging from a 0- to 30-degree angle, to facilitate CSF flow and minimize risk of trapped air (Figure 66-2A).

- A 6–10 mm burr hole is made slightly anterior to the coronal suture and at the level of the midpupillary line.
- The dura mater is coagulated and opened with a no. 11 blade, or with Colorado monopolar cautery (Figure 66-2 B).
- A tract is created and the lateral ventricle is tapped using a ventricular catheter; CSF is collected at this time for analysis.
- There are two main approaches for endoscope placement at this juncture:
  - Approach one:
    - A 14F peel-away sheath is slightly pulled apart and a ring of bone wax is applied at the 3–5 cm mark, depending on age and degree of ventriculomegaly.
    - The peel-away sheath is then placed into the frontal horn of the lateral ventricle.
    - After introduction of the peel-away sheath into the frontal horn of the lateral ventricle, the bone wax ring will seal the burr hole; peel-away sheath serves as the working channel for the endoscope.
  - Approach two:
    - Rather than placement of a peel-away sheath, we prefer to follow the tract created by the ventricular catheter into the frontal horn; this avoids the utilization of the sheath and the significant increase in diameter when compared with the ventricular catheter.
    - Irrigation through the endoscope is initiated and allows for the direct dilation of the catheter tract, under constant visualization by the endoscope, as the endoscope is passed into the lateral ventricle.
- The 0-degree angle endoscope is introduced into the lateral ventricle. In some scenarios it may be important to introduce the endoscope promptly to avoid rapid egress of CSF and partial collapse of the ventricular system. The surgeon then visualizes the choroid plexus, which will lead to the foramen of Monroe entering the third ventricle. The floor of the third ventricle will appear in faint bluish color; the infundibular recess and the mammillary bodies will be visible. The tip of the basilar artery, and sometimes perforators, can be visualized through the ventricular floor (Figure 66-2 C and D).
- There are numerous modalities that can be utilized to fenestrate the floor at this juncture. Using the stiff end of the guidewire, or the catheter tip, the floor of the third ventricle can be fenestrated anterior to the mammillary bodies. This methodology is the most common and preferred scenario where the floor is transparent and/or the vascular anatomy is well visualized. In the scenario were the floor is opacified, distorted, or the vascular anatomy is difficult to visualize, we prefer a secondary technique. In these cases, microforceps or a microsuction attachment are used to elevate the floor, which is then opened. This minimizes potential for vascular compromise. One should never utilize a monopolar filament while electrified ("hot") to perforate the floor.
- The ventriculostomy is now performed using the balloon catheter. The balloon (Fogarty no. 3) catheter is placed through the ostomy, inflated, and slowly pulled through, resulting in progressive dilation. Uncontrolled inflation of the balloon, inferior to the floor, with risk of vessel injury, should be avoided. Any bleeding at the ostomy site is usually controlled by continued inflation of the balloon and associated tamponade for the course of 1 to 2 minutes. The ventriculostomy should be approximately 5–6 mm in diameter. Failure to produce a significant opening will jeopardize the third ventriculostomy and potentially result in a scenario where the ostomy can heal and become occluded.
- Following fenestration, the endoscope is passed into the prepontine cistern to check for arachnoid membranes, which may be inhibiting CSF flow. If needed, these membranes may be separated with the balloon catheter.
- In a successful procedure, the CSF flow through the ventriculostomy can usually be seen by the flapping of the tissue around the hole. It is counterintuitive, but in most successful scenarios CSF flow will be toward the endoscope with associated initial fogging as a result of turbulent CSF flow. The endoscope and sheath are then removed, the burr hole is filled with absorbable gelatin sponge (Gelfoam), and the scalp is closed in layers (Figure 66-3).

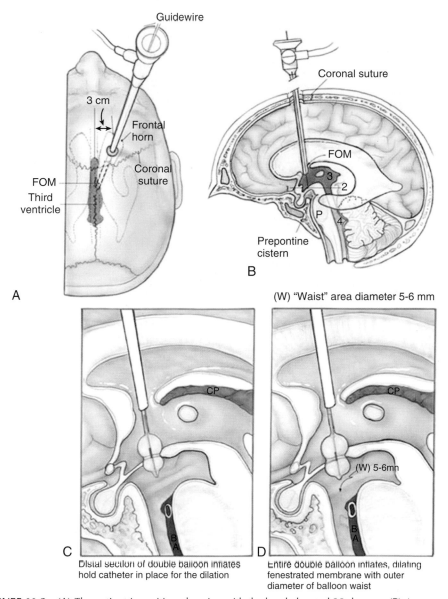

Guidewire

3 cm

Frontal horn

Coronal suture

FOM
Third ventricle

A

Coronal suture

FOM

3
2

P
4

Prepontine cistern

B

(W) "Waist" area diameter 5-6 mm

CP

C

Distal section of double balloon inflates hold catheter in place for the dilation

CP

(W) 5-6mn

D

Entire double balloon inflates, dilating fenestrated membrane with outer diameter of balloon waist

FIGURE 66-2 **(A)** The patient is positioned supine with the head elevated 30 degrees. **(B)** A precoronal skin incision in the midpupillary line and a burr hole are made. Insertion of the peel-away sheath and the endoscope are shown. The choroid plexus (CP) entering the foramen of Monroe (Fom), the thalamostriate, and the septal vein are visualized, guiding the way into the third ventricle. The tip of the basilar artery (BA), the mammillary bodies, and the infundibular recess are shown: 1. infundibular recess; 2. guidewire fenestration. **(C, D)** After perforating the floor of the third ventricle with the guidewire, the balloon catheter is introduced and inflated. In the neuro-double-balloon catheter, the more proximal balloon inflates first. It is gently pushed against the floor of the third ventricle, and then the second balloon is inflated. *P*, pons; *3*, third ventricle; *4*, fourth ventricle. *(Reprinted with permission from Nader R, Gragnaniello C. Neurosurgery Tricks of the Trade: Cranial. Thieme; 2013.)*

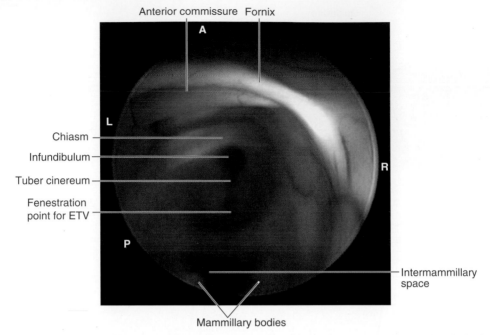

Anterior commissure Fornix

FIGURE 66-3 The floor of the third ventricle is usually attenuated, and the basilar artery may be visualized. The fenestration site should be selected immediately posterior to the infundibular recess. *(Reprinted with permission from Jandial R, et al. Core techniques in Operative Neurosurgery. Elsevier; 2011.)*

Complication Avoidance and Management

- Endoscopic third ventriculostomy
  - The width of the 3rd ventricle should be at least 5mm. Sufficient space between the basilar artery and the clivus should be determined on sagittal preoperative MRIs.
  - Fenestration should be performed at the most transparent portion of the third ventricular floor to minimize the risk of vascular injury.
  - In the scenario of an opacified floor, a distraction technique should be utilized.
  - Always use a blunt instrument for the initial fenestration, instead of cautery or sharp instruments, to minimize the risk to underlying vascular structures that are not directly visualized.
  - Bleeding of any degree can be a significant hindrance and can significantly increase operative time. If hemorrhage is encountered during the procedure, persistent irrigation should be used until the bleeding stops and the CSF clears. If the blood can be cleared through copious irrigation, monopolar or bipolar endoscopic cautery can be used to coagulate the bleeding point.
  - If blood in the CSF compromises visibility and continuous irrigation is not effective, the procedure should be aborted to prevent injury to neurovascular structures that cannot be visualized.
  - If bradycardia occurs and does not respond to stopping irrigation, insert a ventricular catheter or needle to drain CSF.
  - A misplaced fenestration can result in complications, including injury to the hypothalamus, basilar artery, or basilar perforating vessels. If the basilar is perforated, visualization will be lost immediately. The best chance of minimizing complications comes from removing the endoscope and allowing the blood to tamponade the bleeding point prior to angiography. In any scenario of potential injury to the basilar artery, pseudoaneurismal formation must be ruled out. Blind inflation of the Fogarty balloon in the interpeduncular cistern prior to withdrawing the balloon into the third ventricle may inadvertently tear small perforating vessels. It is safer to inflate the balloon with the epicenter at the level of the fenestration.

- Excessive manipulation of the endoscope while in the third ventricle can lead to damage to the structures surrounding the foramen of Monroe, including the fornix, with resultant short-term memory deficits.
- In complicated cases with significant tissue manipulation and/or bleeding, a ventriculostomy catheter can be left in place to allow for postoperative drainage and ICP monitoring.
- Always allow for continuous irrigant outflow from the endoscope, either through the peel-away sheath or endoscope channel itself. Rapid increases in pressure result from aggressive irrigation and can result in bradycardia with associated hypertension. The utilization of aggressive irrigation while minimizing outflow to enlarge the third ventricle is not recommended in our practice.
- Always attempt to determine the site of bleeding (i.e., basilar artery, basilar perforators, ostomy site, choroid plexus, choroidal vein, or parenchymal entrance of endoscope) to allow for the formulation of an appropriate strategy to achieve hemostasis.

KEY PAPERS

Drake JM. Ventriculostomy for the treatment of hydrocephalus. *Neurosurg Clin N Am*. 1993;4:657-666.

Drake JM, Kulkarni AV, Kestle J. Endoscopic third ventriculostomy versus ventriculoperitoneal shunt in pediatric patients: a decision analysis. *Childs Nerv Syst*. 2009;25(4):467-472.

Farin A, Aryan HE, Ozgur BM, et al. Endoscopic third ventriculostomy. *J Clin Neurosci*. 2006;13(7):763-770.

Rekate HL. Selecting patients for endoscopic third ventriculostomy. *Neurosurg Clin N Am*. 2004;15(1):39-49.

Teo C, Jones R. Management of hydrocephalus by endoscopic third ventriculostomy in patients with myelomeningocele. *Pediatr Neurosurg*. 1996;25:57-63.

Case 67

Slit Ventricle Syndrome

Michael L. Levy, MD, PhD ● John R. Crawford, MD, PhD ●
David S. Hong, MD ● Alexa Smith, MD

Presentation

A 12-year-old boy presents to the emergency room with a headache, some intermittent nausea, and not "being himself" today. He has a history of intraventricular hemorrhage as an infant for which he had a ventriculoperitoneal shunt placed at 2 weeks of age. He has a history of seven revisions since that time, including a second shunt placement on the opposite side. A CT scan obtained in the ER shows no difference from a previous CT scan obtained 6 months prior.

Differential Diagnosis

- Slit ventricle syndrome
- Shunt infection
- Headache of other etiology

Initial Imaging

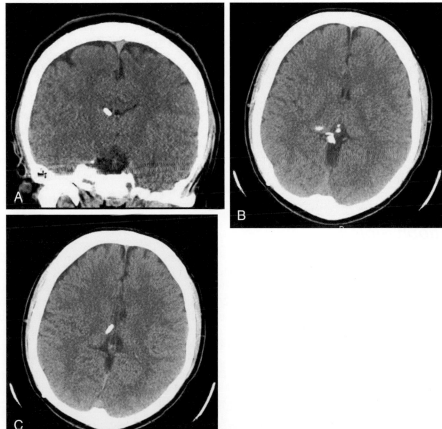

FIGURE 67-1

353

Coronal and axial CT images document slit like ventricles. An occipital originating proximal shunt catheter on the right side is noted to enter the right lateral ventricle.

Imaging Description and Differential

Slit ventricle syndrome describes the CT and/or are the imaging findings of small or "slit-like" ventricles. Of note, most patients with small ventricles on CT or MRI do not have slit ventricle syndrome. They must be symptomatic. Slit ventricle syndrome occurs only in a minority of patients who have been shunted. Diminished elasticity of the ependymal lining of the ventricular chamber, which enlarges either minimally or not at all in the presence of a shunt malfunction and is associated with increased intracranial pressure, is not the same entity. One should not mistake the lack of enlargement of the ventricles on CT and/or MRI at the time of admission as being indicative of a functioning shunt if the patient is symptomatic.

Further Workup

- Labs
  - CBC, ESR, CRP, urinalysis, and blood cultures if febrile to rule out a classic infection; note that the incidence of shunt infection longer than 3 months following shunt surgery is minimal.
- Shunt series
  - X-ray of skull, chest, and abdomen to show no discontinuity at another location in the body of the shunt system
- Shunt tap
  - Sterilely tapping the shunt reservoir with a 25 gauge butterfly needle may yield information regarding the likelihood of either a proximal or distal malfunction and allow one to assess intracranial pressure at that time. Any CSF obtained can be submitted to rule out infection. We utilize either a 1 mL or 3 mL syringe for the shunt tap to maximize the chance of obtaining CSF and not collapsing the ventricle. The inability to obtain CSF from a collapsed ventricle makes it more difficult to determine whether a proximal occlusion is present or not. Smaller syringes allow one to verify patency in the scenario of slit ventricles.
- Shuntogram
  - A nuclear medicine dye study can be performed to verify shunt patency by documenting the movement of CSF for the shunt system. A small amount of radioisotope is injected into the valve reservoir and images are obtained at timed intervals. Though a shuntogram will verify patency of the shunt hardware, it yields little to no information regarding the rate of CSF flow, which is also an important variable in determining shunt function.

Pathophysiology

Although no one is certain of the etiology of slit ventricle syndrome, the proposed mechanism is that of cranial cerebral disproportion. The primary determinants of growth of a child's cranial vault, during approximately the first 20 months following birth, include progressive growth and maturation of the cerebrum, the volume of intracranial cerebral spinal fluid, and the varying intravascular volume. It is believed that the initial diminished volume of CSF during this period of growth, followed by normal increases in CSF production and volume of ventricular chambers and subarachnoid space, results in a calvarial vault that is not of adequate size to hold both the ventricles and CSF. This cranial cerebral disproportion can result in increased intracranial pressure (can become significantly elevated) that is associated with headaches and other symptoms that mimic shunt malfunction. The "slit" part refers to the very tiny appearance of the ventricles. The shunt is usually nearly blocked and has minimal flow.

Treatment Options

- Observation – only if the symptoms are very mild and primarily related to headache; a patient with lethargy and emesis symptoms should not be observed, but further evaluated is needed to rule out shunt malfunction versus potential slit ventricle syndrome.
- Anti-headache medications – may include either abortive or prophylactic headache therapies
- Shunt revision – is essential in the scenario of a true shunt malfunction. In the treatment of patients with symptomatic slit ventricle syndrome, surgical strategies include replacement of the ventricular catheter, placement of a valve incorporating an anti-siphon device, or revision of the existing valve to a programmable variant to assess the impact of different settings on the patient's symptoms. An endoscopic stylet technique can be utilized as an aide to assist in revision of the ventricular catheter. The utilization of stereotaxy for proximal shunt revision is rare. An option that eliminates the need for ventricular catheter placement is the conversion of the existing system to a lumboperitoneal shunt.
- Progressive occlusion of the existing shunt – deliberate externalization and progressive occlusion of the peritoneal catheter can be utilized to expand the ventricles in the ICU setting. This can be undertaken in conjunction with delayed ventricular catheter revision or endoscopic third ventriculostomy. In a paucity of patients, progressive occlusion may result in the ultimate removal of the existing shunt system and the subsequent lack of shunt dependency. In this subset of patients, the existing hardware is externalized in the ICU and fiber optic intracranial pressure monitoring initiated. Progressive occlusion, in the scenario of an asymptomatic patient with normal ICP measurements, may allow for permanent removal of the hardware.
- Endoscopic third ventriculostomy – a subset of patients may have associated aqueductal stenosis and are potential candidates for endoscopic third ventriculostomies. The safe introduction of the endoscope into the lateral ventricle, in the scenario of slit ventricles, can be very challenging in a child. Placement can be maximized by progressive enlargement of the ventricles or, rarely, via the utilization of frameless stereotaxy.
- Bilateral subtemporal decompression–rarely utilized given the morbidity of the procedure, the potential complications, and the success of the aforementioned strategies.

Surgical Technique

In the scenario of slit ventricle syndrome and a functioning shunt, externalization of the VPS can be performed either in the operating room or in the ICU. We prefer to create a small incision just above the clavicle with either a no. 15 scalpel or monopolar cautery. The catheter is elevated from the distal end of the wound and attached to an external ventricular drainage bag as in a standard EVD setup. A purse-string stitch is placed around the exit site. Elevating the level of drainage to at least 20 cm H_2O above the tragus is recommended initially, followed by progressive increments in pressure in the monitored setting. If tolerated, we then clamp the EVD for 24 hours. If successful, the patient can be scheduled for complete removal of all existing hardware, ETV, or both. (See Case 66.)

The surgical techniques of proximal and/or distal shunt revision, valve revision, endoscopic third ventriculostomy, or placement of a fiberoptic ICP monitoring device are discussed elsewhere.

Complication Avoidance and Management

- Complications regarding slit ventricle syndrome are related more so to patient management as opposed to the surgical technique itself. One of the most important variables in determining management is to initially rule out a shunt malfunction. The presence of a slit ventricle system does not obviate the potential for shunt obstruction. Additionally, one must be aware of the fact that the lateral ventricles may not become enlarged in the scenario of a level blocked shunt. All observation and management of these patients should be in a monitored ICU setting. Progressive occlusion of an externalized catheter must be based upon concurrent symptoms and ICP measurements in the patient. Should an ETV placement be considered, one must be mindful of the difficulties and potential complications associated with the placement of an endoscope into a slit-like ventricular chamber.

KEY PAPERS

Cheok S, Chen J, Lazareff J. The truth and coherence behind the concept of overdrainage of cerebrospinal fluid in hydrocephalic patients. *Childs Nerv Syst.* 2014;30:599-606.

Maldonado IL, Valery CA, Boch AL. Shunt dependence: myths and facts. *Acta Neurochir (Wien).* 2010;152:1449-1454.

Olson S. The Problematic slit ventricle syndrome. *Pediatr Neurosurg.* 2004;40:264-269.

Rekate HL. Shunt-related headaches: the slit ventricle syndromes. *Childs Nerv Syst.* 2008;24:423-430.

Sandler AL, Goodrich JT, Daniels LB, et al. Craniocerebral disproportion: a topical review and proposal toward a new definition, diagnosis, and treatment protocol. *Childs Nerv Syst.* 2013;29:1997-2010.

Case 68

Neural Tube Defect-Tethered Cord Syndrome

Hal S. Meltzer, MD ● Michael L. Levy, MD, PhD ●
Alexa Smith, MD ● Salman Abbasifard, MD

Presentation

A 6-month-old was referred by a pediatrician for concern of a sacral dimple. On history, mother does not report any neurologic deficits that she has noted. On physical examination, in addition to the sacral dimple, a dark tuft of coarse hair is noted as well as a small hemangioma in the midline. Imaging consists of an ultrasound at 4 months of age. An MRI of the lumbar spine is ordered. Images are now available for your review.

Differential Diagnosis

- Neural tube defect
  - Open
    - Myelomeningocele
    - Myelocele
  - Closed
    - Subcutaneous mass present
      - Lipoma with dorsal defect: lipomyelomeningocele, lipomyelocele
      - Myelocystocele: terminal or cervical
      - Meningocele
      - Cervical myelomeningocele
    - Subcutaneous mass *not* present
      - Simple dysraphism: spina bifida, persistence of terminal ventricle, intraspinal lipoma (intradural or filum terminale), tight filum terminale (fibrous thickening)
      - Complex dysraphism: dorsal dermal sinus, caudal regression syndrome, segmental spinal dysgenesis, split notochord syndrome (dorsal enteric fistula and neurenteric cyst), split cord malformation (type I or II)

Initial Imaging

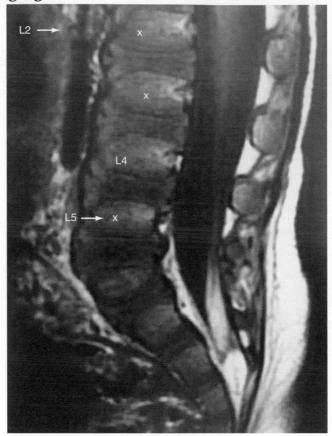

FIGURE 68-1

Imaging Description and Differential

- MRI – fatty filum

Further Workup

- Careful clinical assessment of progressive neurologic, orthopedic, or urologic issues
- Consider baseline urodynamic studies (Table 68-1)

TABLE 68-1	
SYMPTOMS AND SIGNS OF OCCULT SPINAL DYSRAPHISM	
Symptoms/Signs	**Frequency**
Foot deformity	39%
Scoliosis	14%
Gait abnormality	16%
Leg weakness	48%
Sensory abnormality	32%
Urinary incontinence	36%
Recurrent urinary tract infections	20%
Fecal incontinence	32%
Cutaneous abnormality	48%

(Adapted from Pang D. Sacral agenesis and caudal spinal cord malformations. Neurosurgery. 1993;32:755-758.)

Pathophysiology

Thought to be a result of disorder of secondary neurulation, which occurs postovulatory day 25 to day 27. Exact mechanism is unclear, but may be related to improper migration of mesodermal precursors/caudal cells. Abnormally thickened adipose tissue containing filum terminale prevents traction-free movement of the spinal cord during normal growth and can lead to ischemic neuronal changes, resulting in clinical observation of progressive neurologic, orthopedic, and/or urologic disorders. Prophylactic division of the abnormal filum terminale is felt to likely prevent these issues from occurring. Cutaneous markers of spinal dysraphism, such as dimples, hemangiomas, tufts of hair, lipomas, and asymmetric gluteal clefts, are noted in the majority of patients with closed neural tube defects/tethered cord syndrome. Lipoma of the filum terminale, noted on MRI, can be found in over 80% of individuals with tethered spinal cord clinical syndrome. However, approximately 5% of normal individuals may have adipose tissue containing filum terminale, of which the vast majority never develop any tethered cord symptomatology. The treatment of the asymptomatic patient is therefore controversial. Some experts advocate for expectant management and others advocate for prophylactic surgical intervention. We tend to offer prophylactic surgical treatment for younger children/infants and favor expectant management for older children/adolescents. Symptomatic children of any age warrant surgical intervention.

Treatment Options

Division of filum terminale via lumbar laminectomy versus expectant management for the asymptomatic patient

Surgical Technique

After intubation and general anesthesia, the patient is positioned prone for detethering surgery. Lateral rolls are used to elevate the patient and minimize thoracic and abdominal pressure. The lower back and flanks are prepared and draped.

Sectioning of the filum is carried out with a microscopic approach through the L5 and S1 interspace, minimizing laminectomies of L5 and S1 to assist in exposure. After removal of the ligamentum flavum and opening of the dura mater, the midline abnormal adipose tissue containing filum is identified and any associated nerve fibers are carefully teased away from this structure using microdissection. Electrophysiological monitoring, using both a threshold-based interpretation system and continuous electromyography monitoring, provides for intraoperative guidance and should eliminate the possibility of iatrogenic injury. Bipolar electrocautery is performed and the filum transected. The dura mater and overlying soft tissues are then closed in routine fashion.

Complication Avoidance and Management

- CSF cutaneous fistula is best prevented by meticulous dural and fascial closure; we favor nonabsorbent monofilament suture for these layers.
- Nerve root damage is avoided by meticulous dissection and the use of intraoperative neurophysiologic monitoring.
- Wound infection is best addressed in the infant/toddler population by frequent scheduling of diaper changes and aggressive family education on proper wound care.

KEY PAPERS

Cochrane DD. Occult spinal dysraphism. In: Albright AL, ed. *Principles and Practice of Pediatric Neurosurgery*. 3rd ed. Thieme: Medical Publishers; 2014:308-324.

Cools MJ, Al-Holou WN, Stetler WR Jr, et al. Filum terminale lipomas: imaging prevalence, natural history, and conus position. *J Neurosurg Pediatr*. 2014;13:559-567.

George TM, Adamson DC. Normal and abnormal development of the nervous system. In: Albright AL, ed. *Principles and Practice of Pediatric Neurosurgery*. 3rd ed. Thieme: Medical Publishers; 2014:308-324.

Case 69

Craniosynostosis – Plagiocephaly

Hal S. Meltzer, MD ● Michael L. Levy, MD, PhD ●
Alexa Smith, MD ● Dillon Levy ● Salman Abbasifard, MD

Presentation

A new mother and father are concerned about the shape of their baby's head. They point out a flat area of the head on the left side and have many questions about "craniosynostosis surgery," which they read about on the Internet. They have already scheduled a consultation with a plastic surgeon next week and are concerned about potential brain damage to their baby.

Differential Diagnosis

- Craniosynostosis
- Plagiocephaly

Initial Imaging

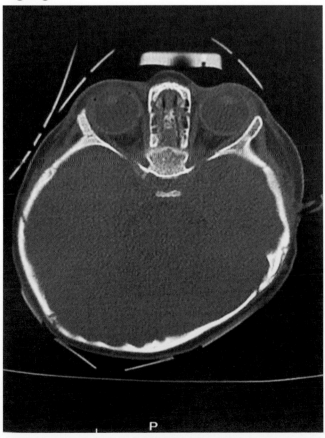

FIGURE 69-1

Imaging Description and Differential

- X-ray skull
- CT scan
  - Show lack of early suture closure or asymmetric closure

Further Workup

A thorough physical examination from multiple angles of the patient's head will allow one to recognize distinguishing signs of positional plagiocephaly from true craniosynostosis. In plagiocephaly, the flattened area, for example left occipital flattening, will have ipsilateral left frontal prominence. This can be noted by comparing the position of the ears. Having the parents hold the child in a sitting position and standing over the child, the examiner can easily tell if the ears and forehead are advanced on the ipsilateral side of the occipital flattening. The head shape will assume the classic parallelogram appearance. This is to be differentiated from the much rarer unilateral lambdoid suture craniosynostosis, where the head shape assumes a trapezoid appearance. In difficult cases a CT scan may be obtained to differentiate between the two entities.

Pathophysiology

Positional plagiocephaly is most frequently secondary to positioning the child's head repetitively in the same location, causing the skull to flatten out on one side. Given the pediatrician's education with regards to prevention of sudden infant death syndrome, babies are positioned on their backs in some cases exclusively. The flattening can be exacerbated by neonatal torticollis, which will result in preferential head turning to one side. If not corrected early by repositioning or physical therapy, in the case of torticollis, clinically significant cranial deformity may occur (Figures 69-2–69-7).

Treatment Options

- All treatments are controversial as the efficacy of any intervention, compared with the natural history of expectant management, has not been definitively determined.
- Repositioning – alternating head position while sleeping on back; ideally minimizing back time while awake
- Physical therapy for children with neonatal torticollis
- Cranial orthosis – worn 23 hours a day for maximal effect for a total of 3 to 6 months

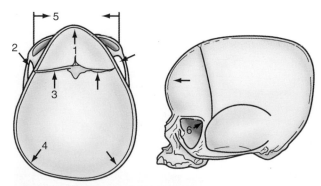

FIGURE 69-2   Features of the trigone-shaped skull of metopic synostosis (trigonocephaly). 1, Ridging of the fused suture; 2, temporal narrowing; 3, patent coronal suture displaced anteriorly; 4, compensatory bulging of the parietooccipital region, contributing to the skull's pear-shaped appearance; 5, narrowed bizygomatic dimension; and 6, posterior displacement of the superolateral orbital rim. Also treated with fronto-supraorbital advancement. *(Reprinted with permission from Winn HR. Youmans Neurological Surgery. 6th ed. Elsevier; 2011.)*

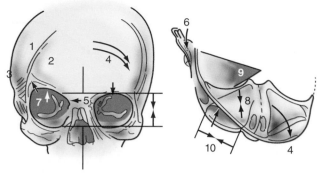

FIGURE 69-3   Unilateral coronal synostosis (anterior plagiocephaly) characteristics. 1, Fused suture; 2, flattening of ipsilateral frontal bone; 3, bulging of the right squamous temporal bone; 4, bulging of the contralateral frontal bone; 5, nasal radix deviated to the ipsilateral side; 6, ear ipsilateral to the fused suture, displaced anteriorly; 7, Ipsilateral Harlequin deformity (seen on radiographs), the superiorly displaced ipsilateral greater wing of the sphenoid bone; 8, shortening of the ipsilateral anterior cranial fossa; 9, narrowed ipsilateral sphenopetrosal angle; and 10, narrowing of the ipsilateral mediolateral dimension of the orbit. Treated with craniectomy of the fused suture and unilateral orbital bar advancement. *(Reprinted with permission from Winn HR.* Youmans Neurological Surgery. *6th ed. Elsevier; 2011.)*

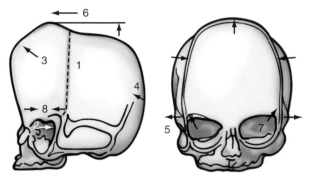

FIGURE 69-4   Features of bilateral coronal synostosis (brachycephaly). 1, Fused coronal suture; 2, recessed superior orbital rim; 3, prominent frontal bone; 4, flattening of occiput; 5, anteriorly displaced skull vertex; 6, shortened anterior cranial fossa; 7, Harlequin deformity of greater wing of sphenoid; 8, protrusion of squamous portion of the temporal bone. Treated with bilateral fronto-supraorbital advancement. *(Reprinted with permission from Winn HR.* Youmans Neurological Surgery. *6th ed. Elsevier; 2011.)*

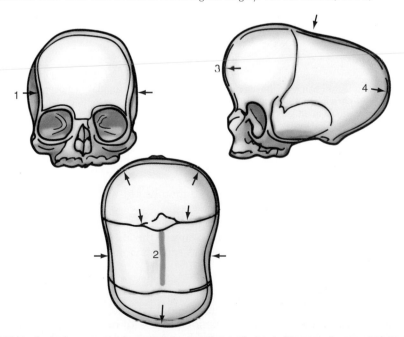

FIGURE 69-5   Sagittal synostosis characteristics (scaphencephaly). 1, Bitemporal narrowing; 2, ridging of fused sagittal suture; 3, frontal bossing; and 4, occipital bossing. A simple linear craniectomy of the suture can be used up to 5 months of age. *(Reprinted with permission from Winn HR.* Youmans Neurological Surgery. *6th ed. Elsevier; 2011.)*

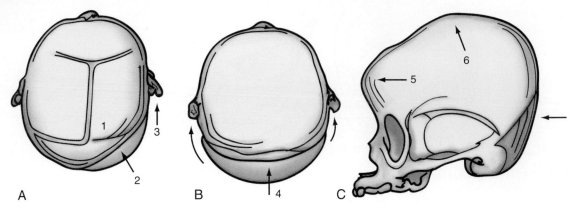

FIGURE 69-6 Features of lambdoid synostosis. **(A)** Unilateral lambdoid fusion: unilateral fusion (posterior plagiocephaly) (1); occipital flattening (2); and anteriorly displaced ear ipsilateral to fusion (3). **(B and C)** Bilateral lambdoid fusion with bilateral occipital flattening (4); prominence of frontal bone (5); and elevation of skull vertex (6). *(Reprinted with permission from Winn HR.* Youmans Neurological Surgery. *6th ed. Elsevier; 2011.)*

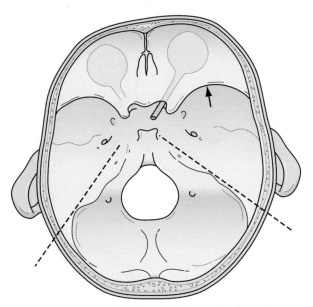

FIGURE 69-7 Skull base changes in the setting of right posterior deformational plagiocephaly, or positional molding. Note the parallelogram-shaped head, anterior displacement of the right ear, and right frontal bossing. This is in contrast to unilateral lambdoid synostosis, which is marked by a trapezoid-shaped skull, posterior displacement of the ipsilateral ear, and contralateral occipital bossing. *(Reprinted with permission from Ellenbogen RG, Abdulrauf SI, Sekhar LN.* Principles of Neurological Surgery. *3rd ed. Elsevier; 2012.)*

- Usually effective in younger infants – 4 to 8 months old when they are at their fastest cranial growth rates
- Surgical intervention is reserved for extreme and refractory cases of positional plagiocephaly. For true synostosis, a strip craniectomy of the affected suture at 3-6 months is often sufficient. Surgery maybe performed as early as 3 months if ICP is increased.

Surgical Technique

Multiple procedures have been used for unilambdoid synostosis from isolated strip craniectomies to extensive total cranial vault cranioplasties with barrel-stave osteotomies. The following describes a limited cranioplasty with reversal and rotation of bone segments.

The patient is positioned prone in a horseshoe headrest. An ear-to-ear incision is made after infiltrating the scalp with a suitable local anesthetic agent. The posterior scalp is dissected in the subgaleal plane to minimize blood loss. A biparietooccipital cranial "monobloc" flap is created with the high-speed craniotome, after placing burr holes over the posterior sagittal sinus and on either side of the sagittal sinus, just proximal to the torcula. Great care must be taken when dissecting the cranium from the dura adjacent to these vascular structures. The posterior cranial flap is then remodeled, often by rotating the flap 180 degrees, and replaced using an absorbable cranial plate fixation system.

Complication Avoidance and Management

- Infection – postoperative drain and perioperative antibiotics
- Blood loss – meticulous surgical technique and communication with anesthesiologist
- Leptomeningeal cyst – immediate repair of inadvertent durotomy noted at surgery

KEY PAPERS

Di Rocco F, Marchac A, Duracher C, et al. Posterior remodeling flap for posterior plagiocephaly. *Childs Nerv Syst.* 2012;28:1395-1397.

Goh JL, Bauer DF, Durham SR, et al. Orthotic (helmet) therapy in the treatment of plagiocephaly. *Neurosurg Focus.* 2012;35(4):1-6.

Ridgway EB, Weiner HL. *Skull Deformities*. Pediatric Clinics of North America 51: Elsevier Saunders; 2004:359-387.

Case 70

Vein of Galen Malformations

Brandon C. Gabel, MD ● Jeffrey A. Steinberg, MD ●
Michael L. Levy, MD, PhD

Presentation

The patient is a 5-day-old full-term female who presented with heart failure and seizures.

- Examination:
  - Full fontanelle
  - Head circumference 37 cm
  - Systolic cardiac bruit
  - Mild right-sided hemiparesis

Differential Diagnosis

The differential diagnosis of vein of Galen malformations includes true arteriovenous malformations involving the thalamus and nearby structures, and intracranial hemorrhage secondary to germinal matrix hemorrhages and/or dural venous sinus thrombosis.

Initial Imaging

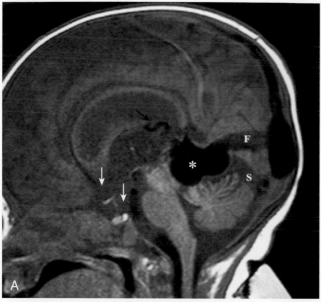

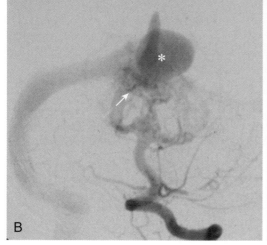
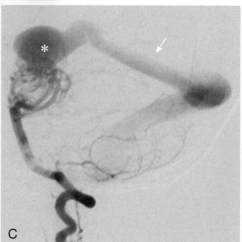

FIGURE 70-1

Imaging Description and Differential

Imaging reveals an arteriovenous malformation centered around the deep cerebral venous structures. There is a persistent falcine sinus and an enlarged straight sinus. The midline venous pouch is consistent with a vein of Galen malformation; however, not all midline engorged venous structures are vein of Galen malformations. The differential diagnosis includes a true brain arteriovenous fistula of the thalamus and/or surrounding structures.

Further Workup

- Laboratory
  - Routine labs
  - ECG and echocardiogram
  - Continuous EEG

- Imaging
  - MRI/MRA/MRV to aid in assessment of vascular anatomy
  - Noncontrast head CT is often useful to assess for hydrocephalus.
  - Formal catheter angiography

Pathophysiology

The term vein of Galen malformation is a misnomer. The malformation actually involves a persistent fetal vessel known as the median prosencephalic vein (of Markowitz). This vein is present during the third to eleventh weeks of gestation and drains many deep-seated structures. As the brain develops, the anterior portion of the vein regresses and the internal cerebral veins usurp its territory. In healthy term infants, the internal cerebral veins drain into the posterior portion of the previously termed median prosencephalic vein, now called the "vein of Galen."

In vein of Galen malformations the anterior portion of the vein does not regress as it normally should. The arterial supply to these malformations is oftentimes a combination of persistent fetal vessels that also fail to regress. Branches of the anterior cerebral artery, anterior choroidal arteries, posterior communicating arteries, and posterior choroidal arteries may terminate directly into the persistent vein, creating a large arteriovenous "pouch." A vein of Galen malformation therefore represents a true arteriovenous fistula.

It is important to realize that arteriovenous malformations of the thalamus and surrounding structures may drain into a dilated "normal" vein of Galen; these may be mistaken for vein of Galen malformations. Catheter angiography is usually able to delineate between the two.

Vein of Galen malformations pose several problems to the newborn. High output cardiac failure is most worrisome in the acute setting. The fistula acts as a venous sump, pulling a significant portion of the infant's circulating blood volume through. The second worrisome feature is a phenomenon known as "melting brain syndrome." The high venous pressures associated with the lesion interfere and white matter development can cause secondary leukomalacia and severe mental retardation. Seizures and hydrocephalus may also develop in many infants and children.

According to the Yasargil classification, there are four classes of vein of Galen malformations. The type of arteriovenous shunting present in vein of Galen malformations can predict the clinical presentation.

- Primary type 1 – choroidal or direct: there exists a small cisternal fistula act, high flow shunting within the wall of the venous aneurysm between the vein of Galen and the anterior pericallosal arteries, the posterior pericallosal arteries, or the posterior cerebral artery
- Primary type 2 – mural or network like: an arterial network of multiple fistulas exist between the vein of Galen and thalamoperforating vessels; an interposed arterial network is usually situated in the quadrigeminal plate cistern and is associated with lower blood flow then found in the type 1 malformation.
- Type 3: represents a combination of type 1 and type 2 vein of Galen malformations, which are high flow in nature.
- Type 4: represents a diffuse parenchymal arteriovenous malformation with primary drainage into the vein of Galen (vein of Galen aneurysmal dilatation).

Clinical Presentation

Neonates

Neonates will usually present significant cardiorespiratory failure at or following birth. Frequently, these children will demonstrate cardiac compromise in utero and hydrops. These symptoms are usually associated with a type 1 high-flow vein of Galen malformation, with the vast majority of neonates exhibiting signs of high-output cardiac failure. Many will additionally experience severe pulmonary hypertension.

Infants

As a result of cerebral steal phenomena in type 2 vein of Galen malformation, most infants will have progressive macrocephaly or hydrocephalus. Many may additionally experience new onset of seizures. The development of hydrocephalus may be noncommunicating (secondary to aneurysmal compression of the aqueduct) or communicating (resultant from intracranial venous hypertension, the presence of subarachnoid blood, or both).

Children and Older

Older children usually have symptoms of headache associated with a subarachnoid bleed; otherwise these lesions are usually asymptomatic and found by MRI. These malformations are usually small with limited shunting. Frequently, type 4 malformations will be included in this group.

Treatment Options

Most of these lesions are treated endovascularly. Both transarterial and transvenous approaches may be used. Oftentimes a combination of both is necessary to decrease flow through the fistula. The goal of treatment is not always complete obliteration of the fistula, but rather the amelioration of symptoms secondary to high-output cardiac failure.

Transarterial embolization is performed through the umbilical artery in neonates, or the femoral artery in older infants. Liquid embolics such as N-butyl-cyanoacrylate (NBCA) and ethylene vinyl alcohol copolymer (Onyx) are commonly used to embolize feeding arterial pedicles. Additionally, coil embolization may be used as an adjunct in some cases.

Transvenous embolization may also be used. Coil embolization of the venous pouch (i.e., the dilated prosencephalic vein) helps reduce flow through the malformation, but this approach is usually reserved for when transarterial options have been exhausted.

Surgical techniques, such as clip ligation of arterial feeders and resection of the malformation itself, have largely been abandoned secondary to high morbidity and mortality. Surgery plays a role in the treatment of hydrocephalus (i.e., ventriculoperitoneal shunting or endoscopic third ventriculostomy) related to aqueductal stenosis caused by compression from the malformation.

Complication Avoidance and Management

- Comorbid conditions such as seizures and heart failure should be treated aggressively.
- CSF shunting procedures may be necessary to treat coexistent hydrocephalus and mitigate further insult to the brain.
- Treatment may be delayed in stable infants to prevent complications from blood loss and contrast load. Delayed treatment also allows easier arterial access for endovascular treatment.
- Treatment of complex lesions should be staged to allow a more controlled devascularization; this can help prevent complications, such as perfusion breakthrough and/or venous thrombosis.

KEY PAPERS

Lasjaunias P, Hui F, Zerah M, et al. Cerebral arteriovenous malformations in children. Management of 179 consecutive cases and review of the literature. *Childs Nerv Syst*. 1995;11:66-79.

Lasjaunias P, Rodesch G, Terbrugge K, et al. Vein of Galen aneurismal malformations. Report of 36 cases managed between 1982 and 1988. *Acta Neurochir (Wien)*. 1989;99:26-37.

Mortazavi MM, Griessenauer CJ, Foreman P, et al. Vein of Galen aneurysmal malformations: critical analysis of the literature with proposal of a new classification system. *J Neurosurg Pediatr*. 2013;12(3):293-306.

Pearl M, Gomez J, Gregg L, et al. Endovascular management of vein of Galen aneurysmal malformations. Influence of the normal venous drainage on the choice of a treatment strategy. *Childs Nerv Syst*. 2010;26(10):1367-1379.

Case 71

Pilocytic Astrocytoma

Michael L. Levy, MD, PhD ● John R. Crawford, MD, PhD ● Alexa Smith, MD ● Ali H. A. Muhammad Altameemi, MD

Presentation

The patient is a 10-year-old male who presents with a 4-month history of headache, without vomiting, and a 4-week history of difficulties with balance. His family reports some weight loss over the past several weeks. He stopped being able to ride a bicycle or skateboard about a month prior to admission, reports having been very tired for the past couple of weeks, and has been sleeping a lot during the day. Despite this, he continues to do well in school. He has had no nausea or vomiting. There are no reports of seizures, syncope, and bowel or bladder changes. By report he was shopping on the day of admission when he developed problems with his vision, which prompted a visit to the emergency room by his grandmother. A head CT was performed and showed a large cyst in the posterior fossa with associated mass effect and occlusion of the fourth ventricle, complete effacement of the basilar cisterns, and markedly enlarged lateral and third ventricles with associated transependymal flow. An MRI of his brain noted a contrast-enhancing mass in the posterior fossa within the large cyst.

Differential Diagnosis

- Anaplastic astrocytoma
- Medulloblastoma
- Ependymoma
- Atypical rhabdoid teratoid tumor
- Hemangioblastoma

Initial Imaging

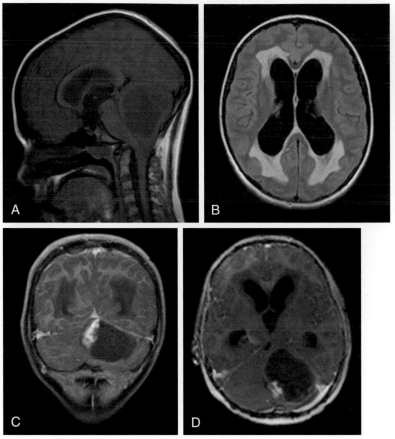

FIGURE 71-1

Imaging Description and Differential

MRI of the brain with and without contrast documented that the lateral and third ventricles are moderately enlarged. The fourth ventricle is nearly completely effaced. Interstitial edema can be seen within the white matter of both cerebral hemispheres. A large cystic and solid mass arises from the left cerebellar hemisphere extending from the tentorial incisura to the foramen magnum. The mass measures slightly less than 6 cm in maximum dimension and demonstrates an enhancing solid mural nodule, and a thin enhancing rim. Basal cisterns and the fourth ventricle are nearly completely effaced. The cerebellar tonsils are inferiorly displaced. Signal characteristics of the brain are otherwise normal. No other intraaxial or extraaxial masses are identified. Normal intracranial vascular flow voids are noted.

Radiological differential diagnosis includes a benign or malignant posterior fossa tumor. Benign brainstem tumor is favored by the long history without multiple cranial nerve involvement, a respect of the boundaries of the medulla, and a medullary location as opposed to a pontine location. Benign masses in this location can include pilocytic astrocytoma. Less likely diagnoses include hemangioblastoma, pleomorphic xanthoastrocytoma, and a brain abscess. Malignant tumors in this location include anaplastic astrocytoma, glioblastoma multiforme, metastases, and lymphoma.

Further Workup

- Laboratory
  - Routine labs
  - ESR, CRP
- Imaging
  - Brain CT, with and without contrast
  - Brain MRI, with and without contrast and thin slice cuts to be utilized for intraoperative stereotactic localization
  - Spine MRI, with and without contrast
- Biopsy versus resection
  - Given the probable benign nature of this lesion, we recommend craniotomy and complete resection of the lesion.

Pathophysiology

PA (or juvenile pilocytic astrocytoma) is a slow-growing, often cystic, and generally circumscribed astrocytoma affecting children and young adults. It is characterized by Rosenthal fibers, loose multipolar cells, and eosinophilic granular bodies. PA is the most common primary brain tumor in children. It represents 85% of cerebellar and 10% of cerebral astrocytomas. Approximately 15% of patients with NF1 develop PA. Gains have been observed in chromosomes 7 and 8 in a third of PAs. In addition to the cerebellum, PA can arise in the optic nerve (optic nerve glioma) or chiasm, hypothalamus, thalamus and basal ganglia, brainstem, cerebral hemispheres, and spinal cord.

Clinical Features

- Clinical signs and symptoms depend on the location of the tumor.
- Posterior fossa PAs most often have signs and symptoms of raised intracranial pressure or hydrocephalus (headache, nausea, vomiting, and increasing head circumference) given the effacement of the fourth ventricle; truncal ataxia is also common in midline lesions.
- Optic pathway PAs can be associated with vision loss or proptosis.
- Although rare, leptomeningeal dissemination of PAs may occur; those with hypothalamic tumors appear to be at greatest risk for dissemination.

Treatment Options

- Surgical
  - Gross total resection of PA provides the best cure rates, otherwise mass debulking (subtotal removal). We do not recommend percutaneous cyst drainage. biopsy, stereotactic or otherwise.
- Radiotherapy and chemotherapy
  - Radiotherapy is usually considered as a final option in tumors with multiple recurrences where further surgery would be associated with significant morbidity. Chemotherapy as an adjunct has not proven to be useful in the treatment of these tumors.

Surgical Technique

For posterior fossa approaches we prefer to position the patient in the lateral position. If the tumor is in the midline, we usually position with right side up. Otherwise position the patient with the tumor-involved cerebellar hemisphere side up. This patient was placed in the lateral position with the left side up. Prior to positioning, place a Mayfield head holder; once positioned, enter the stereotactic coordinates. The head is flexed with the patient's chin resting approximately 1 to 2 cm from the chest. Clip the patient's hair solely around the incision site.

We prefer to make our initial incisions using pinpoint monopolar electrocautery on the cut setting. Any scalp bleeding at this point is addressed with bipolar coagulation. For lateralized tumors, we position our incisions so that they directly overly the lesion; otherwise, we utilize midline incisions. In this case, incision was lateralized over the tumor. Self-retaining retractors were placed and a craniotomy performed to allow for a direct approach to both the enhancing mural nodule and the cystic tumor component. In the scenario of a tight cerebellum, a ventricular catheter can be placed into the cyst to reduce pressure.

For midline approaches, we take the incision down through the underlying muscle in the midline, and specifically, the avascular midline raphe. The inferior extent of this incision is just below C1 and the superior extent usually ending approximately 2 to 3 cm above the foramen magnum. Once the foramen is identified, free the underlying dura circumferentially from the confines of the foramen. We have found that widening the foraminal aperture, using a high-speed drill, facilitates our approach. This allows for the introduction of the craniotome, which we prefer for posterior fossa bone flaps in children. Following dural closure, the flap can be repositioned in the midline using a titanium plating system. We additionally use the craniotome to perform a laminectomy at the C1 level. The dura is then opened in a Y-shaped fashion with a no. 11 scalpel and surgical scissors. The dural leaves are then reflected laterally and superiorly using interrupted Nurolon suture. We prefer to use malleable retractor arms that attach directly to the Mayfield pin headrest (Fukushima type) to minimize clutter in the operative field. Given this approach, we are able to minimize manipulation and/or resection of the vermis while maximizing our operative.

In general, the tumor nodules are grayish in color and somewhat gelatinous in appearance. The ultrasonic aspirator can readily discern between tumor and normal cerebellar parenchyma. Once the tumor has been removed, all tumor margins need to be visualized to verify a complete resection. We couple visualization of the surgical cavity with the lining of the cavity using Surgicel to prevent postoperative clot formation. In pilocytic astrocytomas, the tumor cyst is drained at the time of surgery, but does not need to be resected. The contrary is true for cystic anaplastic astrocytomas.

With either approach, a watertight dural closure (either with or without graft) is the ultimate goal. We do not agree with the approach of leaving the dura open to allow for pseudomeningocele formation and facilitation of future surgeries.

- The approach should be done in the lateral position with neck flexion and the use of a suitable pediatric head frame to stabilize the head for surgery.
- Obtaining accurate neuronavigation information is essential.
- Multimodality-evoked potential monitoring can be utilized with midline lesions.
- Far lateral approaches may be required for large anterior lesions and for lateral growths.
- In a presumably acceptable and distinct appearing tumor, complete resection is the primary goal.
- In the scenario of juvenile pilocytic astrocytoma, the cyst walls (non-enhancing) do not need to be resected, because they are displaced from the cerebellar parenchyma. If the cyst wall enhances thickly, resection is necessary.
- In larger tumors with significant extension into the CP angle and anteriorly, a staged approach to minimize morbidity may be the best option.

Complication Avoidance and Management

- Intraoperative
  - Blood loss should be minimized throughout the procedure; aggressive use of bipolar electrocautery for muscular bleeding, and bone wax for bone bleeding, help maintain a dry field.
  - In young children, the C1 lamina is partly cartilaginous and thus subperiosteal dissection may not be possible; it is also incompletely fused in the midline so care must be taken not to accidentally open dura during the laminectomy.
  - Coagulation of dural venous channels before cutting not only provides good hemostasis, but also decreases the possibility of air embolism.
  - If brisk venous bleeding is encountered during dural opening, small titanium vascular clips provide a useful tool to control bleeding.

- During the procedure, the reflected dural flaps should be copiously and frequently irrigated to prevent drying and shriveling of the dura.
- Postoperative
  - Postresection hydrocephalus: endoscopic third ventriculostomy or ventriculoperitoneal shunting
  - Pseudomeningocele formation and CSF leakage: revision of dural closure, wound closure, CSF shunting, or lumbar CSF drainage may be required
  - Postoperative pneumocephalus: increase in inspired oxygen concentration to 100% using a nonrebreathing mask temporarily; the patient should lay flat
  - Posterior fossa syndrome (cerebellar mutism/ akinetic mutism): high-dose steroids, maintaining adequate mean arterial pressure, and rehabilitation

KEY PAPERS

Bowers DC, Krause TP, Aronson LJ, et al. Second surgery for recurrent pilocytic astrocytoma in children. *Pediatr Neurosurg.* 2001;34:229-234.

Daszkiewicz P, Maryniak A, Roszkowski M, et al. Long-term functional outcome of surgical treatment of juvenile pilocytic astrocytoma of the cerebellum in children. *Childs Nerv Syst.* 2009;5:855-860.

Osborn AG. *Diagnostic Neuroradiology.* St Louis: Mosby; 1994.

PDQ Cancer Information Summaries. *Childhood Astrocytomas Treatment.* June 20, 2014. <http://www.ncbi.nlm.nih.gov/books/NBK65944/>.

Section VI Stereotactic and Functional Neurosurgery

Case 72

Trigeminal Neuralgia

Andrew L. Ko, MD ● Kim J. Burchiel, MD

Presentation

A 58-year-old woman presents with right-sided facial pain described as a shocking sensation that shoots from her ear to her jaw. The first episode occurred without warning 4 years ago. She had several episodes at that time, but the pain went away without intervention. It returned several months later, lasting seconds to a few minutes at a time, then subsiding completely. It can be triggered by eating, talking, and touching her cheek. She was prescribed carbamazepine, which initially eliminated her symptoms. In the last few months, however, she has had more frequent episodes despite increasing the dose. She is now unable to talk without triggering the pain.

- PMH:
  - No surgery or trauma to the head and neck
  - No history of visual or sensory changes
  - No history of transient neurological deficits or difficulty walking
- Exam: normal neurological exam

Differential Diagnosis

- Neoplastic
  - Tumor (atypical face pain that is constant, unilateral and associated with numbness)
- Infectious
  - Postherpetic neuralgia (pain is constant, not paroxysmal)
- Vascular
  - AVM
- Other
  - Multiple sclerosis (bilateral and diminishes sensation)
  - Trigeminal neuropathic pain (responds to tegretol)
  - Tooth problems

Initial Imaging

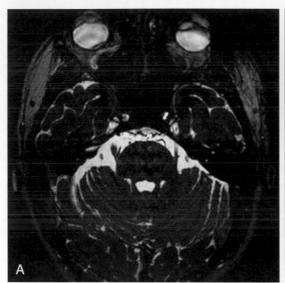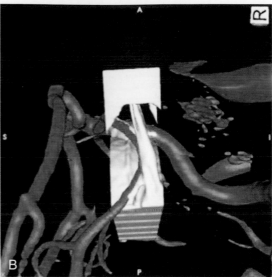

FIGURE 72-1

Imaging Description and Differential

Figure 72-1A shows neurovascular compression of the right trigeminal nerve root entry zone, caused by a loop of the superior cerebellar artery (SCA), seen on high-resolution BFFE sequence.

Figure 72-1B shows a 3D reconstruction of fused anatomic and vascular imaging. This can be helpful in delineating the relationship between nerve and compressive structures.

Further Workup

- Laboratory
  - Routine preoperative labs only

Pathophysiology

Trigeminal neuralgia (TN) is a clinical diagnosis based on the spontaneous development of pain within the distribution of the trigeminal nerve (V2 or V3 most common). Type 1, or classic TN, is characterized by lancinating, shock-like pain, whereas type 2 TN is predominantly a constant and aching pain. The "ignition theory" of TN describes a focus of hyperactivity within the retrogasserian root, associated with focal demyelination. Focal injury leads to hyperexcitability of afferents, resulting in after-discharges significant enough to be perceived as pain. Such injury is often associated with neurovascular compression (NVC), although TN occurs and recurs in the absence of NVC. The most common artery involved in TN is the SCA, but any artery or vein in contact with the nerve can cause TN. Other causes of facial pain must be ruled out, including multiple sclerosis and other demyelinating diseases, tumor, and vascular malformation. TN caused by vascular compression mostly spares facial sensation whereas MS and tumors do not.

Treatment Options

- Medical
  - Antiepileptic medications, such as carbamazepine or gabapentin, are first line treatments.
- Radiation
  - Gamma knife radiosurgery is a safe treatment, although evidence indicates it is less effective than other surgical options; pain relief is not immediate and does not occur

for days, weeks, or even months after treatment. Therefore SRS is good for poor surgical candidates not in severe pain.
- Surgical
  - Percutaneous: ablative procedures directed at the gasserian ganglion are safe and effective; chemoablation with alcohol or glycerol, mechanical disruption with balloon compression, and radiofrequency (RF) thermoablation are commonly used approaches.
  - Craniotomy: microvascular decompression (MVD) is the most effective and durable treatment for TN when NVC is present; when no NVC is present, ablative procedures such as partial sensory rhizotomy and internal neurolysis are effective, but are likely to be less durable than MVD and have a higher incidence of postoperative sensory deficit.

Surgical Technique

Percutaneous Procedures

These procedures are performed under fluoroscopic guidance with IV sedation. RF ablation is the most commonly performed procedure (especially for pain in V2/V3 – not V1) and is described here. A 22 gauge, 10 cm RF cannula is introduced at a point 2–3 cm lateral to, and 1 cm inferior to, the commissura labialis. It is directed toward the pupil at a point 3 cm anterior to the external auditory meatus. A submentovertex, or oblique submental fluoroscopic view, can be used to visualize the foramen ovale. Once within the foramen, a straight lateral view is used to confirm location within Meckel's cave. The cannula is advanced such that the tip of the electrode is located at the junction of the petrous ridge and the clivus (Figure 72-2). Stimulation at 50 Hz and a 1 millisecond pulse width should produce paresthesias at 0.1–0.5 V within the desired distribution of the nerve. Needle repositioning may be necessary. When location is confirmed, thermoablation at 70° for 90 seconds is performed with the patient sedated. Adequate lesioning is confirmed by loss of pinprick discrimination in the target distribution, and the needle is withdrawn. Intraoperative hypertension is not infrequent.

Microvascular Decompression

Positioning can be supine or lateral, with the ear parallel to the floor and the head flexed slightly. BAERs and facial nerve monitoring are confirmed prior to incision. A retrosigmoid craniotomy or craniectomy is performed to expose the junction of the transverse and sigmoid sinuses. The dura is opened in a curvilinear fashion parallel to these structures, and CSF egress is encouraged to relax the cerebellum and minimize need for retraction. Under microscopic visualization, a retractor is advanced along the junction of the

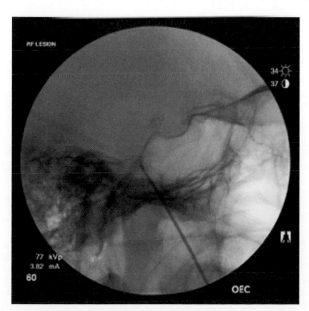

FIGURE 72-2   The tip of the electrode is located at the junction of the petrous ridge and the clivus.

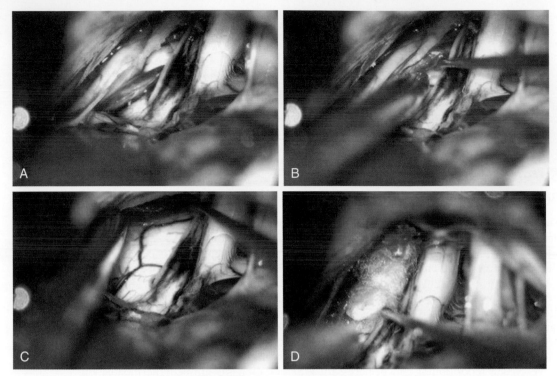

FIGURE 72-3 Arterial compression.

tentorium and the petrous bone. The arachnoid is opened to allow for further CSF egress and to visualize the medial structures. The superior petrosal vein complex may obstruct the view of the trigeminal nerve; these veins may be coagulated and divided. Arterial compression is most commonly due to a loop of the SCA (Figure 72-3A and B, top left and top right). This is often bifurcated, and care must be taken to visualize and mobilize all vascular structures impinging on the root entry zone of the trigeminal nerve (Figure 7-3C, bottom left). Teflon pledgets are used to hold these structures away from the root entry zone (Figure 72-3D, bottom right).

Complication Avoidance and Management

- Percutaneous procedures
  - Complications such as inadvertent carotid puncture and formation of cavernous-carotid fistulae can be avoided by accurate localization of the needle using fluoroscopy. Loss of corneal reflex (V1) and masseter weakness are seen in about 5% of patients, but are often temporary. Dysesthesia and anesthesia dolorosa are rare but dreaded complications. Risk can be mitigated by tailoring the degree of lesioning toward loss of pinprick discrimination, rather than producing numbness.
- Microvascular decompression
  - BAERs and facial nerve monitoring help prevent hearing loss or facial weakness; excessive traction on the cerebellum should be avoided. Care should be taken to obliterate any exposed mastoid air cells with bone wax, and dural closure should be watertight to avoid CSF leak.

KEY PAPERS

Barker FG, Jannetta PJ, Bissonette DJ, et al. The long-term outcome of microvascular decompression for trigeminal neuralgia. *N Engl J Med*. 1996;334(17):1077-1084.

Burchiel KJ. A new classification for facial pain. *Neurosurgery*. 2003;53(5):1164-1167.

Devor M, Amir R, Rappaport ZH. Pathophysiology of trigeminal neuralgia: the ignition hypothesis. *Clin J Pain*. 2002;18(1):4-13.

Kanpolat Y, Savas A, Bekar A, et al. Percutaneous controlled radiofrequency trigeminal rhizotomy for the treatment of idiopathic trigeminal neuralgia: 25-year experience with 1600 patients. *Neurosurgery*. 2001;48(3):524-534.

Case 73

Hemifacial Spasm

Thomas J. Gianaris, MD ● Aaron Cohen-Gadol, MD ●
Nicholas Barbaro, MD

Presentation

A 62-year-old white female presents with a 3-year history of left-sided, uncontrollable, and painless facial spasm at irregular and frequent intervals. This twitching began in her eye, but then spread to the rest of the left side of her face and neck, persisting during sleep. These spasms frequently interfere with her vision. She takes no medications and has no history of facial trauma or psychiatric illness. Botulinum toxin (Botox) injections were initially effective, but more recently the spasms have become more refractory and recur earlier at the end of each injection cycle and before the next Botox injection is due.

Differential Diagnosis

- Blepharospasm
  - Bilateral
  - Synchronous and symmetric
- Oromandibular dystonia
  - Typically more sustained than hemifacial spasm
  - Favors the lower part of face and oropharynx
- Facial tic
  - Often more complex
  - Multifocal and often bilateral
  - Can be suppressed
- Facial synkinesia
  - After paralysis of the facial nerve, facial muscles may contract due to synesthesias with voluntary movement
- Hemimasticatory spasm
  - Painful
  - Masticatory muscles only
- Hemifacial spasm
  - Causes of facial nerve irritation/compression include:
    - PICA (30%)
    - AICA (37%)
    - Vertebral artery
    - Neoplasm
    - Vascular malformation
    - Ectatic veins
  - Noncompressive processes
    - Multiple sclerosis and other focal demyelinating diseases
    - Bell's palsy leading to facial nerve injury
    - Brainstem infarction

Initial Imaging

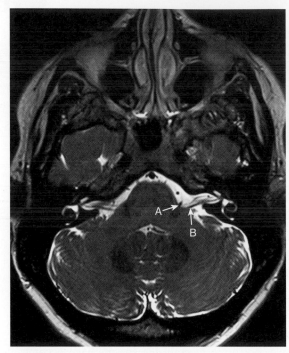

FIGURE 73-1   *(With permission, from the* Neurosurgical Atlas *by Aaron Cohen-Gadol 2015.)*

Imaging Description

- Brain MRI: a dilated ectatic artery (A) compressing the left facial nerve at its exit zone (B) can be appreciated.

Further Workup

- Laboratory
  - Laboratory testing is typically unhelpful, as diagnosis is largely based on clinical grounds.
- Imaging
  - Brain MRI with contrast to assess for neoplastic processes that may be impinging on the facial nerve at its exit point; numerous radiographically evident etiologies have been described, including epidermoids, meningiomas, gliomas, schwannomas, and lipomas.
- Consultants
  - Neurology

Pathophysiology

Hemifacial spasm is typically caused by compression of the facial nerve at its root exit zone at the level of the brainstem by an aberrant or ectatic vascular loop, typically the anterior inferior cerebellar artery (AICA), posterior inferior cerebellar artery (PICA), or vertebral artery (neurovascular conflict). The increased incidence of this disorder among the elderly and hypertensive patients suggests that progressive development of ectatic vessels is a prerequisite. Though not well understood, compression of the facial nerve likely leads to focal demyelination of nerve fibers, causing ephaptic transmission at the compressed site, which may then trigger ectopic impulses (peripheral hypothesis). Additionally, unknown factors may lead to hyperexcitability of the facial nucleus in certain patients (central hypothesis). The lack of epineurium or septa between the nerve fascicles at the nerve root exit zone makes this area the more common site of compression or conflict. Hemifacial spasm is characteristically unilateral, persists in sleep and there is often synkinesis between different muscle groups.

Treatment Options

- Pharmacologic
  - Although medical treatment is first line therapy for hemifacial spasm, it is historically associated with poor results. This mode of therapy mainly consists of benzodiazepines, with side effects including sedation and dependence.
- Botulinum toxin
  - Direct injection of botulinum toxin at the facial nerve irreversibly blocks cholinergic signal transmission at presynaptic nerve endings, resulting in reduction of spasm in 85%–95% of patients. This effect is transient, however, and serial injections must be performed every 3 to 6 months, with repeated injections lasting for shorter time periods. Botulinum toxin can serve as an invaluable tool for patients with medical comorbidities that make open surgery too risky. Although controversial, recent research suggests that prior serial botulinum injections do not lower the effectiveness of later definitive microvascular decompression surgery.
- Surgery
  - Microvascular decompression of the facial nerve root with interposition of a polytetrafluoroethylene (otherwise known as PTFE or Teflon) implant to mobilize the offending vascular loop

Surgical Technique

Lateral or "semilateral" positioning is typically used, and some clinicians prefer the use of a lumbar puncture or subarachnoid catheter to increase brain relaxation. Neuromonitoring of CN VIII, to reduce the danger of hearing loss, and CN VII, to look for changes in the lateral spread reflex (LSR), is strongly recommended. The LSR measures hyperactivity of the facial nerve/nucleus and is evaluated via electrical stimulation of the zygomatic or temporal branch of the facial nerve while recording from the mentalis muscle. When decompression of the nerve is accomplished, the LSR response may disappear, confirming that abnormal compression has been addressed.

Retromastoid craniotomy or craniectomy is used to approach the CN VII/VIII complex from the inframedial direction through an infrafloccular route, which begins with identification of CN IX and X. Adequate exposure of the root exit zone is the key for success in this procedure, as compressive vascular loops may be hidden along the difficult-to-reach cerebellomedullary fissure. Generous dissection of arachnoid membranes along the cranial nerves can relieve traction on these nerves and allow for safe exposure of the region of interest. Once the offending vessel is identified and mobilized, shredded PTFE gauze may be carefully placed in between the compressing vessel(s) and the facial nerve at the level of the brainstem. The use of small pieces of shredded PTFE allows for molding of the implant to the anatomy of the region of neurovascular conflict, therefore minimizing the risk of delayed dislodgement of the implant. Some surgeons add fibrin glue or other biological materials to maintain implant location (Figures 73-2 and 73-3).

Complication Avoidance and Management

- Microvascular decompression: approximately 90% of patients experience resolution of their spasms over a 2.9-year median follow-up period, with recurrence in about 2.4% of patients.
  - Hearing loss:
    - Incidence of 1.5% to 8%. It is important to distinguish true sensorineural hearing loss from postoperative middle ear effusion, which typically presents more as a sense of "fullness in the ear" and is typically temporary
  - Facial paralysis:
    - Temporary facial nerve paralysis occurs in 3%–8% of patients, sometimes in a delayed fashion (10–14 days postoperatively); immediate loss of function is caused

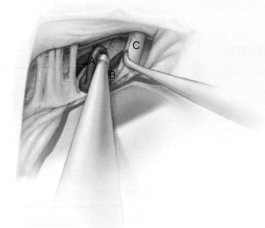

FIGURE 73-2 Offending vessel **(A)**, compressing CN VII at its root exit zone **(B)**, CN VIII being retracted and overlying CN VII **(C)**. Suction being advanced over rubber dam on cottonoid to retract cerebellum. *(With permission, from the* Neurosurgical Atlas *by Aaron Cohen-Gadol 2015.)*

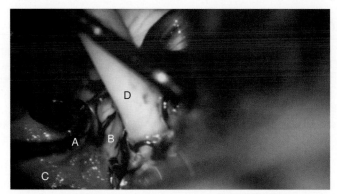

FIGURE 73-3 A dilated, tortuous branch of PICA **(A)**, compressing the facial nerve at its root exit zone **(B)**, being mobilized. Shredded PTFE gauze **(C)** is placed between the vessel and the nerve's root exit zone. CN VIII **(D)**, overlying CN VII.

by direct facial nerve trauma, and delayed palsy may result from reactivation of herpes zoster virus following surgery; permanent facial paralysis has an incidence of 0.7%–0.9%
- Cerebrospinal fluid leak:
  - Incidence of 1.4%; managed similarly to other CSF leaks

KEY PAPERS

Barajas RF Jr, Chi J, Guo L, et al. Microvascular decompression in hemifacial spasm resulting from a cerebellopontine angle lipoma: case report. *Neurosurg.* 2008;63(4):E815-E816.

Cohen-Gadol A. Microvascular decompression surgery for trigeminal neuralgia and hemifacial spasm: nuances of the technique based on experiences with 100 patients and review of the literature. *Clin Neurol Neurosurg.* 2011;113:844-853.

Miller LE, Miller VM. Safety and effectiveness of microvascular decompression for treatment of hemifacial spasm: a systematic review. *Br J Neurosurg.* 2012;26(4):438-444.

Rosenstengel C, et al. Hemifacial spasm: conservative and surgical treatment options. *Dtsch Arztebl Int.* 2012;109(41):667-673.

Xuhui W, et al. Effect of previous botulinum neurotoxin treatment on microvascular decompression for hemifacial spasm. *Neurosurg Focus.* 2013;34(3):E3.

Case 74

Parkinson's Disease

Doris D. Wang, MD, PhD ● Philip A. Starr, MD, PhD

Presentation

A 70-year-old right-handed male presents with progressively worsening right hand tremor that began 5 years ago, now with right leg and left hand involvement. He also has a slowed and shuffling gait with mild memory loss over the last year.

- PMH: former smoker, 40 pack per year, but otherwise unremarkable
- Exam:
  - Hypophonia and word-finding difficulties
  - 5 Hz resting tremor right > left hand
  - Bradykinesia, decreased amplitude of finger taps
  - Cogwheel rigidity
  - Small, shuffling gait

Differential Diagnosis

- Degenerative
  - Parkinson's disease
  - Essential tremor
  - Generalized dystonia
  - Multiple system atrophy
  - Vascular dementia
  - Lewy body dementia
- Neoplastic
  - Brain tumor (history of smoking)
- Vascular
  - Cardioembolic stroke
  - Lacunar syndromes
- Metabolic
  - B_{12} deficiency
  - Thiamine deficiency
  - Wilson's disease
- Other
  - Normal pressure hydrocephalus

Initial Imaging

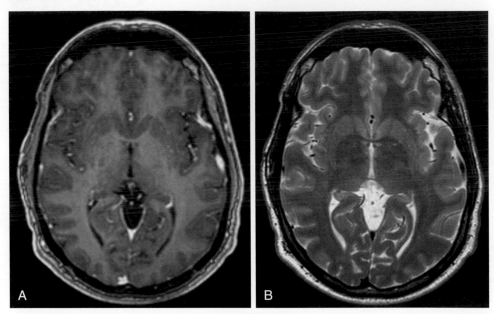

FIGURE 74-1

Imaging Description and Differential

- Axial brain MRI T1 with contrast (Figure 74-1A) and T2 (Figure 74-1B) demonstrating no focal abnormality in the brain. There is no mass lesion, vascular territory infarct, volume loss, striatal gliosis, or hydrocephalus. These sequences are at the level of the AC (anterior commissure) and PC (posterior commissure) plane, which is used for target planning of stereotactic DBS placement.
- Differential: Parkinson's disease, generalized dystonia, or essential tremor

Further Workup

- Laboratory
  - Routine labs
  - LFTs
  - B_{12}
  - Thiamine
- Medical
  - Levodopa trial (improves symptoms of Parkinson's disease)
- Imaging
  - None required
- Consultants
  - Neurology
- Other
  - Unified Parkinson's disease rating scale (UPDRS)

Pathophysiology

Parkinson's disease is a synucleinopathy of unknown origin, affecting multiple neuronal systems. A prominent pathological feature of mid-stage disease is death of dopamine-generating cells in the pars compacta of the substantia nigra (SNc) within the basal ganglia. The basal ganglia are connected to the rest of the brain via four major pathways serving different functions: motor, oculomotor, associative, and limbic. The basal

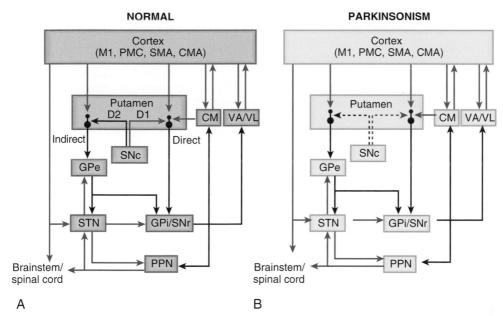

NORMAL

PARKINSONISM

A   B

FIGURE 74-2 Schematic diagram of the direct and indirect pathways of the basal ganglia motor circuits in normal **(A)** and parkinsonian **(B)** states. Red arrows are inhibitory projections, and blue arrows indicate excitatory projections. The changes in the thickness of the arrows in the parkinsonian state indicate the proposed increase (large arrow) or decrease (thin arrow) in firing rate activity of the specific connections. The dashed arrows are used to label the dopaminergic projection from the SNc to the putamen in Parkinson's and indicate partial lesion of that system in this condition. *CM*, centromedian nucleus; *CMA*, cingulate motor area; *GPe*, globus pallidus, external segment; *GPi*, globus pallidus, internal segment; *M1*, primary motor cortex; *PMC*, pre-motor cortex; *PPN*, pedunculopontine nucleus; *SMA*, supplementary motor area; *SNc*, substantia nigra pars compacta; *SNr*, substantia nigra pars reticulata; *STN*, subthalamic nucleus; *VA/VL*, ventral anterior/ventral lateral nucleus. *(Reproduced from Smith Y, Wichmann T, Factor SA, et al. Parkinson's Disease Therapeutics: new developments and challenges since the introduction of levodopa. Neuropsychopharmacology Review. 2012;37:213-216.)*

ganglia-thalamocortical motor circuit is a well-studied network in Parkinson's disease. The basal ganglia have been shown to modulate the amplitude and velocity of movement and to coordinate the activation and suppression of agonist and antagonist muscle groups, respectively. The striatum and subthalamic nucleus are the major input structures of the basal ganglia; the output is through the internal segment of the globus pallidus (GPi). There are two major intrinsic pathways: direct and indirect (Figure 74-2A). In the direct pathway, GABAergic striatal neurons project to the GPi, which in turn sends GABAergic projections to the thalamus. Therefore, activation of the direct pathway disinhibits the thalamus and facilitates movement. The indirect pathway is comprised of GABAergic projections from the striatum to the globus pallidus externa (GPe), which inhibit the subthalamic nucleus (STN). STN has excitatory effects on the GPi, which in turn inhibit the thalamus. Therefore, the indirect pathway suppresses movement. Striatal dopamine excites the direct pathway and inhibits the indirect pathway. Depletion of dopamine from the SNc will cause hypoactivity of the direct pathway and hyperactivity of the indirect pathway (Figure 74-2B). In addition, Parkinson's disease is associated with excessive neuronal synchronization throughout the basal ganglia and thalamocortical motor circuit, which limits the network's ability to respond to change.

Treatment Options

- Medical
  - Levodopa/carbidopa (dopamine precursor)
  - Entacapone (catechol-O-methyl transferase inhibitor)
  - Dopamine agonists such as ropinirole

- Surgical
  - Deep brain stimulation (DBS) of the GPi or STN. DBS has the advantage of being adjustable, reversible, and safe to use bilaterally, but has added cost and higher device-related complications such as infection and skin erosion. Requires regular follow-up after surgery for device programming and surgical battery replacement. Bilateral implantation, either simultaneous or staged by weeks/months, is usually indicated as most patients have bilateral symptoms. Both STN and GPi reduce tremor, rigidity, bradykinesia, gait disturbance, and dyskinesia. STN DBS is associated with a lower dopaminergic medication requirement compared to that of GPi, but may have a higher risk of exacerbating preexisting mood depression or cognitive impairment (contraindications).
  - Pallidotomy: lesional surgery has largely fallen out of favor, because it is permanent, nonadjustable, and has a significant complication rate when performed bilaterally. However, infection risk is lower than DBS and essentially no post-op care is required, therefore pallidotomy has a role in some circumstances.

Surgical Technique

DBS

For STN, the intended target is the center of the motor territory in the dorsolateral part of the nucleus. Approximate coordinates in relation to midcommissural point are lateral 12 mm, A-P -3 mm and vertical -4 mm (Figure 74-3A). For GPi, the intended target is the posterolateral motor territory of the nucleus, 3–4 mm from the internal capsule. Approximate coordinates are lateral 17.5 mm from the third ventricular wall, A-P -2 mm and vertical -5 mm (Figure 74-3B). T2-weighted fast spine echo (T2-FSE) sequence provides the best visualization of the STN and GPi.

A stereotactic frame is placed. The entry point is usually at or just anterior to the coronal suture, and trajectories should avoid any passage through the ventricles, sulci, or cortical veins as visualized on gadolinium-enhanced volumetric T1-weighted images. The patient is placed in a semi-sitting position and sedated for opening and burr hole preparation. After opening the dura and placement of the guide tube for microelectrode recording, the patient is returned to a fully awake state. Microelectrodes are placed on a micropositioner system and passed through the guide tube. Characteristic neuronal discharges are shown for the STN and GPi (Figure 74-3C). STN neurons discharge at 20–50 Hz, while GPi neurons have discharge rates of 60–100 Hz. Borders of the nuclei are defined by microelectrode recording.

DBS leads are then placed. For GPi, the end of the lead is typically 1 mm superior to the lateral border of the optic tract. The leads are connected to a hand-held pulse generator to confirm lead position clinically. Voltages are slowly raised to monitor for threshold of adverse effects. For STN, paresthesias (lemniscal pathway posterior), dysarthria/tonic facial contractions (internal capsule anterolateral), or contralateral gaze deviation (CN III nuclei medial) may be observed above 6 V. For the GPi, dysarthria or facial contractions are typically elicited above 6 V and indicative of activation of the internal capsule medial to GPi. Transient visual phenomena (phosphenes/scintillations) may also occur due to activation of the optic tract at the base of the pallidum (too low). Arm rigidity, if present, should be reduced by test stimulation in either target.

After confirmation with test stimulation, the DBS leads are secured using a burr hole mounted anchor, and the leads are tunneled under the scalp with closure of the incision. Placement of the infraclavicular, subcutaneous pulse generator is performed either immediately or as an outpatient procedure several weeks later.

Complication Avoidance and Management

- Intracerebral hemorrhage (ICH)
  - The risk of any ICH from DBS implantation is around 5%, with asymptomatic hemorrhage occurring in 1%–2% and symptomatic hemorrhage in 1%–2% of patients. To reduce the risks of ICH, blood pressure should be controlled (SBP <160) during DBS surgery, and trajectories should be made to avoid any visible vessels and sulci.

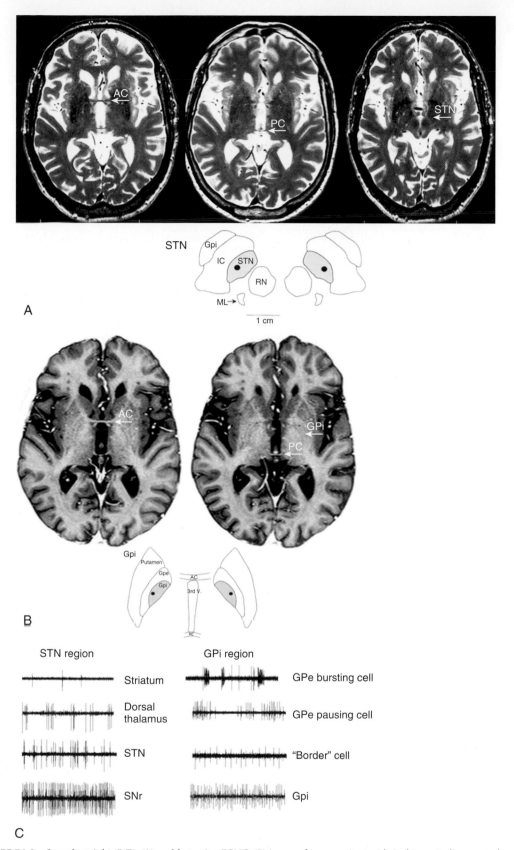

FIGURE 74-3 Sample axial MR T2 **(A)** and fast spine ECHO **(B)** images from a patient with Parkinson's disease undergoing preoperative planning for STN **(A)** and GPi **(B)** targets. Schematic of axial cuts of the nuclei at the bottom represent ideal lead positions for STN **(A)** and GPi **(B)**. Extracellular microelectrode recordings **(C)** showing characteristic firing patterns of different cell types encountered during trajectory to the STN and GPi. These recordings are useful in mapping of the basal ganglia nuclei to identify target of interest. *AC*, anterior commissure; *GPe*, globus pallidus, external segment; *GPi*, globus pallidus, internal segment; *IC*, internal capsule; *ML*, medial lemniscus; *PC*, posterior commissure; *STN*, subthalamic nucleus. *(Reproduced from Starr PA. Placement of deep brain stimulators into the subthalamic nucleus or globus pallidus internus: technical approach.* Stereotact Funct Neurosurg. *2002;79:118-145.)*

- Infection
  - The risk of any infection from DBS implantation varies greatly, between 2% and 10%. Strict adherence to sterile technique is critical in reducing infection risks.

KEY PAPERS

Bergman H, Wichmann T, DeLong MR. Reversal of experimental parkinsonism by lesions of the subthalamic nucleus. *Science*. New York 1990;249:1436-1438.

Follett KA, Weaver FM, Stern M, et al. Pallidal versus subthalamic deep brain stimulation for Parkinson's disease. *New Engl J Med*. 2010;362:2077-2091.

Kravitz AV, et al. Regulation of parkinsonian motor behaviours by optogenetic control of basal ganglia circuitry. *Nature*. 2010;466:622-626. doi:10.1038/nature09159.

Lang AE, Lozano A, Montgomery E, et al. Posteroventral medial pallidotomy in advanced Parkinson's disease. *N Engl J Med*. 1997;337:1036-1042.

Starr PA. Placement of deep brain stimulators into the subthalamic nucleus or globus pallidus internus: technical approach. *Stereotact Funct Neurosurg*. 2002;79:118-145.

Case 75

Progressive Spastic Paraparesis and Decreased Mobility in a Young Patient

Tsinsue Chen, MD ● Andrew Shetter, MD ● Peter Nakaji, MD

Presentation

A 49-year-old male is evaluated for intractable spasticity. During early childhood, the patient was noted to have spastic paraparesis; however, he was able to ambulate until around 18 years of age. His symptoms gradually worsened, and he became wheelchair bound at age 30. He was given a diagnosis of hereditary spastic paraplegia (HSP) and was followed closely by a neurologist. He takes baclofen, 20 mg qHS; however, higher doses of the PO medication have resulted in intolerable sedating side effects. Botulinum toxin injections in the lower extremities have provided minimal relief.

- Past surgical history: repair of nasal septal deviation in early 20s
- Family history: five paternal relatives (including his father) diagnosed with hereditary spastic quadriparesis
- Social history: works part-time; attending school with the intention of becoming a medical coder
- Exam:
  - Calm, cooperative male who appeared of stated age and in no acute distress
  - Oriented to self, date, location, and context
  - Severe rigidity on passive movement of lower extremities; knees were unable to be fully extended
  - Sustained bilateral ankle clonus
  - Any lower extremity movement resulted in extensor spasms at hips and knees

Differential Diagnosis

- Congenital/degenerative
  - Hereditary spastic paraparesis
  - Structural abnormalities involving the brain or spinal cord (e.g., mass lesion compressing the spinal cord, tethered cord syndrome)
  - Cerebral palsy
- Vascular
  - Stroke
- Infectious
  - HIV
  - Neurosyphilis
- Other
  - Traumatic brain or spinal cord injury
  - Leukodystrophies: progressive multiple sclerosis or B_{12} deficiency
  - Spinal cerebellar ataxias

- Early onset dementia
- Other motor neuron disorders (amyotrophic lateral sclerosis or primarily lateral sclerosis)

Initial Imaging

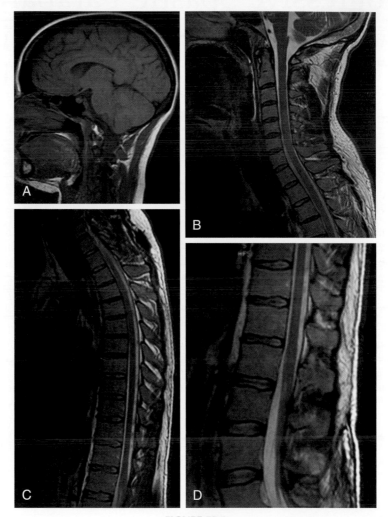

FIGURE 75-1

Imaging Description and Differential

- Figure 75-1A shows sagittal T1-weighted MRI of the brain and sagittal T2-weighted images of the cervical (Figure 75-1B), thoracic (Figure 75-1C), and lumbar (Figure 75-1D) spine demonstrating no structural abnormalities.
- Differential: HSP with no additional HSP-associated CNS findings, such as atrophy of the corpus callosum or cerebellum, or white-matter changes

Further Workup

- Laboratory
  - Routine labs for preoperative evaluation: CBC, BMP, coagulation factors, UA
  - Metabolic labs to rule out metabolic etiologies: free T4, TSH, B12, VRDL, ESR

- Consults
  - Neurology: for evaluation and optimization of medical treatment of spasticity, if not already consulted. Typically patients are referred to the neurosurgeon's office by a neurologist after thorough evaluation and medical therapy has been exhausted.

Pathophysiology

HSP is a category of inherited diseases, involving progressive stiffness and spasticity in the lower extremities. Symptoms result from axonal degeneration that primarily affects the distal portion of the corticospinal tracts and, to a lesser degree, the dorsal columns. Mild loss of anterior horn cells can occur. Inheritance can be autosomal dominant, autosomal recessive, or X-linked recessive. More than 56 HSP loci and HSP-related genes have been identified.

Other types of spasticity typically result from upper motor neuron or cortical spinal tract dysfunction, leading to the inability of distal gamma amino butyric acid (GABA) receptors to correctly absorb GABA, which presynaptically inhibit excitatory neurotransmitter release. The affected nerves lack inhibition and stimulate target muscles constantly, and this results in tonic contraction and muscle spasticity. The inciting upper motor neuron dysfunction can be due to intrauterine maldevelopment or perinatal cerebral injury (e.g., cerebral palsy) or secondary injury (e.g., stroke, traumatic brain injury, or spinal cord injury).

Treatment Options

- Medical: no pharmacotherapy is known to reverse the effects of, or halt the progression of, spasticity. Thus, drug therapy focuses on reducing the severity of symptoms and improving physical comfort, mobility, and quality of life.
  - GABA agonists: oral baclofen (binds GABA receptors in the dorsal horn to presynaptically inhibit the release of excitatory neurotransmitters); most widely used oral pharmacotherapeutic agent for treatment of spasticity
  - Alpha 2 adrenergic agonists: tizanidine (for nocturnal or intermittent spasms)
  - Benzodiazepines: diazepam or clonazepam to decrease spasm intensity
  - Antimuscarinic: tolterodine decreases bladder spasm
  - Botulinum toxin: neurotoxin injected intramuscularly to affected areas
  - Physical therapy
- Surgical
  - Orthopedic operations for contracture release and to correct joint deformities
  - Baclofen pump placement: direct intrathecal administration of baclofen
  - Rhizotomy
  - Myelotomy (last option)
- Observation
  - Patients with spasticity who are observed typically do no exhibit improvement and their spasticity can progress to the point where their mobility, gait, and quality of life become significantly affected.

Surgical Technique
Baclofen Pump Placement

Indications

When a patient is determined to have intractable spasticity despite multiple medical treatments, or suffers significant side effects from medical therapies (e.g., tolerance to or over-sedation from PO baclofen, ineffectiveness of Botox injections), he or she is considered for continuous administration of baclofen into the lumbar subarachnoid space. Delivery via this route creates a lumbar-to-brain concentration gradient of $4:1$, and significantly decreases the risk of extra-spinal baclofen side effects.

Patients first undergo a trial of intrathecal baclofen injection to assess for a positive response. Through the standard lumbar puncture technique, a bolus of baclofen is injected (typically 50 μg). A clinical response, graded by the modified Ashworth scale, is usually seen by 2 hours and lasts up to 6 hours. If there is a decrease in spasticity in response to the bolus, a permanent subarachnoid catheter is placed in a later scheduled operation for continuous delivery of the drug.

Procedure

The patient is placed in the standard lateral decubitus position with the knees moderately flexed to expand the interspinous space for percutaneous puncture. Attention must be made to allow adequate exposure of the abdominal area for a transverse incision necessary for the drug pump. The side of the pump placement can be decided based on patient preference, or the incision should be made contralateral to the side of any external drains (e.g., feeding tubes or colostomies). A transverse incision is made approximately at the level of the umbilicus, or slightly lower, based on the size of the baclofen pump. Blunt dissection can be performed with the surgeon's fingers or Metzenbaum scissors to create a subcutaneous pocket large enough for the pump. Fibrous bands are released with Bovie electrocautery.

A small linear incision is made in the midline posteriorly, over the L4 and L5 interspace. A large-bore spinal needle is used to puncture the spinal subarachnoid space. The spinal catheter is advanced to approximately the T10-T12 level (less chance of respiratory depression) for patients with lower extremity spasticity or to the mid thoracic level for patients with upper extremity spasticity. A larger diameter catheter is tunneled around the flank to connect the drug pump to the thinner spinal catheter. The two catheters are connected with a small metal connector and snapped in place with a plastic securing device, or sometimes secured with a 2.0 silk tie, depending on the device brand. The pump is then aspirated from the side port to check for distal CSF flow prior to closure. Both incisions are thoroughly irrigated and closed. The pump is programmed externally to deliver continuous baclofen, typically at a starting dose of 50 to 100 μg/day, and gradually titrated upward based on symptomatic improvement.

Percutaneous Thermal Rhizotomy

Indications

This operation is well suited for treatment of lower extremity spasticity in patients with complete or near-complete spinal cord lesions, or for patients with supraspinal pathology who are nonambulatory. It is safe and easily accessible, and should be the first choice for an ablative operation. For diffuse lower extremity spasticity, rhizotomy can be completed bilaterally from L1-S1, or unilaterally for hemiplegic spasticity. If spasticity recurs, more invasive procedures can be considered (open rhizotomy, dorsal root entry zone [DREZ]-otomy, and myelotomy). Techniques for cervical rhizotomy are available, but there are limited studies on their safety and efficacy.

Procedure

The procedure is typically performed under local anesthesia in the prone position. General anesthesia and/or the use of lateral decubitus position may be necessary in patients whose positioning is limited by fixed joint contractures or severe flexor spasms. In the lumbar area, a 12 gauge spinal needle is inserted approximately 5–7 cm lateral to midline at the level of, or slightly inferior to, the target nerve root foramen. The needle is subsequently advanced under anteroposterior fluoroscopy in an oblique fashion toward the junction of the pedicle and transverse process.

Once the transverse process or lamina is reached, the needle tip is advanced ventrally and medially into the foramen adjacent to the dorsal root ganglion. The tip of the needle should not penetrate medial to the medial aspect of the pedicle, to prevent violation of the thecal sac. A lateral X-ray is obtained to ensure that the needle tip is contained in the dorsal one third of the neural foramen. A thermistor electrode with a 1-cm uninsulated tip is inserted through the needle and subsequently withdrawn 2 cm over the shaft of the electrode. Next, 2-Hz pulse electrical stimulation is performed, and motor activity in the corresponding muscle groups should occur at ≤0.5 V. If not, the electrode might require repositioning. When the electrode is in the appropriate anatomical and physiological location, a 120-second radiofrequency lesion (90°C) is made. This is then repeated sequentially for each level of desired rhizotomy.

Myelotomy

Indications

Good long-term success rates are achieved with myelotomy when it is used to treat lower extremity spasticity due to severe spinal cord etiology. However, it is a large and invasive surgical procedure when compared with other techniques. It may be a good alternative in patients with complete or near complete spinal cord lesions without automatic bladder function.

Procedure

A standard midline incision in the lower thoracic spine is made based on X-ray localization, and a laminectomy from T10 to T12 or L1 is performed. After the dural opening, the root of T12 is identified by following its dorsal rootlets medially from exiting foramen. The point where the lowest T12 dorsal rootlets and the spinal cord meet is the rostral landmark of the myelotomy. The S1 nerve root is identified by counting caudally and it marks the inferior extent of the myelotomy. With microscopic dissection, the posterior spinal vein and dorsal median sulcus are identified. The vein is preserved and retracted from midline. The midline sulcus is then sharply divided to a 3 mm depth over a 3 mm superior–inferior segment of the spinal cord. A myelotomy knife with a 3 mm length right-angle blade is inserted 4 mm below the spinal cord surface at the level of the central canal. The knife handle is rotated 360 degrees at the lower and upper extents of the midline incision. This process is repeated every 5 mm between L1 to S1. Subsequently, the dura and fascial layers are closed in the usual meticulous fashion.

Complication Avoidance and Management

- Baclofen pump
  - The most common complications associated with baclofen pump placement are breakage or blockage of the spinal catheter and drug overdosage. Thus, meticulous technique when connecting and securing the spinal catheter to the distal pump catheter is critical. Attention must be focused on removing the spinal needle from the intrathecal space in a fashion that will not shear or injure the spinal catheter. Pump failure can cause baclofen withdrawal which is associated with headaches, fever, worsening spasticity, seizures, cardiac instability and pruritis. Temporize with i.v. or p.o. baclofen and benzodiazepines. Drug overdosage can lead to nausea, emesis, dizziness, weakness or oversedation. These symptoms can be addressed by reprograming the pump to a lower delivery rate. Severe overdosage can lead to respiratory depression and coma, and these patients must receive immediate ventilatory support, have their pump rates decreased or emptied, and may be treated with physostigmine. Care must be taken to start at a low delivery rate and gradually titrate upward. Infrequently, a granuloma can occur at the tip of the catheter. If asymptomatic, stopping the pump will usually resolve the granuloma. However, if severe symptoms are evident, some advocate decompression especially with mass effect.
- Percutaneous thermal rhizotomy
  - Complications are rare and may include infection or worsening of sensory or motor function in intact patients. However, most patients undergoing thermal rhizotomy for spasticity have severe deficits at baseline. Some authors have reported a high recurrence rate; however, given the ease of the procedure and relatively low complication rate, the operation can be repeated a second time without difficulty.
- Myelotomy
  - Given the invasive nature of this procedure, inherent risks include worsening sensory or motor deficit, CSF leak, infection, and postoperative pain. Careful patient selection is critical and should be reserved for patients with severe spinal cord pathologies with complete or near complete loss of lower extremity motor and sensory function, and without preserved automatic bladder function.

KEY PAPERS

Benini R, et al. Updates in the treatment of spasticity associated with cerebral palsy. *Curr Treat Options Neurol.* 2012;12(6):650-659.

Putty TK, et al. Efficacy of dorsal longitudinal myelotomy in treating spinal spasticity: a review of 20 cases. *J Neurosurg.* 1991;75:397-401.

Shetter AG. The neurosurgical treatment of spasticity. *Neurosurg Q.* 1996;6(3):194-207.

Case 76

Mesial Temporal Sclerosis

Nathan C. Rowland, MD, PhD ● Edward F. Chang, MD

Presentation

A 31-year-old right-handed female with a history of one febrile seizure at 7 months of age, followed by complex partial seizures beginning at age 12, was seen. She has had a total of three generalized seizures, the most recent occurring 4 years prior. Her typical seizures consist of bad odor sensation preceding loss of awareness, lip smacking, and bimanual automatisms, and have persisted despite taking levetiracetam, topiramate, lacosamide, and lamotrigine. She has had two normal EEG evaluations. She is unable to drive or work and is on disability. She has a maternal grandfather with seizures.

- PMH:
  - Otherwise unremarkable
- Exam:
  - Normal-appearing female of stated age, accompanied by mother, gives appropriate historical account of present illness
  - No speech abnormalities
  - Recall of three objects within normal limits
  - Cranial nerves intact
  - Normal, symmetric strength and sensation
  - No cutaneous stigmata

Differential Diagnosis

- Idiopathic/Congenital
  - Mesial temporal sclerosis (MTS)
  - Malformation of cortical development
- Neoplastic
  - Mass lesion (less likely, given the nonfocal exam and chronicity of seizures)
  - Vascular malformation (e.g., AVM)
- Infectious: less likely, given the absence of infectious sequelae, though should remain in differential if history suggests indolent process
  - Encephalitis/cerebritis
  - Meningitis
  - Abscess
- Traumatic: chronic seizures may be associated with mild head trauma, though lack of history places this lower on differential.
- Syndromic: typically occurring when much younger and is associated with severe cognitive delay
  - Tuberous sclerosis (Bourneville's disease)
  - Sturge-Weber (encephalotrigeminal angiomatosis)

Initial Imaging

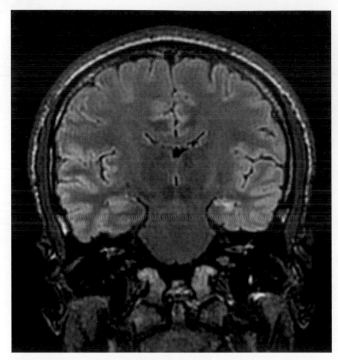

FIGURE 76-1

Imaging Description and Differential

- FLAIR MRI of the brain showing a coronal image through the temporal lobes. The left hippocampal formation shows FLAIR hyperintensity, slight volume loss, and abnormal architecture compared with the right. These findings are consistent with a presumptive diagnosis of mesial temporal sclerosis.

Further Workup

- Monitoring
  - Video-EEG telemetry with goal of capturing three or more typical seizures to confirm lateralization/localization
- Laboratory
  - Routine labs
  - Antiepileptic drug (AED) levels
    - AED levels vary widely based on individual metabolism.
    - Maximal tolerated dose may be more important than absolute levels
- Imaging
  - Structural MRI with neuronavigation sequence, along with coronal reconstructions and/or hippocampal protocols
  - PET (MTS appears as interictal hypometabolic region)
  - may consider MEG
  - WADA as needed
- Consultants
  - Epilepsy neurology
  - Multidisciplinary epilepsy case conference (at some institutions)
  - Neuropsych testing

Pathophysiology

Although mesial temporal sclerosis is the most common cause of temporal lobe epilepsy, its etiology is poorly understood. Additionally, association with risks factors such as febrile seizures remains controversial. Neuropathologic changes in classic hippocampal sclerosis include severe neuronal loss and gliosis predominantly in the CA1 hippocampal sector and less severe changes in CA4. Other changes observed are granule cell dispersion, mossy fiber sprouting, and loss of interneurons. The term "mesial temporal sclerosis" implies damage to the hippocampus, the amygdala, and the parahippocampal gyrus. A randomized trial comparing temporal lobectomy and best medical therapy resulted in seizure freedom in 58% of patients in the surgical group versus 8% in the medical group at 1 year followup.

Treatment Options

- Medical
  - One or two AEDS
- Radiosurgery
  - Remission rate 60%–80% in recent trials
- Surgery
  - Anterior temporal lobectomy (ATL)
  - Selective amygdalohippocampectomy (SelAH)

Surgical Technique

The following describes the surgical technique for ATL with awake speech mapping. Please see Hu et al for a meta-analysis of 13 prospective and retrospective studies comparing ATL and SelAH, in which SelAH was found to have similar or slightly better seizure-free outcomes than ATL in selected patient groups.

The patient is placed in a supine or semilateral position with the head above the chest and parallel to the floor. A local sensory block is performed with 1% lidocaine before immobilizing the head with three-point fixation. A reverse question mark incision is carried down to the bone, taking care to preserve the superficial temporal artery. The posterior aspect of the incision is brought down inferiorly to expose the root of the zygomatic arch. Burr holes are placed (1) near the root of the zygoma, (2) anterosuperiorly at the keyhole, and (3) posterosuperiorly at the superficial temporal line. A bone flap is raised and tack up sutures are placed. A dural flap is incised with the pedicle oriented anteriorly.

Depth electrodes are placed in the hippocampus using neuronavigation. Additionally, electrocorticography is performed on the surface of the exposed cortex to localize seizure foci. For cases involving dominant-side lesions, a bipolar stimulation probe can be used to map speech and sensorimotor areas to define the borders of the resection. Areas of repetition, name, and speech arrest are marked.

The corticectomy is begun at the superior temporal sulcus near the anterior temporal pole. A 0.5 to 1 cm thick section of parenchyma is resected superficially, and this plane is carried down to the floor of the middle cranial fossa. Next, the resection proceeds medially, using the temporal horn of the lateral ventricle as a surgical landmark. This may be accessed through the middle temporal gyrus. The hippocampus will be visualized once inside the ventricle. This should be resected beginning anteriorly with the head, taking care to identify and avoid injuring the anterior choroidal artery (Figure 76-2). Once the hippocampus has been removed, all remaining temporal lobe tissue should be resected, taking care to remain in the subpial plane and not violate the subarachnoid space, which contains the third and fourth cranial nerves, posterior cerebral artery, basal vein of Rosenthal, and cerebral peduncle all in close proximity. The resection cavity should be carried posteriorly until 3–4 cm (left or dominant) or 5–6 cm (right or nondominant) from the temporal pole is reached. Electrocorticography is again performed at the resection interface to confirm absence of further abnormal epileptiform activity.

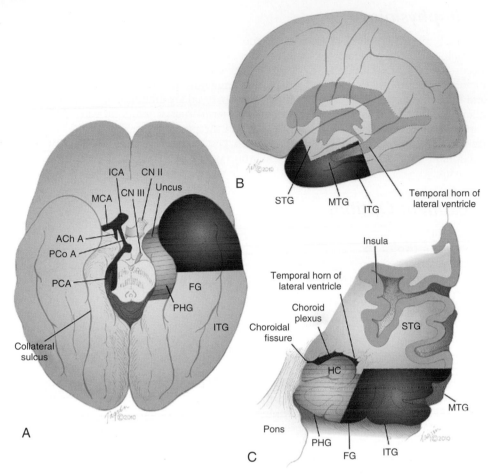

FIGURE 76-2 Schematic of resection. The two-part ATL is shown from basal **(A)**, lateral **(B)**, and coronal **(C)** views. The lateral resection (orange stippled region) includes the MTG and ITG. The posterior extent is generally about 4 cm, but may be modified based on anatomic considerations, ECoG, or functional mapping. The lateral specimen includes the MTG, ITG, and part of the fusiform gyrus (FG). The incision plane approaches, but does not enter, the temporal horn of the lateral ventricle, which lies deep in the MTG. The anterior most 1.5 to 2 cm of the STG is emptied with subpial dissection. The mesial resection (hatched region) includes the remainder of the FG, PHG, hippocampal formation (HC), and amygdala. *AChA,* anterior choroidal artery; *CN II,* optic nerve; *CN III,* oculomotor nerve; *ICA,* internal cerebral artery; *MCA,* middle cerebral artery; *PCoA,* posterior communicating artery. *(Reprinted with permission from Quiñones-Hinojosa A. Schmidek and Sweet Operative Neurosurgical Techniques. 6th ed. Elsevier; 2012.)*

Complication Avoidance and Management

- Language areas
  - It cannot be stated with enough emphasis to avoid resecting more than 3–4 cm on the left (or dominant) or 5–6 cm on the right (or nondominant) side from the temporal pole. Care should also be taken to protect the mid to posterior extent of the superior temporal gyrus (Figure 76-2). Doing so avoids unnecessary risks to language areas in the absence of an awake language mapping procedure. A useful landmark to indicate the absolute posterior limit of the hippocampal resection is the tectum, which can be confirmed with neuronavigation.
- Subpial dissection
  - One must remain subpial to the structures just beyond the subarachnoid space – these include CN III and IV (with IV usually remaining hidden under the tentorium), P2 segment of the PCA, basal vein of Rosenthal, and the cerebral peduncle. Violation of the pia substantially raises the possibility of damaging one or more of these structures, causing significant morbidity.

- Posterior temporal lobe anatomy
  - It is important to remember that the temporal stem is medial to the middle temporal gyrus and that medial to the superior temporal gyrus is the arachnoid, covering the middle cerebral artery (MCA) candelabra. Both of these areas should be cautiously avoided, and it is especially critical to avoid bipolar cautery near the MCA vessels, which could risk hemispheric stroke.

KEY PAPERS

Hu W-H, Zhang C, Zhang K, et al. Selective amygdalohippocampectomy versus anterior temporal lobectomy in the management of mesial temporal lobe epilepsy: a meta-analysis of comparative studies. *J Neurosurg*. 2013;119(5):1089-1097.

Kwan P, Brodie MJ. Early identification of refractory epilepsy. *N Engl J Med*. 2000;342(5):314-319.

Malmgren K, Thom M. Hippocampal sclerosis—origins and imaging. *Epilepsia*. 2012;4:19-33.

Quigg M, Rolston J, Barbaro NM. Radiosurgery for epilepsy: clinical experience and potential antiepileptic mechanisms. *Epilepsia*. 2011;53(1):7-15.

Wiebe S, Blume WT, Girvin JP, et al. Effectiveness and efficiency of surgery for Temporal Lobe Epilepsy Study Group. A randomized, controlled trial of surgery for temporal-lobe epilepsy. *N Engl J Med*. 2001;345(5):311-318.

Case 77

Corpus Callosotomy

Thomas L. Beaumont, MD, PhD ● Matthew D. Smyth, MD

Presentation

A 17-year-old male with Lennox-Gastaut syndrome presents with medically refractory atonic seizures. He has experienced multiple extremity fractures and repeated mild head trauma related to daily drop attacks. He underwent vagal nerve stimulator (VNS) placement 3 years prior, with some improvement in his mood and alertness, but no significant reduction in seizure frequency.

- PMH: acute lymphocytic leukemia (ALL), status post bone marrow transplant
- Exam: grossly neurologically intact
  - Somewhat cooperative, no distress
  - Cranial nerves intact
  - Moving all extremities with 5/5 strength
  - Ambulates without assistance, stable gait

Differential Diagnosis

- Medication noncompliance
- VNS malfunction
- Focal epilepsy with secondary generalization

Initial Imaging

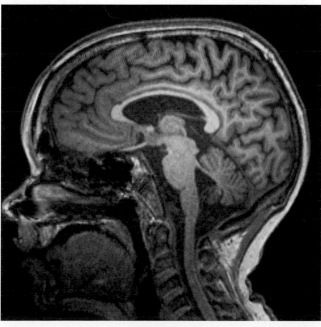

FIGURE 77-1

Imaging Description

- Figure 77-1 shows a preoperative noncontrast T1-weighted MRI of the brain which shows no intracranial lesions.

Further Workup

- Laboratory
  - Routine labs
  - ESR, CRP
  - Antiepileptic drug (AED) levels
- Imaging
  - Brain MRI with and without contrast, including 1 mm slices for stereotactic navigation
- Electrodiagnostics
  - Continuous electroencephalography with video monitoring
- Consultants
  - Epileptology

Pathophysiology

The corpus callosum is composed of 200 million commissural fibers whose primary role is to effect contralateral inhibition. With the exception of the primary motor cortex, which has limited or no callosal projections, the position along the rostrocaudal axis of corpus callosum roughly indicates the brain regions subserved. In the setting of epilepsy, corpus callosum provides a route for bilateral synchronization and rapid generalization of seizure activity leading to atonia and/or loss of consciousness. Corpus callosotomy reduces bilateral synchronization and the rapid generalization of ictal discharges. After callosotomy, interictal discharges can become lateralized to the side of the dominant seizure onset zone. Therefore, callosotomies are effective for drop attacks and seizures with multiple, bilateral foci.

Because the corpus callosum is involved in contextual learning, memory, and associative tasks, a spectrum of disconnection syndromes can occur following callosotomy. In higher functioning patients, an anterior callosotomy (about 2/3rds) that spares the splenium can be performed to preserve parietal interhemispheric connections and minimize the likelihood of a disconnection syndrome (mutism, apraxia and hemiparesis).

Treatment Options

- Medical
  - Multi-agent AED therapy
- Surgical
  - Vagal nerve stimulator
  - Often preferred option over callosotomy
  - Left side decreases cardiac risk
  - Corpus callosotomy
    - Anterior two thirds
    - Complete, with or without sparing of splenium

Surgical Technique
Corpus Callosotomy

The patient is positioned supine with the head neutral, chin flexed, and the torso elevated 10 degrees above the horizontal (Figure 77-2). Mannitol and intravenous antibiotics are given prior to skin incision. A curvilinear, bicoronal incision is located over the coronal suture (Figure 77-3). The bone flap is centered on the coronal suture, extending across midline (Figure 77-4). Frameless neuronavigation can be used to avoid cortical veins and

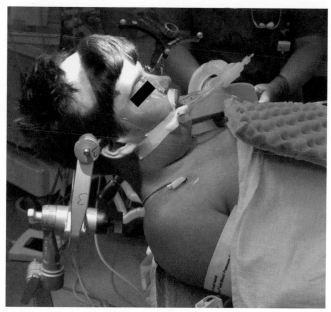

FIGURE 77-2   The patient is positioned supine with the head neutral to facilitate venous outflow and minimize intracranial venous pressure. The chin is flexed and the torso elevated 10 degrees above horizontal. *(Reprinted with permission from Jandial R, McCormick P, Black PM.* Core Techniques in Operative Neurosurgery. *Elsevier; 2011.)*

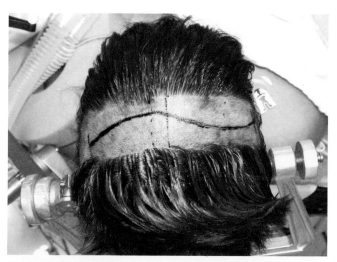

FIGURE 77-3   A gentle curvilinear, bicoronal incision is located over the coronal suture extending between the superior temporal lines bilaterally. *(Reprinted with permission from Jandial R, McCormick P, Black PM.* Core Techniques in Operative Neurosurgery. *Elsevier; 2011.)*

to optimize the trajectory to the anterior and posterior extent of the corpus callosum. Six to eight burr holes are placed for dural stripping and a 4 × 8 cm craniotomy is turned. Bleeding from the sagittal sinus can be controlled with Gelfoam and cottonoids; bipolar cautery can be used judiciously. A U-shaped dural opening is made and reflected toward the superior sagittal sinus until the interhemispheric fissure is visualized (Figure 77-5). Cortical veins posterior to the coronal suture should be carefully preserved. Cotton strips or Telfa are placed on the mesial frontal lobes to minimize injury over the course of the dissection. Arachnoid bands within the interhemispheric fissure are dissected and retractor blades are advanced to deepen the exposure. Frontal lobe retraction is limited to the minimum necessary to expose the corpus callosum, approximately 10–15 mm (Figure 77-6). The pericallosal arteries are identified and should be carefully separated to find the

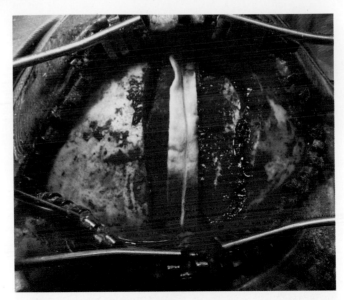

FIGURE 77-4 A 4 × 8 cm craniotomy centered over the coronal suture and extending across midline is performed with six to eight burr holes for dural stripping and to ensure protection of the sagittal sinus. Bleeding from the dura overlying the sagittal sinus is controlled with Gelfoam and cottonoids. *(Reprinted with permission from Jandial R, McCormick P, Black PM.* Core Techniques in Operative Neurosurgery. *Elsevier; 2011.)*

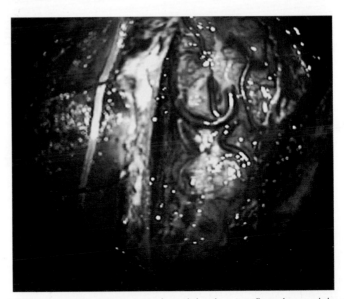

FIGURE 77-5 A U-shaped dural opening is made and the dura is reflected toward the superior sagittal sinus until the interhemispheric fissure is visualized. Care should be taken to preserve all bridging veins, particularly when posterior to the coronal suture. *(Reprinted with permission from Jandial R, McCormick P, Black PM.* Core Techniques in Operative Neurosurgery. *Elsevier; 2011.)*

avascular midline. The characteristic white appearance of the corpus callosum is visualized between the pericallosal arteries after sharp dissection of adherent arachnoid bands (Figure 77-7). The length of the intended disconnection is completely exposed before beginning callosotomy. It is helpful to confirm midline with neuronavigation before beginning the resection. Callosotomy is performed with a combination of low-power bipolar cautery and suction or ultrasonic aspiration. Dividing the callosum, by entering between the midline, will leave the septum, preserve the ependymal lining, and minimize the risk of

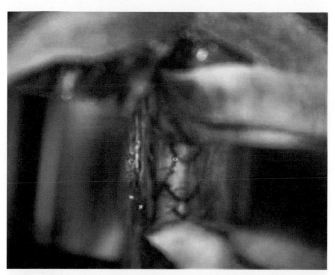

FIGURE 77-6   Cotton strips or Telfa are placed on the mesial frontal lobes to minimize injury during dissection. Arachnoid bands within the interhemispheric fissure are sharply divided and retractor blades are advanced to expose the pericallosal arteries and corpus callosum. Frontal lobe retraction is limited to the minimum necessary, approximately 10–15 mm. *(Reprinted with permission from Jandial R, McCormick P, Black PM.* Core Techniques in Operative Neurosurgery. *Elsevier; 2011.)*

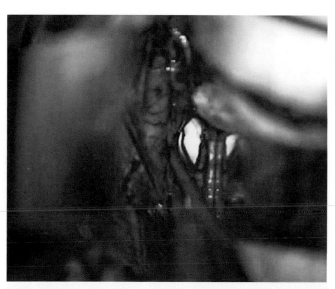

FIGURE 77-7   The characteristic white appearance of the corpus callosum is visualized between the pericallosal arteries after arachnoid dissection. Frameless stereotactic navigation can be used to confirm the midline before beginning callosotomy to prevent entry into the ventricle. *(Reprinted with permission from Jandial R, McCormick P, Black PM.* Core Techniques in Operative Neurosurgery. *Elsevier; 2011.)*

postoperative CSF leak. Posterior callosotomy can be challenging, because the angle of the splenium falls away from the surgeon (Figure 77-8). During this final maneuver, the table is placed in relative Trendelenburg position and the microscope is directed posteriorly to facilitate intracallosal disconnection from the posterior body to the splenium. Care is taken to preserve the pial membrane just posterior to the splenium to prevent injury to the internal cerebral veins and vein of Galen. Postoperative MRI (Figure 77-9) demonstrates complete corpus callosotomy.

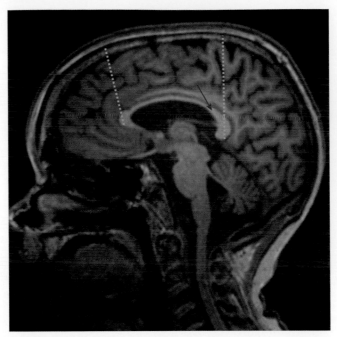

FIGURE 77-8   During posterior callosotomy, the table is placed in relative Trendelenburg position and the microscope is directed posteriorly (arrow) to facilitate intracallosal disconnection from the posterior body to the splenium. Hashed lines indicate the operative corridor.

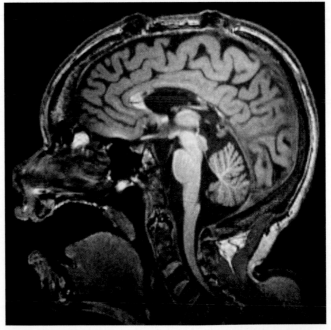

FIGURE 77-9   Postoperative noncontrast T1-weighted MRI demonstrating complete disruption of the corpus callosum.

Complication Avoidance and Management

- Injury to cortical veins causing venous infarction
  - Preserve all bridging cortical veins posterior to coronal suture
- Retraction injury to medial frontal lobes
  - Administer mannitol early and use mild hyperventilation (pCO_2 30 mmHg)
  - Place cotton or Telfa strips along the frontal lobes
- Injury to pericallosal arteries
  - Perform interhemispheric dissection with operative microscope
- Entry into ventricles resulting in CSF leak
  - Verify midline using neuronavigation and identify leaflets of septum pellucidum
- Incomplete callosotomy
  - Completely expose corpus callosum before beginning callosotomy
  - Perform intracallosal sectioning of the splenium when performing single stage, and then complete callosotomy
- Injury to internal cerebral veins or vein of Galen
  - Preserve pial membrane posterior to the splenium

KEY PAPERS

Fuiks KS, Wyler AR, Hermann BP, et al. Seizure outcome from anterior and complete corpus callosotomy. *J Neurosurg.* 1991;74(4):573-578.

Jalilian L, Limbrick DD, Steger-May K, et al. Complete versus anterior two-thirds corpus callosotomy in children: analysis of outcome. *J Neurosurg Pediatr.* 2010;6(3):257-266.

Kasasbeh AS, Smyth MD, Steger-May K, et al. Outcomes after anterior or complete corpus callosotomy in children. *Neurosurgery.* 2014;74(1):17-28.

Sunaga S, Shimizu H, Sugano H. Long-term follow-up of seizure outcomes after corpus callosotomy. *Seizure.* 2009;18(2):124-128.

Tanriverdi T, Olivier A, Poulin N, et al. Long-term seizure outcome after corpus callosotomy: a retrospective analysis of 95 patients. *J Neurosurg.* 2009;110(2):332-342.

Case 78

Normal Pressure Hydrocephalus

Michael Bohl, MD ● David S. Xu, MD ● Peter Nakaji, MD

Presentation

A 67-year-old woman with gait difficulties, progressively decreased cognition, and an inability to carry out her ADLs is seen. Her family says that her walking has become progressively slower over time and she shuffles instead of taking long strides. Dementia workup reveals mild psychomotor slowing; otherwise she is normal.

- PMH:
  - Right internal carotid stenosis treated with thromboendarterectomy 6 months ago
  - Hypertension
  - Hyperlipidemia
- Family Hx: Alzheimer's disease in mother
- Exam:
  - Oriented to self and location, has trouble with the date
  - Gait is broad based, without turned feet and a magnetic/glued foot shuffle
  - No apraxia
  - Otherwise intact

Differential Diagnosis

- Neurodegenerative
  - Cortical dementias
    - Alzheimer's disease (coexistent in up to 75% of iNPH patients)
    - Frontotemporal dementia (personality and psychiatric abnormalities more prevalent)
  - Subcortical dementias
    - Parkinson's disease (often asymmetric symptoms, apraxia, rest tremor, gait is not broad-based, and feet are not externally rotated)
- Vascular
  - Vascular dementia (asymmetrical symptoms and step-wise progression; up to 75% coincidence)
- Metabolic/toxic
  - Wernicke-Korsakoff syndrome/alcoholic encephalopathy (ophthalmoplegia, ataxia, amnesia, confabulation)
- Psychiatric
  - Age-related depression (depressive thought content, responsive to antidepressants)
- Other
  - Age-related cognitive decline
  - Aqueductal stenosis
  - iNPH

Initial Imaging

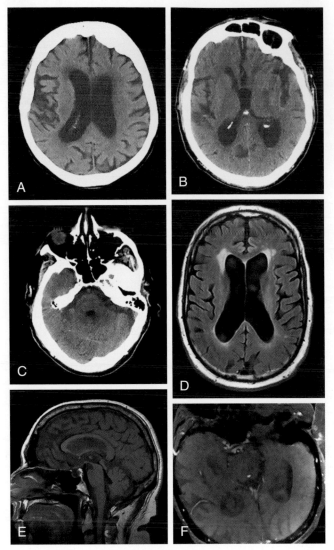

FIGURE 78-1

Imaging Description and Differential

- Figure 78-1A-C shows axial CT images of a patient with lateral and third ventriculomegaly, but with a relatively normal sized fourth ventricle. Aqueductal stenosis, age-related atrophy, and ex vacuo ventricular dilatation secondary to ischemic vascular disease should all be considered. Mild periventricular hypodensity is consistent with increased interstitial fluid and microvascular white matter disease. Figure 78-1D shows a corresponding axial FLAIR MR image of ventriculomegaly and transependymal flow of CSF surrounding the frontal horns. (Images used with permission from Barrow Neurological Institute.)

- On sagittal T1-weighted MRI (Figure 78-1E), increased flow through the cerebral aqueduct can be seen in the form of a flow void jet into the fourth ventricle. Real-time cine phase contrast MRI (Figure 78-1F) can be used to quantify the flow rate of CSF through the aqueduct. Hyperdynamic flow and elevated stroke volumes (in many studies >42 μL/stroke) have been described as being diagnostic of NPH and predictive of good response to CSF diversion. The diagnostic and prognostic utility of this study remains controversial. (Images used with permission from Barrow Neurological Institute.)

- Differential: age-related atrophy, ex vacuo dilatation secondary to ischemic vascular disease, or obstructive hydrocephalus (e.g., aqueductal stenosis)

Further Workup

- Laboratory
  - Routine labs
  - Dementia workup (TSH, vitamin B_{12}, ESR, VDRL)
- Consults
  - Neurology for neurocognitive evaluation, spinal tap, and Tinetti gait and balance testing
- Confirmatory testing
  - Large volume (30–40 mL) lumbar tap, or temporary external CSF drainage, which has a high positive predictive value (>95%) for clinical improvement after ventriculoperitoneal shunt (VPS)

Pathophysiology

The pathophysiology of iNPH remains poorly understood. Many prominent theories highlight the role of the loss of blood vessel and parenchymal viscoelasticity, resulting in decreased periventricular compliance that can transmit CSF "water hammer" pulsations; this decreased periventricular compliance subsequently alters venous compliance and disrupts the egress of CSF into the dural sinuses. Less compliant white matter that is subject to higher CSF pulsations is furthermore at greater risk for ischemia, thereby offering a possible explanation for the association between vascular dementia and iNPH. It has also been hypothesized that decreased CSF turnover may lead to the buildup of toxic metabolites and plaques, such as beta-amyloid, which would explain the association between iNPH and Alzheimer's disease.

Treatment Options

- Surgical
  - Permanent CSF diversion remains the treatment of choice for NPH; gait disturbance symptoms are the most frequent to respond, with improvements in memory and bladder occurring less frequently.
    - VPS is most commonly used because of its relatively low complication rate and ease of insertion.
    - Other distal locations for a ventricular shunt include the pleura and right atrium for patients with extensive prior abdominal surgery or high intraperitoneal pressure (ascites and morbid obesity).
    - Endoscopic third ventriculostomy is not an appropriate treatment for NPH.
- Observation
  - Variable rates of progression; nearly all patients eventually develop the full clinical triad of gait disturbance, memory impairment, and urinary incontinence; life expectancy among nontreated patients with NPH is less than that of treated patients.

Surgical Technique

For a right VPS the patient is positioned supine with the head turned to the left. The incision site can be planned with stereotactic navigation or based on anatomic landmarks (Kocher's point or Keen's point). A small incision is made, a subgaleal pocket is bluntly dissected with a Kelly clamp, and then a small burr hole is made with the underlying dura coagulated. Attention is then turned to the abdomen where intraperitoneal access can be obtained with a trocar or by direct visualization. The distal catheter is then tunneled from the scalp incision to the abdomen and placed in the peritoneal cavity. The shunt valve is attached to the distal catheter and placed in the subgaleal pocket in the scalp. The proximal shunt catheter is then inserted into the lateral ventricle and secured to the proximal valve inlet.

Complication Avoidance and Management

- Peritoneal access
  - Verification of intraperitoneal placement can be performed by testing runoff through the distal catheter with a manometer.
  - In patients with a history of extensive abdominal surgery, assistance by general surgery should be sought to minimize risk of bowel injury.
- Over/under shunting
  - Use of adjustable valves can allow titration of CSF drainage in order to pursue greater clinical response through increased CSF drainage or to ameliorate complications related to overdrainage, such as development of bilateral hygromas or subdural hematomas

KEY PAPERS

Bradley WG Jr, Scalzo D, Queralt J, et al. Normal-pressure hydrocephalus: evaluation with cerebrospinal fluid flow measurements at MR imaging. *Radiology*. 1996;198(2):523-529.

Hakim CA, Hakim R, Hakim S. Normal-pressure hydrocephalus. *Neurosurg Clin N Am*. 2001;12(4):761-763.

McGirt MJ, Woodworth G, Coon AL, et al. Diagnosis, treatment, and analysis of long-term outcomes in idiopathic normal-pressure hydrocephalus. *Neurosurgery*. 2008;62(suppl 2):670-677.

Relkin N, Marmarou A, Klinge P, et al. Diagnosing idiopathic normal-pressure hydrocephalus. *Neurosurgery*. 2005;57(suppl 3):S4-S16.

Toma AK, Stapleton S, Papadopoulos MC, et al. Natural history of idiopathic normal-pressure hydrocephalus. *Neurosurg Rev*. 2011;34(4):433-439.

Case 79

Idiopathic Intracranial Hypertension (Pseudotumor Cerebri)

Benjamin D. Elder, MD, PhD ● C. Rory Goodwin, MD, PhD ●
Thomas A. Kosztowski, MD ● Daniele Rigamonti, MD

Presentation

A 35-year-old female with a history of migraines presents with a worsening headache, nausea, and pulsatile tinnitus in the right ear. She reports acutely worsening blurred vision and double vision for the past several days.

- PMH: otherwise unremarkable
- Exam:
  - Severe papilledema bilaterally (Figure 79-1A)
  - Concentric field constrictions bilaterally (Figure 79-1B)
  - Right sixth nerve palsy
  - 20/100 vision (previously 20/20)
  - Otherwise neurologically intact

Differential Diagnosis

- Neoplastic
  - Mass lesion
  - Leptomeningeal carcinomatosis
- Vascular
  - Sinus thrombosis
  - AVM or dural AV fistula
  - Superior vena cava syndrome

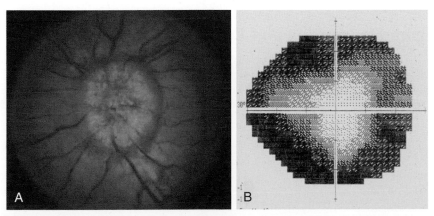

FIGURE 79-1 **(A)** Fundoscopic exam shows severe papilledema. **(B)** Formal visual field testing demonstrates concentric visual field cut.

- • Bilateral jugular vein thrombosis or ligation
- • Post hemorrhagic hydrocephalus
- • Infectious
  - • Meningitis
  - • Postinfectious hydrocephalus
- • Inflammatory
  - • Sarcoidosis
- • Other
  - • Idiopathic intracranial hypertension (IIC)
  - • Secondary pseudotumor cerebri

Initial Imaging

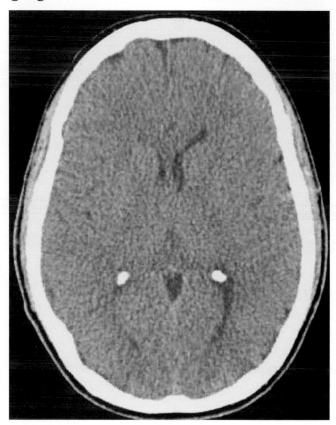

FIGURE 79-2

Imaging Description and Differential

- • The head CT in Figure 79-2 demonstrates no focal abnormality in the brain paren-chyma. The ventricles are normal in size and position. There is no mass effect or abnor-mal extraaxial collection. The basilar cisterns are patent.
- • Differential: idiopathic intracranial hypertension, less likely sinus thrombosis or venous outflow obstruction

Further Workup

- • Laboratory
  - • Routine labs
  - • CSF for glucose; cell count; bacterial, fungal, and mycobacterial cultures; and cytology
    - • CSF sent once mass lesion ruled out on initial imaging

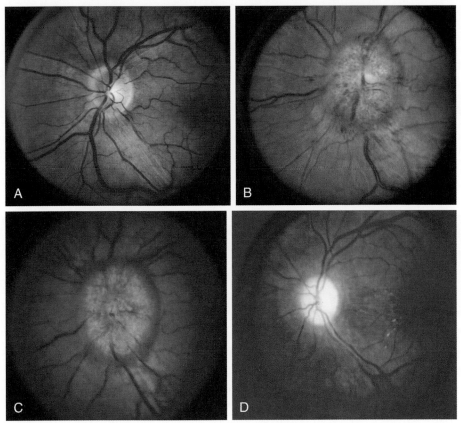

FIGURE 79-3 Varying degrees of papilledema (Frisén scale). **(A)** Grade I papilledema with a C-shaped halo and a temporal gap. Grade II papilledema has a circumferential halo (not shown). Grade III papilledema shows many major vessels as they leave the disc (not shown). **(B)** Grade IV papilledema characterized by a loss of major vessels on the disc. **(C)** Grade V papilledema meets grade IV criteria, plus partial or total obscuration of all vessels of the disc. **(D)** A normal fundus is included for comparison.

- Imaging
  - MRI/MRV to evaluate for sinus thrombosis or transverse sinus stenosis, neoplastic lesions, or signs of infection/inflammation of the leptomeninges
- Procedural
  - Lumbar puncture for opening pressure and aforementioned studies if mass lesion is ruled out
- Consultants
  - Ophthalmology (Figures 79-3 and 79-4)
  - Neurology

Pathophysiology

IIC, formerly known as pseudotumor cerebri, is a rare disorder characterized by signs and symptoms of elevated intracranial pressure, normal CSF composition, elevated ICP (>250 mm H_2O in the lateral decubitus position), no identifiable cause on imaging, such as ventriculomegaly, mass, structural, or vascular lesion, and no other cause including medication of intracranial hypertension.

The exact mechanism of IIC is unclear, but several theories have been introduced. First, it is believed to be related to stenosis of the transverse sinus (Figure 79-5). Increased intracranial venous pressure results from stenosis of the distal portion of the transverse sinus. It is unclear if the elevated intracranial pressure causes the transverse sinus stenosis or if the sinus stenosis results in elevated intracranial pressure; likely a combination of the two in a self-perpetuating cycle. As CSF is passively resorbed into the sinus, via arachnoid

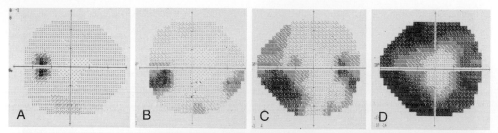

FIGURE 79-4 Automated visual field testing. **(A)** Enlargement of the physiologic blind spot. **(B)** Enlarged physiologic blind spot and inferior nasal loss. **(C)** Worsening nasal and temporal field loss. **(D)** Severe concentric field loss.

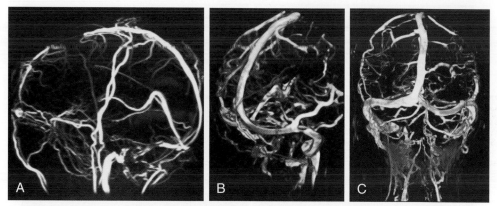

FIGURE 79-5 **(A)** CT venogram demonstrates sagittal sinus thrombosis. **(B)** Contrast-enhanced MR venogram demonstrates right transverse sinus stenosis lateral to the vein of Labbé. **(C)** Contrast-enhanced MR venogram demonstrates a hypoplastic right transverse sinus.

granulations, sinus stenosis can impair venous drainage and CSF absorption. Additionally, the occurrence of microthrombosis in cerebral veins may impair venous drainage and CSF absorption. Evidence also exists of increased brain water content and brain compliance, which prevents ventricular dilation on imaging; thus, small ventricles remain as the total volume within the cranial vault remains constant due to an equilibrium between CSF and blood flow. Furthermore, there may be excess CSF production or reduced CSF absorption. There is an association with abnormal vitamin A metabolism and lower body adiposity. Finally, new data suggest a relationship with aquaporin-4, involved in brain water homeostasis, and abnormal serotonin/norepinephrine regulation, which has an effect on the choroid plexus.

Treatment Options

- Medical
  - Weight loss (associated with improvement in papilledema and headaches)
  - Carbonic anhydrase inhibitors (acetazolamide)
    - Decrease secretion of CSF from choroid plexus
    - Effective in 75% of patients with IIC
    - Effective dose is 1–4 g daily in divided doses
  - Furosemide
    - Reduces CSF secretion from choroid plexus
  - Corticosteroids
    - Rapidly decrease ICP, but not suitable for chronic use
    - May have rebound intracranial hypertension

- Surgical
  - Optic nerve sheath fenestration (ONSF)
    - Opens "window" in sheath of edematous nerve
    - Treatment of choice for patients with failing vision as main symptom, but does little to treat headache
    - Mechanism poorly understood, but likely increases blood flow to optic nerve
    - More effective in acute papilledema than chronic papilledema
    - ~35% chance of failure from 3–5 years post-op
    - Complications include failure, ischemic optic neuropathy, and transient blindness
  - CSF shunting
    - Ventricles not enlarged, so lumboperitoneal shunting often performed over ventriculoperitoneal shunting, though either treatment is acceptable
    - Curative procedure, but many complications
      - >50% of patients require revision within 2 years of treatment, often sooner
      - LP shunt failure rate at least 50%, with complications of Chiari formation, infection, obstruction, intracranial hypotension, lumbar radiculopathy, and abdominal pain
- Interventional
  - Transverse sinus stenting
    - Between 30% and 90% of patients with some degree of transverse sinus stenosis
    - 78% of patients had improvement of headache and 85% with improvement of papilledema with stenting
    - Typically require only unilateral stenting
    - ICPs decrease from mean 322 mmH$_2$O to 220 mmH$_2$O
    - Mean pressure gradient across stenosis decreases from 20 mmHg to <1 mmHg
    - 12% of patients require restenting at an average of 20 months, from adjacent segment stenosis
    - Requires dual aspirin/Plavix antiplatelet therapy with 3–5 day load

Surgical Technique
Lumbar Catheter Insertion

The patient is positioned in the lateral position on a beanbag with an axillary pad. (Figure 79-6) A midline incision is made in the lower lumbar region, and the fascia is exposed. A Tuohy needle is inserted between the spinous processes into the subarachnoid space, the stylet is removed, and the proximal catheter is advanced into the subarachnoid space for at least 5 cm and the needle is then removed. The catheter is tunneled to a flank incision where a pocket for the valve is created and a third incision is made in the abdomen for the distal shunt.

Ventricular Catheter Insertion

The catheter can be inserted in the frontal or parietooccipital region, though due to the small ventricles in IIC patients, the frontal approach is preferred. For a frontal catheter, a curvilinear incision overlying Kocher's point is made, and the pericranium is preserved. A subgaleal pocket is made to house the valve and reservoir, a burr hole is made, dura opened, and the catheter is passed to a depth of 5 ± 2 cm for a frontal approach. The tubing is tunneled to the peritoneal site and the valve is advanced into the pocket and secured to the pericranium with 4-0 sutures.

Peritoneal Insertion

A paramedian incision is made just lateral to midline, rectus fascia is exposed and incised parallel to the muscle fibers, after which the inner muscle fascia and parietal peritoneum are incised and a blunt dissector is inserted into the peritoneum to verify the proper location.

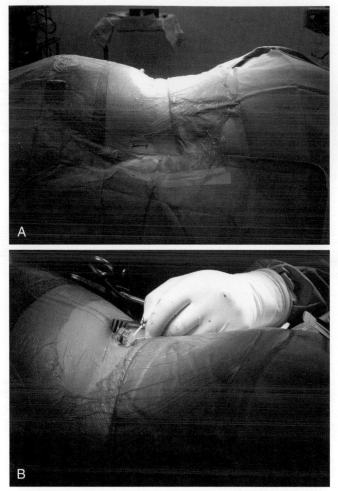

FIGURE 79-6 The patient is positioned in the lateral position on a beanbag with an axillary pad. **(A)** A midline incision is made in the lower lumbar region. **(B)** The catheter is tunneled to a flank incision where a pocket for the valve is created and a third incision is made in the abdomen for the distal shunt.

Complication Avoidance and Management

- IIC patients who present with acute vision loss are a small subset, but are the patients that require much earlier neurosurgical involvement, as medical therapy does not provide rapid enough treatment to prevent further visual decline. These patients require emergent surgical intervention, including emergent optic nerve sheath fenestration (if available at the institution), or shunt placement. Alternatively, if transverse sinus stenosis is present, the patient can be temporized with lumbar drain placement to stabilize vision loss as a bridge to further definitive stenting treatment. Although serial lumbar punctures are an option, this treatment often may not remove enough CSF unless performed multiple times each day and may not prevent further visual decline.
- When performing ventricular catheterization in IIC patients, catheter misplacement is a common complication. Using image guidance during catheter placement is the best way to mitigate the risk of catheter malposition. We generally opt to perform LP shunting in this patient population due to this risk of ventricular catheter misplacement and a risk of shunt malfunction from collapsed ventricles, though either procedure is acceptable. When using LP shunts, we prefer horizontal-vertical (H-V) valves, which have two valve components that allow for controlled drainage when supine or upright. This prevents the siphoning effect when a patient elevates from supine to upright, which can be especially pronounced in LP shunts. However, these valves must be implanted in the correct orientation to function properly.

- Finally, there is a substantial infection risk with all shunt placements. Some modifications that have significantly decreased the infection risk include a wide shave, 5-minute prescrub with povidone-iodine solution, wide draping, minimizing traffic within the operating room, and minimizing handling of the shunt or its contact with the patient's skin. These practices are recommended in all shunt surgeries.

KEY PAPERS

Ahmed RM, Wilkinson M, Parker GD, et al. Transverse sinus stenting for idiopathic intracranial hypertension: a review of 52 patients and of model predictions. *AJNR Am J Neuroradiol*. 2011;32(8):1408-1414.

Arac A, Lee M, Steinberg GK, et al. Efficacy of endovascular stenting in dural venous sinus stenosis for the treatment of idiopathic intracranial hypertension. *Neurosurg Focus*. 2009;27(5):E14.

Friedman DI. Pseudotumor cerebri. *Neurol Clin*. 2004;22(1):99-131vi.

Tarnaris A, Toma AK, Watkins LD, et al. Is there a difference in outcomes of patients with idiopathic intracranial hypertension with the choice of cerebrospinal fluid diversion site: a single centre experience. *Clin Neurol Neurosurg*. 2011;113(6):477-479.

Case 80

Intractable Oncologic Pain

Nelson Moussazadeh, MD ● Michael G. Kaplitt, MD, PhD

Presentation

A 66-year-old woman with endometrial cancer, metastatic to her pelvis, hip, and recently irradiated right leg has had 1 month of intractable pelvic, hip, low back, and bilateral leg pain severely limiting her mobility and is refractory to optimal medical therapy.

- PMH: hip replacement for lytic metastasis; otherwise unremarkable
- Exam:
  - Right hip and leg tenderness to palpation
  - Pain-limited bilateral LE motor exam
  - Neurologically nonfocal
  - Normal sensory exam and rectal tone

Differential Diagnosis

- Neoplastic
  - Intractable oncologic pain referable to metastatic lesions
  - Spinal/radicular metastases
- Degenerative
  - Spinal stenosis or lumbar disk herniation (in the setting of chronic low back pain or sudden onset radicular pain, respectively)
  - Pathologic or osteoporotic lumbar compression fracture
- Other
  - DVT (high suspicion in cancer patients with unilateral leg pain)
  - Neuropathy (often from chemotherapy or other medications)
  - Retroperitoneal hematoma or infection (increased risk from chemotherapy-induced thrombocytopenia or neutropenia)

Initial Imaging

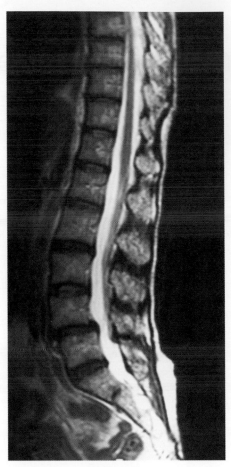

FIGURE 80-1

Imaging Description and Differential

- Sagittal T2-weighted thoracolumbar MRI demonstrates absence of spinal metastasis, canal-obstructing deformity, or other mass lesion.
- Differential: intractable oncologic pain not referable to, and ITP not contraindicated by, spinal involvement

Further Workup

- Laboratory
  - Routine labs including coagulation profile and platelet count to rule out bleeding dyscrasias (common in the setting of myelosuppression in oncologic patients)
- Imaging
  - Complete spinal MRI with contrast to rule out spinal/leptomeningeal metastases
- Consultants
  - Pain management for potential epidural opiate catheter trial
  - Medical oncology for life expectancy assessment and coordination of care

Pathophysiology

Pain can affect up to half of all cancer patients, and intractable pain in terminally ill patients can severely limit quality and quantity of remaining life. Both nociceptive and neuropathic mechanisms related to tissue damage, paraneoplastic inflammatory mediator secretion, nerve damage, and a variety of cancer treatments contribute.

Treatment Options

- Medical
  - Oral/transdermal analgesia
  - Intravenous patient-controlled anesthesia (usually requires institutionalization)
  - Epidural analgesia (generally reserved for dosing titration prior to intrathecal drug delivery system/IDDS implantation or for outpatients with very short life expectancies)
- Interventional and radiation therapies
  - Ablative therapy for symptomatic/progressive osseous or soft tissue metastases
  - Cementoplasty (vertebroplasty/kyphoplasty/sacroplasty) for selected spinal compression fractures
  - Neurolytic block (e.g., celiac/hypogastric plexi, splanchnic nerve, stellate, and dorsal root ganglia)
- Surgical
  - Neurectomy/cordotomy
  - Spinal cord stimulator: generally useful for neuropathic pain and possibly back pain, but unusual to use for cancer pain, which is often mixed
  - Intrathecal pump/IDDS: approved for morphine, baclofen, and ziconotide; shown to confer reduced pain and drug toxicity, and potentially improved survival in RCT; preoperative neuraxial epidural trial is not necessary for prediction of IT dose requirement; off-label mixing of opiates with local anesthetics or other neuropathic agents is often used in specialty settings

Surgical Technique
Intrathecal Pump

After the induction of general anesthesia, the patient is positioned laterally, with the side amenable to the pump pocket up (right side up in this case, given the patient's leg and hip disease). In cancer patients, take care when positioning not to dislocate artificial or diseased hips/shoulders. Axillary roll is placed, beanbag is deflated to hold the patient in position, and fluoroscopy is used to mark a parasagittal incision just inferior to e.g., the L3 and L4 interspace. Abdominal incision is marked just below the costal margin, taking care to ensure that the pump will neither irritate the rib cage nor prevent hip flexion. Cancer patients also often have a variety of ostomies, or prior abdominal/flank incisions, which must be considered when planning incisions and tunneling paths to avoid hardware contamination or wound/skin complications. The lumbar back, flank, and abdomen are prepped and draped, and incision marks are infiltrated with anesthetic.

The back incision is taken to the lumbodorsal fascia, and a Tuohy needle is passed via an inferior-to-superior and lateral-to-medial approach into the mid spinal canal as guided by AP and lateral fluoroscopy. This approach reduces the risk of kinking from bending a catheter placed through a midline, in a straight-on approach. Upon demonstration of CSF egress, a U-stitch is placed through the fascia, around the needle, and clamped out of the way. Performing this prior to needle removal avoids risk of needle penetration of the catheter.

The distal catheter is passed superiorly until approximately T10 and the needle and central stylet are removed (Figure 80-2). The final tip location may vary more in cancer patients compared with degenerative patients, depending on the primary location of pain. Isolated pelvic pain often responds best with a lower catheter tip location, and chest wall or upper thoracic pain benefits from a higher location. Note that drugs such as opiates diffuse well, so exact catheter position relative to pain is less critical. Other drugs are most effective with a precisely placed catheter tip. The tip position is reconfirmed by fluoroscopy and CSF flow is rechecked prior to tightening the U-stich and again rechecking CSF flow. The anchoring device is slid over the catheter, its neck secured to the fascia to prevent catheter migration, and CSF flow again reconfirmed.

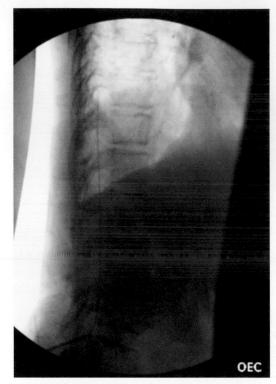

FIGURE 80-2   Intraoperative fluoroscopy.

Following abdominal incision, a suprafascial pocket is made subcutaneously inferior to the incision. In exceedingly thin cancer patients or children, a subfascial placement can be considered. It is unusual for a cancer patient to be obese, but in those situations, avoid placing the pump deeper than 2 cm below the skin surface, because this can make both refilling the drug reservoir and telemetry communication with the pump difficult. The pump is prepared by first flushing out the storage solution; the filled pump (with drug or preservative-free saline) is then placed into the mesh bag.

The proximal catheter is tunneled from the abdomen to the back wound. Both catheters are then trimmed, connected with a straight connector, covered with a plastic boot, and secured with ties. Excess proximal catheter is drawn into the abdomen until the joined catheter unit is laid flush in back without kinks or right angles, CSF egress is reconfirmed, and the proximal catheter end is attached to the pump and secured with a tie. An alternative longer spinal catheter can be tunneled to the abdomen and is connected to the pump with a small connector.

Excess catheter is looped behind the pump and the excess loops and pump are placed into the subcutaneous pocket, ensuring that the refill valve is facing toward the skin, and that the pump edge is parallel to, and sufficiently free from, the costal margin. The pump can be inserted into a mesh bag and the back of the mesh bag is secured to the fascia with interrupted stitches. Alternatively, metal loops on the pump can be secured directly to the fascia with sutures. The wounds are irrigated with antibiotics; Scarpa's fascia, deep dermis, and skin are reapproximated; and the closed wounds are cleaned and dressed. The patient is extubated supine and immediately examined for lower extremity neurology. The pump is programmed to infuse at the lowest possible initial rate. Do not leave the pump off for a long period of time as the catheter can become easily obstructed due to lack of flow.

Complication Avoidance and Management

- Catheter placement and continuity
  - It is key to position the patient in true lateral with fluoroscopy at the beginning of the case, to monitor catheter migration superiorly upon threading, and to monitor

and correct kinking as necessary. Do not withdraw and reinsert the catheter through a fixed needle as this can shear the catheter. Also, try to position the needle tip in the center of the spinal canal by fluoroscopy. Despite good CSF flow, a needle tip that is off center in either direction could only be partially within the subarachnoid space and could still lead to epidural catheter placement. Ensure clear CSF egress at all manipulative stages. Use particular care to not occlude catheter when securing it and to ensure loops of excess catheter remain behind the pump where it is safe from percutaneous reservoir instrumentation.

- Postoperative care
  - Prompt initial and serial neurologic exams following emergence from anesthesia and initiation of drug infusion are essential given the risk of direct spinal cord injury from hematoma formation. Lower extremity hypesthesia, bowel/bladder dysfunction, and other sensory changes or weaknesses should prompt a detailed physical exam, pump interrogation, and stoppage, given the likelihood of drug overdose if local anesthetics or neuropathic pain agents are included in the drug mix; related symptoms should resolve within 1–2 hours. If there is no prompt resolution, or if the drugs used are opiates alone, imaging and possible exploration are warranted.
  - Cessation of analgesic effect, abdominal or back tenderness, and swelling should all prompt an appropriate malfunction workup, including multiplanar X-ray to evaluate catheter continuity, which can be secondary to device disconnection or occlusion. Infectious symptoms should be worked up immediately given the risk of meningitis. A change in neurological exam after a long period of stable therapy often, but not always, is associated with loss of pain relief, and should prompt consideration of a catheter tip granuloma/inflammatory mass causing cord compression. Intrathecal pumps are generally compatible with MRI, but CT myelography can also demonstrate an intrathecal mass at the catheter tip. This is associated less with opiates than other drugs and is also less common in cancer patients, because it often requires many months or years to develop and the life expectancy of cancer patients requiring neurosurgical pain intervention is generally lower than for other pain patients. While these are known but rare complications that must be considered, the most common cause of loss of efficacy, or change in neurological exam, in cancer patients is disease progression.

KEY PAPERS

Chai T, Bruel BM, Nouri KH, et al. Complications after intrathecal drug delivery due to the underlying malignancy in two patients with intractable cancer pain. *Pain Physician.* 2013;16(2):E107-E111.

Malhotra VT, Root J, Kesselbrenner J, et al. Intrathecal pain pump infusions for intractable cancer pain: an algorithm for dosing without a neuraxial trial. *Anesth Analg.* 2013;116(6):1364-1370.

Marcus DA. Epidemiology of cancer pain. *Curr Pain Headache Rep.* 2011;15(4):231-234.

Smith TJ. An implantable drug delivery system (IDDS) for refractory cancer pain provides sustained pain control, less drug-related toxicity, and possibly better survival compared with comprehensive medical management (CMM). *Ann Oncol.* 2005;16(5):825-833.

Ver Donck A, Vranken JH, Puylaert M, et al. Intrathecal drug administration in chronic pain syndromes. *Pain Pract.* 2014;14(5):461-476.

Case 81

Spinal Cord Stimulation

Daniel M. Birk, MD ● Konstantin V. Slavin, MD

Presentation

A 52-year-old woman presents with a history of persistent chronic lower extremity radiculopathy and axial pain after lumbar laminectomy and discectomy. Her primary complaint is shooting pain along the L5-S1 dermatome bilaterally. The patient has been evaluated by pain specialists and is refractory to conservative measures. She requires increasing doses of oral narcotics to manage her symptoms.

- PMH: diabetes mellitus and a tobacco smoker
- Examination:
  - No tenderness to palpation of the spine
  - Normal examination of upper extremities
  - Right lower extremity: weakness of extensor hallucis longus
  - Decreased sensation to pinprick in L5-S1 dermatomes on the right
  - Antalgic gait

Differential Diagnosis

- Chronic neuropathic pain
  - Failed back surgery syndrome (chronic radicular and axial pain after lumbosacral surgery)
  - Complex regional pain syndrome due to traumatic or surgical peripheral nerve injury (reflex sympathetic dystrophy)
- Vascular
  - Peripheral arterial occlusive disease
- Endocrine
  - Diabetic neuropathy
- Infectious
  - Postherpetic neuralgia
- Other
  - Metabolic disorder

Initial Imaging

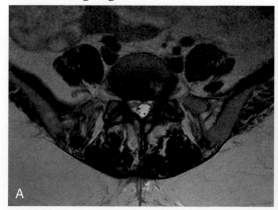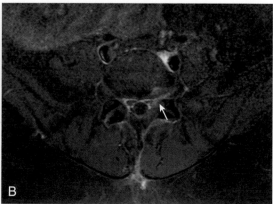

FIGURE 81-1

Imaging Description and Differential

- Lumbar spine MRI in Figure 81-1A and B show pre- and postcontrast axial images with evidence of previous surgery at L4-L5 level, correlating with pain distribution.
- Differential: failed back surgery syndrome versus other pain syndrome

Further Workup

- Laboratory
  - Routine labs
- Psychological screening
  - Widely practiced and required part of routine presurgical evaluation; has high negative predictive value (unfavorable findings correlate with poor outcomes), but an uncertain positive predictive value (no correlation between favorable psychological profile and treatment success)

Pathophysiology

The gate control theory of neuropathic pain describes a balance between large and small sensory fibers in feedback loops that control dorsal horn cells. Large-diameter peripheral nerve fibers, which close the dorsal horn "gate," have a lower threshold for activation by an electrical field. Spinal cord stimulation (SCS) elicits antidromic signals from the dorsal column fibers to neurons in the dorsal horns that release GABA. Orthodromic activation is responsible for the paresthesias experienced during stimulation. SCS can selectively activate the fibers due to their spatial arrangement in the dorsal columns. Other proposed mechanisms involve interneurons in the dorsal horn and descending fibers or sympathetic fibers. Neurohormonal changes may explain poststimulation analgesia effects.

Failed back surgery syndrome is characterized by chronic pain in the back and legs after lumbosacral spine surgery. Along with other studies, the prospective, randomized, controlled multicenter study of patients with failed back surgery syndrome (PROCESS) provides conclusive evidence of better pain relief and quality of life, yet higher costs, for patients with spinal cord stimulators when compared with medical management. SCS with physical therapy was shown to be superior to physical therapy alone in patients with complex regional pain syndrome; however, the difference disappeared at 5 years due to control group improvement.

Treatment Options

- Medical
  - Medical management with pain service consultation
- Surgical
  - Spinal cord stimulation: best option for chronic pain related to failed back surgery syndrome where radicular symptoms are more severe than axial pain; SCS may also be used to treat complex regional pain syndrome or ischemic pain.
  - Intraspinal infusion system: programmable opioid pumps have proven efficacy in patients with cancer-related pain.
  - Repeat lumbar spine surgery: evidence that SCS is more effective than redo spinal surgery in the presence of operable pathology

Surgical Technique

Placement of epidural electrodes can be done percutaneously, or with a single-level laminectomy, for placement of paddle-type electrode. Wire-like (percutaneous), or more recently introduced percutaneously insertable paddle electrode leads, may be freely advanced in a cranial direction. Regular paddle (laminectomy-type) electrode leads may only be placed one to two levels cranial to the laminectomy. For lower extremity pathology a percutaneous electrode lead should be inserted at L1-L2 or L2-L3; targets for stimulation range from T8-T12 based on the location of pain.

Intravenous sedation, local anesthesia, and prone positioning with C-arm fluoroscopy for an AP view of the thoracolumbar junction are utilized. A linear incision is made at the

L3 level with dissection to the fascia after infiltration with lidocaine. Insert the Tuohy needle into the epidural space at the L1-L2 level. CSF flow indicates subarachnoid placement and this should be avoided. The entry into the epidural space is confirmed by loss of resistance with gentle aspiration; if a percutaneous electrode lead is planned, it is then inserted through the Tuohy needle. A guide wire is inserted through the needle and advanced in a cephalad direction under live fluoroscopy (Figures 81-2 and 81-3). Once the needle is removed, the lead delivery device is inserted over the guide wire into the

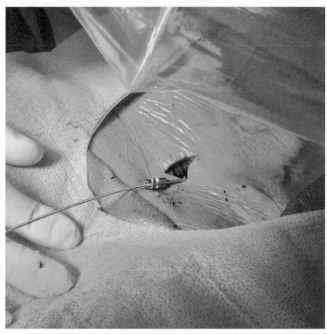

FIGURE 81-2 Tuohy needle with guide wire inserted into the epidural space at L1-L2. *(Courtesy of Dr. Slavin.)*

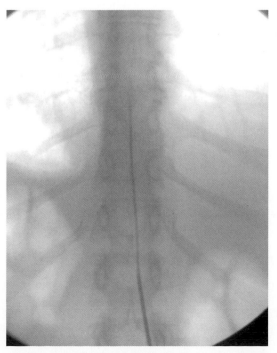

FIGURE 81-3 Guide wire is advanced in a cephalad direction under live fluoroscopy. *(Courtesy of Dr. Slavin.)*

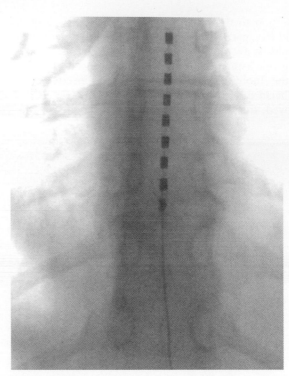

FIGURE 81-4   Electrode is advanced in a cephalad direction under live fluoroscopy. *(Courtesy of Dr. Slavin.)*

epidural space. The guide wire is removed and an eight-contact narrow paddle electrode lead is inserted through the lead delivery device and advanced to the level of T6-T7, either over the midline or slightly off the midline on the side of the pain. During electrode lead insertion, confirm the position of the lead with fluoroscopy and consider turning the C-arm laterally to be sure that the electrode lead is positioned in the dorsal epidural space (Figure 81-4).

Intraoperative stimulation is performed by adjusting the polarity of the electrodes, the pulse width of stimulation, the frequency of stimulation, and the stimulation amplitude to cover the painful areas of the patient with paresthesias. For bilateral symptoms, the same procedure may be repeated on the other side for the second electrode (Figure 81-5).

The electrode leads are secured using anchors partially buried in the fascia with a tension relief loop distal to the anchor. The anchors are secured with nonabsorbable sutures at multiple points. The electrode lead position is reconfirmed and the subcutaneous extension cables are tunneled lateral and in a cephalad direction. Each extension cable is connected to the electrode tail and secured with a set-screw, plastic sleeve, and nonabsorbable ties. Bury the excess of the electrode leads and connectors between the leads and extension cables under the skin. Finally, the incision is closed in layers, using nylon for the skin, and to secure the extension cables (Figure 81-6).

After a successful weeklong trial of stimulation via an external generator, the patient may return for internalization of the electrode leads and implantation of the pulse generator under general anesthesia. If the trial is unsuccessful, remove or revise the electrode leads.

Complication Avoidance and Management

- Spinal cord stimulation has low risks, but occasional complications such as wound breakdown, infection, or lead migration, may require reoperation. Creating a strain relief loop reduces the risk of migration. Hardware durability may limit device longevity. A rarely reported complication is paralysis due to epidural compression or abscess. Most practitioners avoid the use of monopolar cautery to avoid overheating the electrodes and damaging tissue.

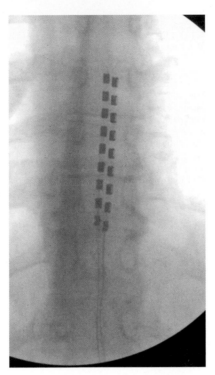

FIGURE 81-5   For bilateral symptoms, a second electrode may be inserted. *(Courtesy of Dr. Slavin.)*

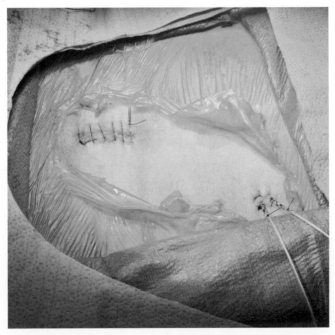

FIGURE 81-6   The incision is closed in layers and tunneled electrodes are secured. *(Courtesy of Dr. Slavin.)*

KEY PAPERS

Kemler M, De Vet H, Barendse G, et al. Effect of spinal cord stimulation for chronic pain complex regional pain syndrome type I: five-year final follow-up of patients in a randomized, controlled trial. *J Neurosurg.* 2008; 108:292-298.

Kumar K, North R, Taylor R, et al. Spinal cord stimulation vs. conventional medical management: a prospective, randomized, controlled, multicenter study of patients with failed back surgery syndrome (PROCESS Study). *Neuromodulation.* 2005;8:213-218.

Melzack R, Wall PD. Pain mechanisms: a new theory. *Science.* 1965;150:971-979.

North RB, Kidd DH, Piantadosi S. Spinal cord stimulation versus reoperation for failed back surgery syndrome: a prospective, randomized study design. *Acta Neurochir Suppl.* 1995;64:106-108.

Slavin KV. Placing neuromodulation in the human body: limiting morbidity. In: Arle JA, Shils JL, eds. *Essential Neuromodulation.* London: Academic Press; 2011:301-320.

Turner JA, Loeser JD, Deyo RA, et al. Spinal cord stimulation for patients with failed back surgery syndrome or complex regional pain syndrome: a systematic review of effectiveness and complications. *Pain.* 2004;108: 137-147.

Section VII Peripheral Nerve Neurosurgery

Case 82

Thoracic Outlet Syndrome

Justin Brown, MD ● Mark A. Mahan, MD

Presentation

A 27-year-old woman is referred for upper extremity pain and numbness. She has noted intermittent pain and numbness in her left arm during the past several years. The course has been notable for occasional "flare-ups" separated by months without symptoms. Over the past year her symptoms have worsened, significantly affecting her ability to perform activities of daily living, such as brushing her teeth, combing her hair, removing bottle lids, and donning her clothes. The pain originates at the lateral border of her neck and medial scapula, and descends medially along the left arm into the fourth and fifth digits of her left hand. She has undergone prior treatment, including physical therapy and chiropractic therapy, but exercise and stretching exacerbated her symptoms.

- PMH: otherwise unremarkable
- Exam:
  - Hand is warm and well perfused when dependent and shoulder adducted; raising her arms over her head results in pallor of the left hand and exacerbation of symptoms; full strength in intrinsic and extrinsic muscles to the fingers
  - Decreased sensation of the ulnar side two digits of the left hand on Semmes-Weinstein monofilament test
  - Tinel's sign at the left wrist, retrocondylar groove, and supraclavicular fossa
  - Palpable fullness in the left supraclavicular fossa; applying direct pressure to this region reproduces the majority of her symptoms into the neck, back, arm, and hand

Differential Diagnosis

- Neoplastic
  - Peripheral nerve sheath tumor
  - Pancoast tumor
- Vascular
  - Aneurysm of subclavian artery
- Degenerative
  - C8 radiculopathy
  - Cubital tunnel syndrome

Initial Imaging

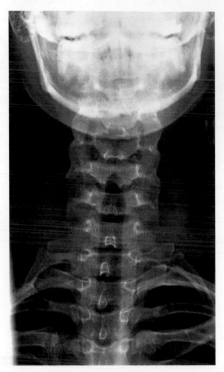

FIGURE 82-1

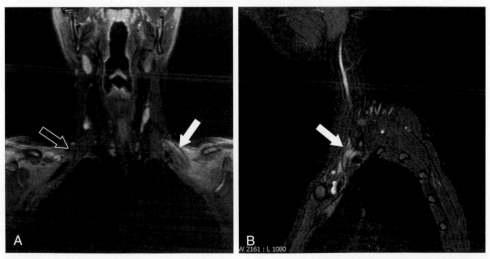

FIGURE 82-2   *(Printed with permission from the University of Utah.)*

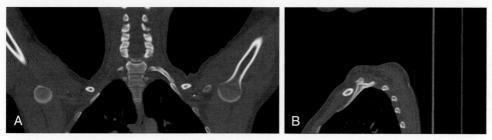

FIGURE 82-3   *(Printed with permission from the University of Utah.)*

Imaging Description and Differential

- EMG /NCS – mildly enlarged motor units with reduced recruitment, indicating chronic axonal loss in the C8-T1 myotomes; smaller medial antebrachial cutaneous sensory response on the left
- Chest X-ray – Figure 82-1 demonstrates bilateral cervical ribs with vertical orientation of the left cervical rib.
- MRI – Figure 82-2A shows coronal fat-suppressed T2-weighted MRI depicting left cervical rib pseudoarthrosis with the left first rib, and elevation and edema of the lower and middle trunks (compare solid arrow versus the outline arrow). Figure 82-2B shows sagittal fat-suppressed T2-weighted MRI demonstrating severe narrowing of the left subclavian artery at the pseudarthrosis, with tortuosity and edema of the lower and middle trunks (indicated by the solid arrow).
- CTA chest – Figure 82-3 demonstrates bilateral cervical ribs with pseudarthrosis between the left cervical rib and the first thoracic rib; with the patient's arms above the head, there is moderate narrowing of the left costoclavicular space.

Further Workup

- Physical therapy
  - Must ensure that nerve glides, scalene stretches, and postural exercises were utilized rather than activities that would exacerbate the symptoms (e.g., exercises that would focus on strengthening the shoulders, chest, and upper trapezius)
- Pain management
  - Scalene injections (e.g., Botox) or C7-T1 TFESI can at times alleviate symptoms such that the patient can better participate in proper therapy.

Pathophysiology

Compression of the nerves of the brachial plexus after they exit the spine and before they enter the axilla is the common denominator in thoracic outlet syndrome. Although cervical ribs are a classic finding, they account for <10% of neurogenic thoracic outlet syndrome cases. Anything that narrows the space for the passage of the nerves, including bony calluses from prior trauma, hypertrophied scalene muscles, aberrant arteries, or tight pectoralis minor, can result in symptoms of neck, chest, and arm pain. In many cases, EMG is negative and MRI may not show a notable mass lesion. Neurography sequences can help detect subtle hyperintensity of the nerves as they pass between the scalenes. The physical examination is paramount in the diagnosis. Symptoms are reproduced with arms overhead; pressure over the scalenes should result in severe local pain and reproduce the symptoms throughout the arm. Assessing Tinel's sign at many distal sites of entrapment (that are less dramatic than at the thoracic outlet) may assist in the diagnosis, as would an examination finding of loss of pulse with arms elevated. There remains considerable debate about the proper diagnosis and management of neurogenic thoracic outlet syndrome, especially when there is a paucity of confirmatory data (e.g., anatomic findings and EMG changes).

Treatment Options

- Conservative
  - Physical therapy, including nerve glides, scalene stretches, and postural correction
  - Scalene blocks
  - Medications, including antiepileptics for neuropathic conditions
- Surgical
  - Scalenectomy
  - Rib resection

Surgical Technique

The patient is placed in a supine position with the arm prepped for surgery and positioned at the patient's side. A roll is placed between the scapulae to retract the shoulder with gravity and the head is turned away from the side of surgery. The head of the bed is elevated to 30 degrees. An incision is made 1 cm above the clavicle, starting at the lateral half of the sternocleidomastoid and extending 2 inches to the mid clavicle. The underlying platysma is divided and the supraclavicular nerves are identified under the platysma, looped, and retracted. The lateral half of the sternocleidomastoid is divided and retracted medially. The supraclavicular fat pad is mobilized superolaterally to reveal the anterior scalene and, typically, the upper trunk of the brachial plexus. On the surface of the anterior scalene, the phrenic nerve is found running longitudinally in a lateral to medial trajectory. With the phrenic nerve protected, the anterior scalene is divided. This provides an excellent view of the brachial plexus. Each trunk is then neurolysed and looped. The upper trunk is mobilized inferiorly and the cervical rib is followed proximally. The rib is divided proximally using a 3-mm Kerrison punch and then followed distally. Typically, the subclavian artery will need to be looped and retracted. Once the insertion of the cervical rib onto the first rib is identified, the punch is once again used to divide the rib. If a large callus remains, an ultrasonic tool can be used to remove it. The first rib can be also removed.

Complication Avoidance and Management

- Neuroma pain
  - During the approach it is important to identify and mobilize the supraclavicular nerve branches. Inadvertent transection leads to anterior chest wall numbness and occasionally, burning paresthesias that may last several weeks. Nerve stumps may develop into painful neuromas.
- Preoperative assessment of extent of resection
  - It should be determined preoperatively whether the decompression requires scalene resection alone, cervical rib resection, first rib resection, or even second rib resection. It can be useful to have a vascular surgeon available if significant vascular mobilization is required with rib resection.

KEY PAPERS

Huang JH, Zager EL. Thoracic outlet syndrome. *Neurosurg.* 2004;55(4):897-903.
Roos DB. Congenital anomalies associated with thoracic outlet syndrome: anatomy, symptoms, diagnosis, and treatment. *Am J Surg.* 1976;132(6):771-778.
Tender GC, Thomas AJ, Thomas N, et al. Gilliatt-Sumner hand revisited: a 25-year experience. *Neurosurg.* 2004; 55(4):883-890.

Case 83

Peroneal Neuropathy

Mark A. Mahan, MD ● Justin Brown, MD

Presentation

A 61-year-old man presented with right lower extremity weakness for approximately 1 year. He has noticed a slapping of his foot during gait and having to lift his right leg higher to avoid tripping on his toes. One month after the onset of his lower extremity weakness, he underwent a lumbar 4/5 microdiscectomy, which provided improvement of prior back pain and radiating right lower extremity pain.

- PMH: denies significant current disease, including diabetes, hypothyroidism, and any history of other peripheral nerve disorders, personally, or in his family; prior surgery for lumbar herniated nucleus pulposus; no neck surgery
- Exam:
  - Excellent (MRC 5/5) and symmetric strength in hip flexion, knee extension, knee flexion, foot plantar flexion, foot inversion, and toe flexion; asymmetric right-sided weakness (MRC 4-/5) in foot dorsiflexion; great toe extension and foot eversion
  - Positive Tinel's inferior to the fibular head
  - Hypesthesia along the lateral aspect of his shin and dorsum of foot
  - Negative straight leg raise

Differential Diagnosis

- Central nervous system
  - Stroke
  - Motor strip convexity meningioma
- Lumbar spine
  - L4, L5 radiculopathy
  - Cauda equina syndrome
- Lumbosacral plexopathy
  - Trauma (i.e., blunt or hematoma)
  - Pelvic masses
  - Iatrogenic (e.g., obstetrical injuries)
- Sciatic
  - Traumatic (e.g., hip dislocation)
  - Iatrogenic (e.g., hip arthroplasty)
- Metabolic
  - Diabetes mellitus
  - Pregnancy
  - Myxoedema
- Neoplastic and nonneoplastic mass lesions
  - Peripheral nerve sheath tumors (e.g., schwannoma or neurofibroma)
  - Ganglion cysts of the tibiofibular joint
- Neuropathy
  - Motor neuron diseases (e.g., ALS or poliomyelitis)
  - Generalized polyneuropathies (e.g., CMT, hereditary neuropathy with liability pressure palsy, inflammatory or vasculitic neuropathies, e.g., CIDP)

- Trauma
  - Tibialis anterior tendon rupture
  - Compartment syndrome
- Less common
  - Myotonic dystrophies
  - Multiple sclerosis
  - Leprosy

Initial Imaging

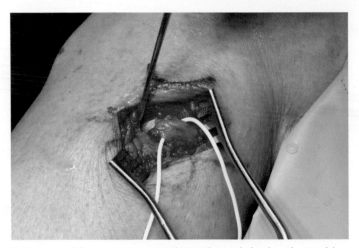

FIGURE 83-1   Entrapment of the common peroneal nerve beneath the deep fascia of the peroneus longus muscle. A Penfield retracts the lateral muscular edge of the peroneus longus, exposing the fascia overlying the common peroneal nerve. The common peroneal nerve (white loop) is visibly kinked immediately lateral to the fascial edge. Fibular head (violet "U" at top); tibial tuberosity (violet dot in upper left corner of image), which is anatomically aligned with the fibular head. *(Reprinted with permission from the Barrow Neurological Institute.)*

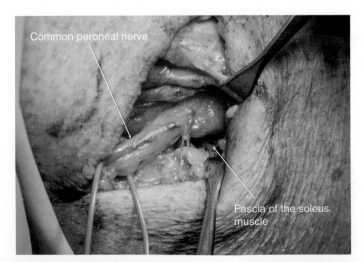

FIGURE 83-2   Compression of the common peroneal nerve by the lateral fascial edge of the soleus muscle. Ragnell retractors mobilize the subcutaneous tissue to visualize the proximal common peroneal nerve. Lower retractor exposes the divided fascial edge of the soleus muscle. The common peroneal nerve is slightly fusiform and swollen adjacent to the lateral fascia of the soleus muscle, indicative of the zone of pathologic compression. *(Reprinted with permission from the Department of Neurosurgery, University of Utah.)*

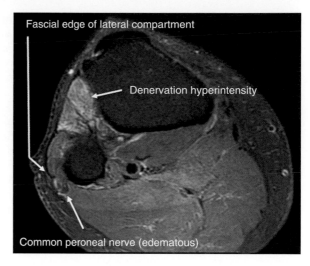

FIGURE 83-3 Proton density axial MRI of the fascial compartments of the lower extremity. Fascia of the lateral compartment and the soleus are well demonstrated to encircle the common peroneal nerve. In this case, the common peroneal nerve is enlarged and edematous. Individual fascicles can be identified – however, at this axial level, the common peroneal nerve makes an anterior turn; the posterior fascicles are diagonal, whereas the anterior fascicles are more horizontal. Denervation hyperintensity of the anterior compartment is well visualized by proton density. *(Reprinted with permission from the Department of Neurosurgery, University of Utah.)*

Further Workup

- Laboratory
  - If diabetes mellitus suspected, A1c
  - Preoperative laboratory studies are not typically necessary unless history is concerning for possible bleeding or clotting diathesis.
- Imaging
  - Imaging is not usually necessary to establish a diagnosis; however, it is appropriate or valuable in the following conditions:
    - Trauma
    - Focal mass or history of peripheral nerve sheath tumor or nerve sheath tumor syndromes, such as neurofibromatosis or schwannomatosis
  - Ultrasound and MRI are the modalities of choice; useful adjuncts to evaluate the health and possible compression of the common peroneal nerve, especially if there is a concern for mass, or if contemplating revision surgery associated with iatrogenic injury.
- Electrodiagnostic studies
  - Nerve conduction velocity – two typical tests: sensory and motor conduction velocity; helpful for identifying decreased conduction, either to axon or myelination loss; practitioner should evaluate for focal slowing of nerve conduction velocity at the fibular head.
  - Electromyography (EMG) – needle EMG is helpful in determining the severity of the lesion and the location (i.e., deep versus superficial peroneal neuropathy); presence of spontaneous firing of the median-innervated muscles, such as fibrillation and positive sharp waves, suggests acute denervation; polyphasic potentials suggest chronic denervation; EMG should include the deep head of the biceps femoris to evaluate for pathology proximal to the fibular head.

Pathophysiology

Common peroneal neuropathy describes a focal mononeuropathy that affects both the deep and superficial peroneal nerves, producing loss of ankle dorsiflexion, ankle eversion, toe extension, and particularly extensor hallucis longus and sensory loss in the cutaneous distribution of the deep and superficial peroneal nerves. CPN is formed after the bifurcation of the sciatic in the mid thigh and continues into the popliteal fossa, medial to the tendon of the biceps femoris. The CPN passes deep to the peroneus longus origin and superficial to the lateral edge of the soleus muscle. The edges of the peroneus longus and soleus are fibrous and frequently pinch the common peroneal nerve at this anatomic location. Within the peroneus muscle, the CPN divides into the superficial peroneal nerve (SPN) and deep peroneal nerve (DPN). The DPN passes through the anterior compartment to supply tibialis anterior, extensor digitorum longus, extensor hallucis longus, and peroneus longus generating ankle dorsiflexion, eversion, and toe extension.

The most common causes for common peroneal neuropathy at the fibular head include trauma, focal entrapment, and compression by local masses. Increased incidence is seen with frequent squatting (roofers and carpet layers). Several traumatic mechanisms frequently cause injury to the common peroneal nerve at the fibular head, with sports-related injuries being perhaps the most common cause of traumatic injury. The mechanisms include focal contusion and stretch or rupture, which may occur with or without knee dislocation, fracture of the fibular head, laceration, and gunshot wound, among others. Iatrogenic injury can occur during knee ligament repair, or knee arthroplasty, especially involving correction of valgus deformities.

Focal entrapment is due to the compression of the common peroneal nerve as it enters the fascia of the lateral compartment (Figure 83-1). The nerve dives under a fascial band on the undersurface of the superficial head of the peroneus longus muscle at the lateral aspect of the lateral compartment. The nerve may also be compressed on the deep surface by the fascia of the posterior compartment (Figures 83-2 and 83-3).

Treatment Options

- Medical
  - There are few proven successful conservative treatments for entrapment of the common peroneal nerve at the fibular head.
  - Posttraumatic stretch injuries should be followed with serial EMG to assess recovery.
- Surgical
  - Entrapment: decompression of the fascia at the fibular head
  - Traumatic, iatrogenic, or other injuries: consider nerve grafting or referral; no nerve transfer options have shown to be successful for common peroneal nerve injuries

Surgical Technique

The most routinely employed technique involves a curvilinear incision centered at the fibular head and approximately 1 cm beneath it (Figure 83-1). The common peroneal nerve lies just deep to the most superficial layer of fascia. The nerve is readily identified by the cord-like movement upon palpation. Once identified, the nerve should be gently neurolysed, proximally, to assess for entrapment by an accessory band of the soleus muscle, the short head of the biceps femoris, the lateral head of the gastrocnemius, or other fascial structures. The superficial investing fascia of the peroneus longus should be elevated and divided without division of the peroneus longus muscle. The muscle belly can then be elevated to expose the deep fascia, which overlies the nerve (Figure 83-2). Gently elevate the nerve to explore if there are fascial ridges beneath. Some practitioners advocate resection of the fascial plate, between the lateral and anterior compartments, for complete decompression of the deep branch.

Complication Avoidance and Management

- The most common complications with common peroneal nerve decompression involve inappropriate localization of the lesion and failure to adequately decompress the nerve. The deep peroneal branch seems the most susceptible portion of the nerve for incomplete decompression, due to the passage from the lateral compartment to the anterior compartment.

KEY PAPERS

Dellon AL, et al. Anatomic variations related to decompression of the common peroneal nerve at the fibular head. *Ann Plast Surg.* 2002;48(1):30-34.

Katirji MB, Wilbourn AJ. Common peroneal mononeuropathy: a clinical and electrophysiologic study of 116 lesions. *Neurology.* 1988;38(11):1723-1728.

Kim DH, et al. Management and outcomes in 318 operative common peroneal nerve lesions at the Louisiana State University Health Sciences Center. *Neurosurgery.* 2004;54(6):1421-1429.

Spinner RJ, et al. Peroneal intraneural ganglia: the importance of the articular branch. A unifying theory. *J Neurosurg.* 2003;99(2):330-343.

Case 84

Nerve Sheath Tumor

Justin Brown, MD ● Mark A. Mahan, MD

Presentation

A 47-year-old woman presents for evaluation of a palpable mass in her left popliteal fossa. She is a runner and has pain in the popliteal fossa that radiates down the anterolateral leg after running. It has become increasingly uncomfortable over the past 6 months.

- PMH: otherwise unremarkable
- Exam:
  - No sensation loss in all major nerves to the lower leg and foot
  - A mobile mass is palpable in the popliteal fossa
  - Percussion of the mass produces mild paresthesias in the anterolateral leg
  - Passive range of motion about the knee and ankle is full
  - Very mild weakness in eversion against resistance, but walks with a normal gait
  - Reflexes – patellar and Achilles reflexes are normal

Differential Diagnosis

- Tumor
  - Lipoma
  - Neurofibroma
  - Schwannoma
  - Neuroma
  - Ganglion cyst
  - Malignant peripheral nerve sheath tumor
- Trauma
  - Hematoma
- Infection
  - Abscess

Initial Imaging

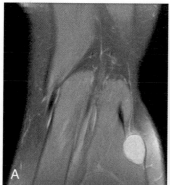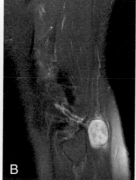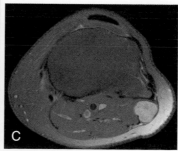

FIGURE 84-1   T1-weighted gadolinium-enhanced **(A)** coronal, **(B)** sagittal and **(C)** axial imaging of the knee demonstrates a cystic mass arising within the common peroneal nerve.

Imaging Description and Differential

- MRI of the knee demonstrates $3 \times 2 \times 2$ cm lesion posterior to the fibular head that is well circumscribed, isointense on T1, and hyperintense on T2, with some cystic component centrally that enhances avidly on contrast administration.

Further Workup

- Laboratory
  - CBC, BMP
  - ESR, CRP
- Imaging
  - Ultrasound
  - PET CT (if suspicion for malignancy to evaluate for metastasis)
- Consultants
  - Pathology (fine needle aspiration if question of malignancy)

Pathophysiology

PNSTs arise from nonnerve cells within the peripheral nerve and are far more common than metastatic lesions to nerves. PNSTs are either schwannomas or neurofibromas, both arising from Schwann cells. Both types of tumor may originate as sporadic and isolated lesions, as a part of a complex, a plexiform lesion, or as a part of a genetic syndrome or mosaic disorder.

The most common PNST is a schwannoma, which typically originates from a single fascicle within the peripheral nerve. They are typically solid and well encapsulated, although they can undergo central necrosis or cystic degeneration. Benign neurofibromas appear quite similar to schwannomas and arise from a nonmyelinating type of Schwann cell. They tend to incorporate additional types of cells and structural elements. Neurofibromas commonly arise from more than one fascicle of a nerve, while plexiform neurofibromas typically arise from multiple fascicles, or the entire nerve, and cannot be resected without significant damage to the nerve of origin. While these tumor types can develop sporadically, neurofibromas are a hallmark feature of NF1 and schwannomas are the predominant tumor type of NF2. Indications for resection of benign tumors include pain or discomfort, or progressive neurological deficit. Severe pain or neurological deficit occur with MPNSTs.

MPNSTs represent 5%–10% of soft tissue sarcomas and typically arise from a neurofibroma, most commonly a plexiform variant. Very rarely they can develop from a schwannoma. They are composed of, at least in part, cells that differentiate toward Schwann cells. Patients with NF1 have an approximately 5%–10% lifetime risk of developing a MPNST. Risk factors that increase the likelihood of a peripheral nerve sheath tumor being malignant include NF1, large size (generally regarded as >5 cm, but <5 cm is not a reliable predictor of benignity), rapid neurologic loss, and pain at rest. They are graded according to the Enneking system (Table 84-1).

TABLE 84-1

BENIGN VS MALIGNANT NERVE SHEATH TUMORS

	Benign	Malignant
Pain	Occasionally painful	Often associated with nocturnal or rest pain
Weakness/numbness	Infrequent	Denervation atrophy frequently present on MRI or EMG
Genetics	Most commonly sporadic	Greater risk in plexiform NF-1 lesions
Size	Frequently small	Frequently >5 cm

Type A tumors are contained within fascial planes, and wide surgical resection can provide cure in some cases.

When addressing PNSTs it is critical to determine whether the lesion is benign or malignant, because the treatment is dramatically different. A benign tumor should be approached with sparing of the nerve as the priority. Surgery for a malignant tumor must consider the patient's overall prognosis and ideally involve a sarcoma tumor board. Open biopsy (intraoperative pathology is insufficient for decision making) with subsequent staged oncologic operation is recommended. If there are diffuse metastases, palliative debulking for neuropathic pain control may be appropriate.

Treatment Options

- Surgery
  - Wide excision
  - Nerve sparing
- Conservative management/monitoring

Surgical Technique

The patient is positioned in the right lateral decubitus position, with the left leg padded and prepped circumferentially. An incision is made starting just inferior to the fibular head, toward the popliteal fossa at the posterior midline. The incision is taken in a Bruner's Z-plasty across the popliteal fossa and ends in the midline, about 1 inch above the popliteal crease. The fascia of the peroneus longus muscle is exposed and is unroofed just proximal to the peroneal nerve. A vessel loop is placed around the nerve and followed proximally. The tumor is encountered about 3–4 cm proximal to the peroneus longus muscle. The nerve is followed further proximally until the bifurcation from the sciatic nerve is identified. Another vessel loop is placed around the nerve, proximal to the tumor. Once the tumor is widely released from the surrounding soft tissue, it is rotated to identify a longitudinal window between nerve fascicles that run over the surface of the tumor. A nerve stimulator is used to confirm that this window contains no excitable nerve tissue. Using a No. 15 blade scalpel, the capsule is divided longitudinally across its entirety making sure not to cross any apparent nerve fascicle. Once the capsule has been divided, a Freer elevator can be used to separate the tumor from the capsule internally. It can often be completely separated from all neural structures, except for a single fascicle entering and exiting the tumor. Once this single fascicle is identified, it is stimulated for motor response. If there is any motor response, the fascicle should be further investigated to be sure it was not simply missed previously, in which case it can be mobilized away from the tumor. Once the tumor has been dissected free from the rest of the nerve, the tumor is then extirpated en bloc (Figure 84-2). The region is irrigated, hemostasis is achieved, and the incision is closed with 3-0 Vicryl and 4-0 Monocryl.

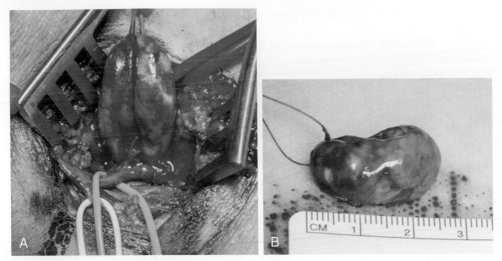

FIGURE 84-2 **(A)** Cystic schwannoma just prior to en bloc removal. Suture is sewn through the tumor to facilitate traction and visualization. Blue vessel loop: parent nerve of the schwannoma. White vessel loop: cutaneous nerve unrelated to parent nerve of the schwannoma. **(B)** Tumor after removal. *(Printed with permission from the University of Utah.)*

KEY PAPERS

Levi AD, Ross AL, Cuartas E, et al. The surgical management of symptomatic peripheral nerve sheath tumors. *Neurosurg.* 2010;66(4):833-840.

Woodruff JM, Selig AM, Crowley K, et al. Schwannoma (neurilemoma) with malignant transformation. A rare, distinctive peripheral nerve tumor. *Am J Surg Pathol.* 1994;8(9):882-895.

Case 85

Cubital Tunnel Syndrome

Justin Brown, MD ● Mark A. Mahan, MD

Presentation

A 53-year-old right hand–dominant woman is referred for evaluation after experiencing approximately 4 months of progressive numbness in the last two fingers of her right hand and aching along the medial forearm. She works as an administrative assistant and notes progressive increase in her symptoms during the workday. Symptoms abate to some degree with rest, but some amount of numbness has persisted for the last couple of months. Additionally, she notes new onset of weakness in grip and difficulty opening jars.

- PMH: otherwise unremarkable
- Exam
  - Hand is warm and well perfused
  - No significant valgus deformity of elbow
  - Decreased sensation in the ulnar-side two digits on Semmes-Weinstein monofilament test
  - Paresthesias in the ulnar-side two digits with maximal elbow flexion
  - Tinel's sign at the retrocondylar groove
  - Weakness
    - Mild intrinsic wasting is visible in the first webspace (first dorsal interosseous muscle)
    - Weakness in abduction of the index finger
    - Positive Froment's sign (thumb interphalangeal flexion to compensate for loss of thumb adduction power from adductor pollicis) (Figure 85-1)
    - Negative Wartenberg's sign (abduction of the fifth finger at rest from unopposed action of the extensor digiti minimi)

Differential Diagnosis

- Neoplastic
  - Nerve tumor
  - Pancoast tumor
- Neuropathic or myopathic
  - Medical conditions: hypothyroidism, diabetes mellitus, alcoholism
  - Hereditary, inflammatory, or other neuropathies
  - Myopathy
  - Amyotrophic lateral sclerosis (lacks sensory findings)
  - Vasculitis
- Degenerative
  - C8 radiculopathy
  - Thoracic outlet syndrome
  - Medial epicondylitis
  - Guyon's canal compression (preserved sensation on dorsomedial hand)

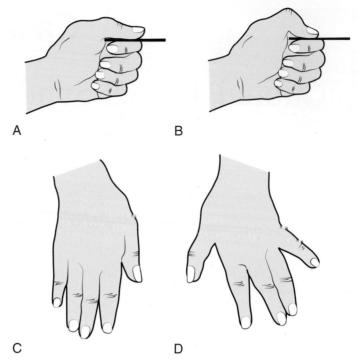

FIGURE 85-1   Special tests for ulna nerve pathology. The importance of Wartenberg's and Froment's signs is in recognizing weakness associated with ulnar nerve compression. Froment's sign: **(A)** normal and **(B)** positive. The patient is asked to grip a piece of paper between their thumb and clench as shown. Flexion of the thumb with resistance indicates significant adductor pollicis weakness (supplied by the ulnar nerve). Wartenberg's sign: **(C)** normal and **(D)** positive. Little finger lies abducted as a result of the unopposed action of the extensor digiti minimi. *(Reprinted with permission from Smith R. Reports on the Rheumatic Diseases. Series 6 Spring 2012. Hands On No. 11.)*

Initial Studies

- NCS demonstrates notable slowing across the cubital tunnel
- EMG demonstrates some insertion activity within the first dorsal interosseous with large appearing motor units

Imaging Description and Differential

- Imaging is uncommonly necessary to establish a diagnosis; however, it is appropriate or valuable in the following conditions:
  - Recurrent or persistent cubital tunnel syndrome after surgical decompression
  - History of peripheral nerve sheath tumors or nerve sheath tumor syndromes, such as neurofibromatosis or schwannomatosis
  - Presence of other mass lesions in the anatomical vicinity
- Ultrasound and MRI are the modalities of choice.
  - MRI of the cubital tunnel (Figure 85-2): the ulnar nerve is enlarged and hyperintense on STIR imaging in the retrocondylar groove (panel A), and returns to normal diameter, without hyperintensity distally in the proximal forearm (panel B); coronal oblique reformat of the STIR imaging depicts ulnar nerve hyperintensity proximal to the entry under Osborne's band, which is the fascial sleeve between the two heads (asterisks) of the flexor carpi ulnaris.

Further Workup

- Laboratory
  - If diabetes mellitus suspected, A1c
  - Preoperative laboratory studies are not typically necessary unless history is concerning for possible bleeding or clotting diathesis.

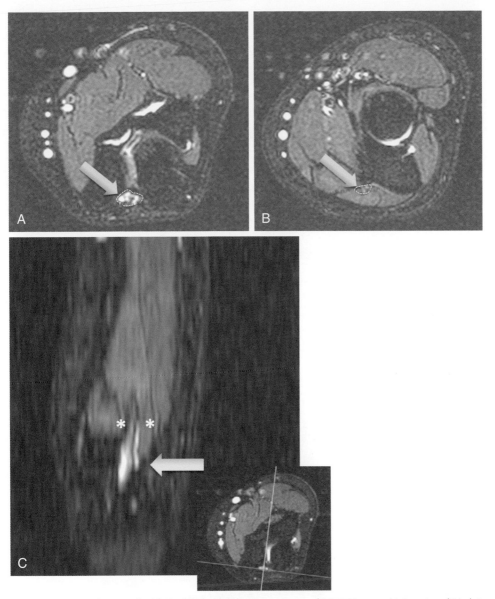

FIGURE 85-2   *(Reprinted with permission of the Department of Neurosurgery, University of Utah.)*

Pathophysiology

Ulnar nerve compression at the elbow is the second most common entrapment neuropathy after carpal tunnel syndrome (Figure 85-3). With elbow flexion, the nerve is subjected to both traction and compression forces. Pressures within the nerve have been measured at >200 mmHg when elbow flexion and flexor carpi ulnaris (FCU) contraction are combined. Commonly, patients exposed to repetitive trauma, including manual labor, athletics, or typical office duties, develop symptoms in a subacute fashion.

Symptoms typically begin with paresthesias in the ulnar-innervated, medial-sided fourth and fifth digits. With ulnar nerve compression at Guyon's canal in the wrist (Figure 85-4), sensation on the dorsomedial hand is preserved because the dorsal cutaneous branch exits proximal to the wrist. This sensory difference, along with Tinel's, can be used to help differentiate ulnar nerve compression at the elbow versus the wrist. Patients frequently complain of aching or cramping in the medial forearm, along the FCU muscle. If the ulnar neuropathy is severe, there may be weakness and atrophy of the ulnar-innervated hand muscles.

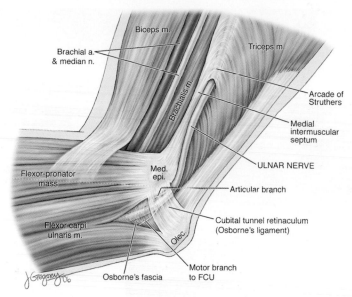

FIGURE 85-3 Anatomy of the ulnar nerve at the elbow. *a*, artery; *FCU*, flexor carpi ulnaris; *n*, nerve; *m*, muscle; *Med. epi*, medial epicondyle; *olec*, olecranon. *(Reprinted with permission from Polatsch DB, et al. Ulnar Nerve Anatomy. Hand Clinics. Volume 23, Issue 3. Pages 283-289.© 2007.)*

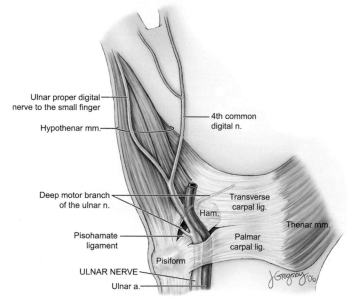

FIGURE 85-4 Anatomy of the ulnar nerve at Guyon canal. *a*, artery; *Ham*, hamate; *lig*, ligament; *mm*, muscles; *n*, nerve. *(Reprinted with permission from Polatsch DB, et al. Ulnar Nerve Anatomy. Hand Clinics. Volume 23, Issue 3. Pages 283-289.© 2007.)*

Treatment Options

- Conservative
  - Elbow pads
  - Nocturnal splinting – straight elbows
  - Physical therapy, including nerve glides
- Surgical
  - Simple decompression
  - Subcutaneous transposition

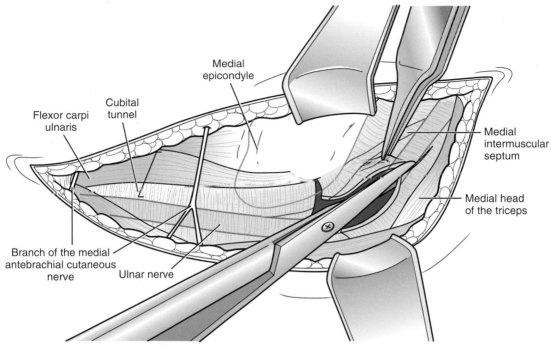

FIGURE 85-5 Simple decompression.

- Submuscular transposition
- Intramuscular transposition

Surgical Technique

The patient is placed in a supine position with the arm abducted on an arm board. The shoulder is abducted and externally rotated. For a simple decompression, an incision is made from 2 inches above the medial epicondyle to 2 inches below, midway between the olecranon and the medial epicondyle, and in line with the course of the ulnar nerve (Figure 85-5). Soft tissue is carefully dissected to avoid transection of the medial antebrachial cutaneous nerve, medial brachial cutaneous nerve, and their branches. Branches of these cutaneous nerves are mobilized by longitudinal soft tissue dissection, and then retracted with vessel loops. The ulnar nerve is identified just posterior to the medial intramuscular septum. The brachial fascia overlying the nerve is divided and the nerve is unroofed through the cubital tunnel (the cubital tunnel retinaculum, arcuate ligament of Osborne) to the level of the FCU. The superficial fascia of the FCU (Osborne's band) is divided, and the plane between the two heads of the muscle (ulnar and humeral head) is spread to reveal the deep fascia of the FCU. This deep fascia is divided until the nerve is fully decompressed.

If a transposition is desired, a skin incision is made from approximately 8 cm proximal to the medial epicondyle to 8 cm distal to the same landmark. All ligamentous structures that retain the nerve posteriorly must be removed or released. This includes the cubital tunnel retinaculum, the FCU fascia, and the medial intramuscular septum between the biceps and triceps. The surgeon may favor a purely subcutaneous transposition, an intramuscular transposition, or a fully submuscular transposition. For a submuscular transposition, the fascia overlying the flexor-pronator mass is divided, and flaps are developed using this divided fascia. The insertion of the flexor-pronator group of muscles is released immediately adjacent to the medial epicondyle to create a trough into which the nerve can be transposed. Care must be taken to release the fascia between the humeral head of the FCU and the flexor digitorum superficialis (FDS) to prevent the ulnar nerve from kinking during flexion. The nerve is mobilized from its surrounding enveloping tissue and transposed into this new trough. The nerve is followed both proximally and distally to ensure there are no additional potential sites of compression. The fascial leaves that were created are loosely reapproximated over the nerve, in its new location, to avoid subluxing out of its new location. A drain is commonly utilized and the skin is closed with Vicryl and Monocryl sutures.

Complication Avoidance and Management

- Transection of medial antebrachial cutaneous nerve
  - During this approach, it is useful to identify and mobilize the overlying medial antebrachial cutaneous nerve. Transection of this nerve can result in a painful incision and the development of a neuroma.
- Iatrogenic luxation
  - With a simple decompression, it is possible to create iatrogenic luxation of the nerve (across the medial epicondyle) when the elbow is flexed. The elbow joint should be passively ranged at the end of decompression to ensure that the nerve does not luxate. This complication may result in recurrence of symptoms and necessitate revision surgery with an anterior transposition.
- Compression of anatomical structures
  - When an anterior transposition is undertaken, a number of normal anatomical structures can become sites of compression. The brachial fascia, the medial intermuscular septum, the proximal most FCU branch from the nerve, and the common aponeurosis of the FCU and FDS all have the potential of tethering or kinking the nerve in its new position and can lead to later recurrence of original symptoms.

KEY PAPERS

Bozentka DJ. Cubital tunnel syndrome pathophysiology. *Clin Orthop Relat Res*. 1998;351:90-94.
Kamat AS, Jay SM, Benoiton LA, et al. Comparative outcomes of ulnar nerve transposition versus neurolysis in patients with entrapment neuropathy at the cubital tunnel: a 20-year analysis. *Acta Neurochir*. 2014;156: 153-157.
Palmer BA, Hughes TB. Cubital tunnel syndrome. *J Hand Surg*. 2010;35A:153-163.

Case 86

Carpal Tunnel Syndrome

Justin Brown, MD ● Mark A. Mahan, MD

Presentation

A 45-year-old automobile mechanic with progressive numbness in his bilateral hands is seen. He describes numbness and tingling in the thumb and radial-sided two digits. The numbness and paresthesias wake him from sleep. He feels worsening numbness while at work and feels that he cannot manipulate tools with dexterity due to the loss of sensation. Mild neck pain. Prior surgery for lumbar herniated nucleus pulposus. No neck surgery.

- Exam:
  - Symmetric and unbreakable strength in all muscles of the bilateral upper extremities; no atrophy of the thenar eminence (compared to contralateral)
  - Positive Phalen's maneuver, reverse Phalen's maneuver, Tinel's at transverse carpal ligament
  - No radiating pain or numbness on percussion of the lower trunk, median nerve in supracondylar fossa, nor at the leading edge of pronator teres
  - Negative Spurling's sign, Lhermitte's phenomenon

Differential Diagnosis

- Cervical spine
  - C6 radiculopathy
  - C7 radiculopathy
  - Myelopathy
- Median nerve entrapment
  - Elbow: supracondylar spur/ligament of Struthers
  - Forearm: pronator syndrome
  - Forearm: anterior interosseous syndrome (Kiloh-Nevin syndrome)
  - Wrist: carpal tunnel syndrome
- Metabolic
  - Diabetes mellitus
  - Pregnancy
  - Myxedema
- Neoplastic and nonneoplastic mass lesions
  - Peripheral nerve sheath tumors (e.g., schwannoma or neurofibroma)
  - Brachial plexopathy
  - Variant muscles
  - Lipomas
  - Ganglion cysts of the carpal tunnel
- Neuropathy
  - Mononeuritis multiplex
  - Ischemic monomelic neuropathy
- Carpometacarpal arthritis
- Less common
  - Ulnar nerve entrapment with Martin-Gruber variant innervation
  - Multiple sclerosis
  - Leprosy
  - Lipomatosis of nerve

Initial Studies

- Electrodiagnostic studies
  - There is some debate about the role of electrodiagnostic studies in carpal tunnel syndrome. They have high correlation to high-quality clinical assessment, and some authors have argued that the results of electrodiagnostic studies do not necessarily correlate with outcome. However, when evaluated prospectively, the results of electrodiagnostic studies have changed management decisions in nearly one fifth of all patients. Electrophysiologic data are compared to ipsilateral ulnar and radial nerves because the contralateral median may be affected. The most sensitive test is prolongation of sensory latency demyelination (measured by stimulating sensory fibers in the palm and recording over the wrist).
  - Nerve conduction velocity: variant innervation patterns, such as the Martin-Gruber anastomosis (communicating nerve branch between median and ulnar nerves in forearm), which is present in approximately 17% of all arms, may partially mimic the typical findings in carpal tunnel syndrome.
  - Electromyography (EMG): needle EMG is helpful in determining the severity of the median neuropathy and localizing the lesion (i.e., forearm compression). Presence of spontaneous firing of the median-innervated muscles in the thenar eminence, such as fibrillation and positive sharp waves, suggest acute denervation; over time, collateral sprouting of residual fibers leads to absence of spontaneous firing and large motor units, in chronic denervation.

Imaging Description and Differential

Median nerve ultrasound: at the distal wrist crease (Figure 86-1A). Median nerve: demonstrates a loss of fascicular pattern, is more hypoechoic, and has an enlarged cross-sectional area (17 mm^2, which is greater than a standard upper limit of 10 mm^2) versus the median nerve in the forearm (Figure 86-1B), which has a cross-sectional area of 6 mm^2.

Further Workup

- Laboratory
  - If diabetes mellitus suspected, A1c
  - Preoperative laboratory studies are not typically necessary unless history is concerning for possible bleeding or clotting diathesis.
- Imaging
  - Imaging is uncommonly necessary to establish a diagnosis; however, it is appropriate or valuable in the following conditions:
    - Recurrent or persistent carpal tunnel syndrome after carpal tunnel release
    - History of peripheral nerve sheath tumor or nerve sheath tumor syndromes, such as neurofibromatosis or schwannomatosis

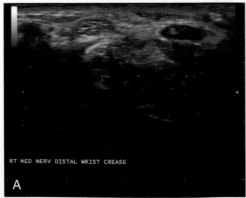
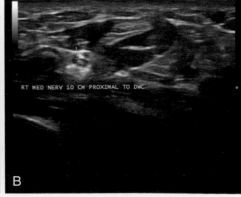

FIGURE 86-1

- Presence of other mass lesions in the anatomical vicinity to the transverse carpal ligament, or other congenital abnormalities, such as macrodactyly
- Ultrasound and MRI are the modalities of choice.
  - Ultrasound: less expensive, more dependent upon the skill and experience of the technician or clinician. Based on meta-analysis, the sensitivity is 78% and specificity 87%, which compares similarly with electrodiagnostic studies in regards to sensitivity, yet with inferior specificity.
  - MRI: more expensive, less reliant on technique

Pathophysiology

Carpal tunnel is formed by the carpal bones and ventrally located transverse carpal ligament (TCL). It contains the median nerve and four tendons of the flexor digitorum superficialis (FDS), profundus (FDP), and the flexor pollicis longus tendon. The median palmar cutaneous branch branches proximal to the TCL, off of the radial side of the median nerve, and courses superficial to the TCL for sensory innervation over the thenar eminence (TCS should not have numb palm) (Figure 86-2). The recurrent motor branch most often comes off of the median nerve, distal to the TCL (anatomic variants that exist with branch arising within TCL), and innervates thenar muscles (opponens pollicis, abductor pollicis brevis, and flexor pollicis brevis) (Figure 86-3).

Carpal tunnel syndrome is a consequence of median nerve compression under the transverse carpal ligament. Additional insults may exist, such as with diabetes mellitus, which may compound problems with osmotic swelling of the finger flexor tendons and susceptibility to neuropathy. For idiopathic cases, numerous theories have been put forth to explain the development of carpal tunnel syndrome. Recently, Amadio and colleagues have published a body of literature explaining that the noninflammatory thickening of the subsynovial connective tissue of the finger flexors appears to be an inciting agent in the development of increased pressure within the carpal tunnel. Finger flexor pathology correlates to the relatively high prevalence of finger triggering in patients with carpal tunnel syndrome.

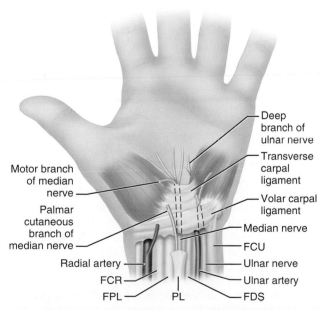

FIGURE 86-2   Care should be taken during wrist incision to avoid cutting the palmar cutaneous branch of the median nerve. *(Reprinted with permission from Canale ST, Beaty JH. Campbell's Operative Orthopaedics. 12th ed. Elsevier; 2013.)*

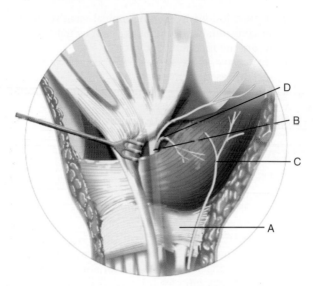

FIGURE 86-3   Artistic drawing demonstrating surgical anatomy of the carpal tunnel: *A*, flexor retinaculum; *B*, median nerve; *C*, palmar cutaneous branch; *D*, recurrent motor branch. *(Reprinted with permission from Huang JH, Zager EL. Mini-open carpal tunnel decompression. Neurosurgery. 2004;54:397.)*

Treatment Options

- Medical
  - Bracing with splints is a primary treatment, especially nocturnal splints.
  - Corticosteroid injections within the carpal tunnel should be considered in advance of surgical decompression.
- Surgical
  - Open transverse carpal ligament release versus endoscopic transverse carpal ligament release; meta-analysis of comparative trials suggests no significant difference at long-term follow-up; however, near-term pain results and earlier return to work favored endoscopic techniques

Surgical Technique

Surgery may be performed while the patient is completely awake, with sedation or general anesthesia, based on surgeon and patient preference. For awake and sedation procedures, procedural anesthesia may be achieved with local anesthesia or regional techniques, such as Bier block. Use of a tourniquet is optional.

The open technique is performed with an approximately 2 cm longitudinal incision in the valley between the thenar and hypothenar eminence – generally in line with the ulnar edge of the fingernail of the folded fourth phalanx (Figure 86-4A). The skin incision should be medial to the palmar crease, and not cross the distal wrist crease, to avoid scar contracture. After the skin is divided, the subcutaneous fat is spread laterally to expose the palmar aponeurosis, which has longitudinally oriented fibers (Figure 86-4B). Deep to the palmar aponeurosis lies the transverse carpal ligament, with transverse fiber arrangement (Figure 86-4C). A palmaris brevis muscle may be superficial to the transverse carpal ligament in some individuals, which should be bipolar coagulated to divide the fibers and expose the transverse carpal ligament (Figure 86-4D). Detection of the constant fat globule, superficial to the median nerve, confirms adequate distal sectioning of TCL. Since the palmar sensory branch is most often on the radial side, sectioning of the TCL should be on the ulnar side of the median nerve to avoid important branches. Once the transverse carpal ligament is sharply divided, the median nerve should be inspected for mass lesions, such as a schwannoma. Scissors may be run proximally and distally to ensure division of the transverse carpal ligament into the palm, and into the distal edge of the antebrachial fascia of the distal forearm.

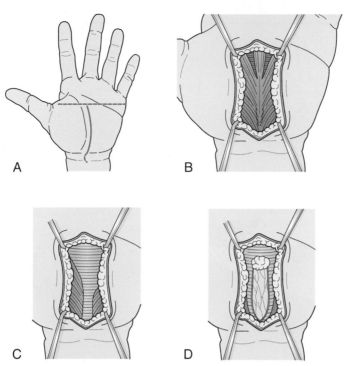

FIGURE 86-4 **(A)** The skin incision extends from the wrist crease to a point in the midpalm in line with the fully extended thumb (*horizontal interrupted line*). An optional extension may be carried out in the distal forearm (*curvilinear interrupted line*) to facilitate exposure of the proximal part of the transverse carpal ligament and the distal part of the deep fascia of the forearm. Note that the main skin incision is not in the palmar skin crease, but just medial to it. **(B)** Exposure of the palmar aponeurosis. **(C)** Exposure of the transverse carpal ligament after midline section and retraction of the palmar aponeurosis. The distal margin of the transverse carpal ligament can faintly be seen blending with the deep fascia of the palm. The proximal part of the transverse carpal ligament is covered by the hypothenar and thenar muscles. In many instances (not shown in this illustration) they may meet and interdigitate in the midline, blocking the transverse carpal ligament from view. **(D)** About 80% of the transverse carpal ligament has been divided, exposing the median nerve. Note the constant fat globule superficial to the median nerve at the distal end of the exposure. *(Reprinted with permission from Ellenbogen RG, Abdulrauf SI, Sekhar LN. Principles of Neurological Surgery. 3rd ed. Elsevier; 2012.)*

The operative technique of endoscopic release requires use of specialized systems, which is well described in other texts. In most systems, the technique involves passage of endoscopic trocar into the carpal tunnel and use of a blade to divide the transverse carpal ligament on withdrawal of the cannulated system.

Complication Avoidance and Management

The most common complications with carpal tunnel release include: incomplete transverse carpal ligament division, injury to the palmar cutaneous branches, injury to the thenar motor branch, accidental decompression of Guyon's canal (contains the ulnar nerve) without decompression of the carpal tunnel, and injury to the median nerve. The most common problem seen by specialists is persistent symptoms (or short-term recurrence) of carpal tunnel syndrome after surgery, which suggests incomplete division of the transverse carpal ligament. There is diversity in the innervation of the palm, and no single surgical incision is without risk of division of the small sensory fibers and consequent potential for the formation of a painful neuroma. In rare circumstances, the thenar motor branch may pass through the transverse carpal ligament, predisposing it to injury. If the surgical dissection proceeds too ulnarly, the surgeon may divide the thin ligament overlying Guyon's canal, which exposes the ulnar nerve and the ulnar artery. The presence of an artery during decompression suggests entrance into Guyon's canal; however, a persistent median artery may be present in up to 10% of individuals.

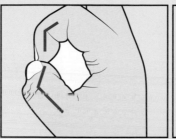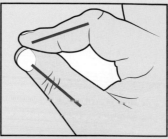

FIGURE 86-5 The "O" sign. Inability to make the "O."

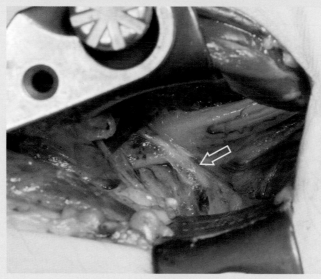

FIGURE 86-6 Ligament above the anterior interosseous nerve, just prior to release. Note the loss of vascularity and blood flow due to compression by the ligament. *(Printed with permission from the University of Utah.)*

- Anterior interosseous syndrome pearls
- AIN originates as branch of the median about 6cm distal to the elbow
- Most AIN dysfunction is inflammatory
- DDx- tendon rupture, proximal median nerve injury, and brachial plexopathy
- Exam: weakness of flexor digitorum profundus (index and middle) and flexor pollicis longus; no sensory findings because AIN has no sensory branches; "O" sign (Figure 86-5)
  - Workup:
    - EMG: inflammatory causes often show changes in muscles outside the AIN distribution
    - MRI: surgical lesions will demonstrate fascicular hyperintensity, often at the tendinous arch of the sublimis muscle (FDS)
- Tx:
  - Spontaneous cases: inflammatory versus compression; if conservative therapy fails (6-months for suspected inflammation and 3 months for suspected compression), consider surgery; inflammation causes more pain, and pain precedes weakness.
  - Closed crush injury: serial clinical and EMG exam; surgery if no improvement at 3 months
  - Penetrating: early exploration
- Surgical technique (Figure 86-6)
  - If decompressing at the sublimis arch, simple linear incision in the proximal forearm, medial to biceps aponeurosis. Identify the plane lateral to the flexor-pronator muscle group and trace the median nerve to the branch of the AIN. Follow the AIN under the sublimis arch and divide the leading edge of the FDS until AIN is decompressed.

KEY PAPERS

Keith MW, Masear V, Chung K, et al. Diagnosis of carpal tunnel syndrome. *J Am Acad Orthop Surg.* 2009;17(6): 389-396.

Phalen GS. The carpal-tunnel syndrome. Seventeen years' experience in diagnosis and treatment of six hundred fifty-four hands. *J Bone Joint Surg Am.* 1966;48(2):211-228.

Scholten RJ, Mink van der Molen A, Uitdehaag BM, et al. Surgical treatment options for carpal tunnel syndrome. *Cochrane Database Syst Rev.* 2007;(4):CD003905, doi:10.1002/14651858.CD003905.pub3.

Brachial Plexus Injury

Justin Brown, MD ● Mark A. Mahan, MD

Presentation

A 24-year-old man presents after recent hospitalization. He was in a high-speed motorcycle accident that resulted in multiple injuries including femur fracture, rib fractures, and traumatic subarachnoid hemorrhage. While he was in rehabilitation, it was discovered that he had no function of his right shoulder or biceps, with numbness of the lateral arm and hand. He was referred to the clinic 3 months after the injury where he presents with no improvement in the weakness and numbness of his arm.

- PMH: otherwise unremarkable
- Exam:
  - Pupils are symmetrical and reactive and face is symmetrical
  - Symmetrical shoulder shrug
  - Notable atrophy of the shoulder and biceps
  - 0/5 shoulder flexion, abduction, and external rotation
  - 0/5 elbow flexion
  - 4/5 triceps and full strength in wrist and fingers

Differential Diagnosis

- Trauma
  - Spinal cord injury
  - Cervical spine trauma with compromise of upper neural foramen
  - Rotator cuff injury
  - Biceps rupture

Initial Imaging

- MRI of the cervical spine and brachial plexus (Figure 87-1A-C)

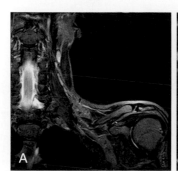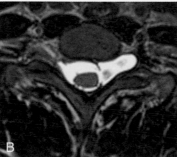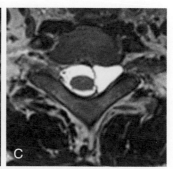

FIGURE 87-1 *(Printed with permission from the University of Utah.)*

Imaging Description and Differential

- MRI of the cervical spine demonstrates no canal compromise, but there is a region of hyperintensity in the right side of the cord between C3 and C6. Additionally, there is an outpouching of cerebrospinal fluid through the neural foramen (pseudomeningocele) on the right, at C4–C5 and C5–C6.
- MRI of the brachial plexus demonstrates redundancy in the upper trunk. Continuity with the spine cannot be confirmed.

Further Workup

- Imaging
  - CT myelogram can be considered to further evaluate for avulsions.
- EMG/NCS
  - EMG confirms loss of motor units to shoulder and elbow flexion muscles. The EMG should also be used to assess potential donor nerves for use in reinnervation. For example, the FCU and FCR should be evaluated for evidence of denervation, as the fascicles to FCU or FCR may be transferred to reinnervate the elbow flexor muscles.
  - NCS can be useful in confirming presence of root avulsions, as sensory nerve conduction will still be present by the continuity of the dorsal root ganglion to the distal nerve.

Pathophysiology

Violent distraction of the shoulder away from the neck, as frequently occurs in high-speed accidents, results in traction of the elements of the brachial plexus. When the traction is severe enough, the elements of the brachial plexus can rupture, or even be avulsed from the spinal cord. Lower trunk spinal nerves (C8 and T1) are less connected to the bone and connective tissue, leading to preganglionic injury (Figure 87-2A, B), and the upper trunk spinal nerves (C5 and C6) are more connected to the bone and lead to postganglionic injury (Figure 87-2C, D).

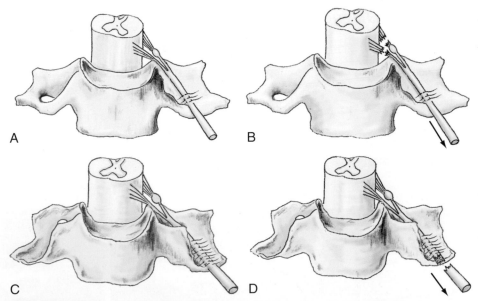

FIGURE 87-2   Severe distracting force can result in nerve stretch injury or even avulsion, depending on local anatomic factors. Note that lower trunk spinal nerves are prone to preganglionic injury. The lower trunk spinal nerves traversing these bony "chutes" are less bound to the bone by connective tissue. Consequently, the C8 and T1 nerves are susceptible to preganglionic injury **(A, B)**, whereas the spinal nerves (C5 and C6), contributing to the upper trunk, tend toward postganglionic injury **(C, D)**. *(Reprinted with permission from Yang LJ-S, McGillicuddy JE. Lower trunk brachial plexus palsy. In: Midha R, Zager E, eds.* Surgery of Peripheral Nerves: A Case Based Approach. *New York: Thieme; 2008:14-17.)*

When nerves are stretched and some degree of motor strength is present immediately after injury, a reasonable recovery can be expected. When paralysis is complete and there is evidence of discontinuity, surgery will be required for recovery. In cases where the proximal end of the nerve is present and in continuity with the spinal cord, nerve grafting is frequently the procedure of choice. When there is no continuity with the spinal cord, grafting is no longer useful and another nerve must be used to reinnervate the target via a nerve transfer.

In this case of avulsion of the C5 and C6 nerve roots, grafting is not an option. Nerve transfers that target the shoulder and elbow flexion function are pursued. A commonly used set of nerve transfers in this case would be transfer of (1) the distal spinal accessory nerve to the suprascapular nerve, (2) triceps branches of the radial nerve to the axillary nerve, and (3) a motor predominant fascicle of the median nerve (primarily innervates the flexor carpi radialis) to the musculocutaneous nerve.

Treatment Options

- Conservative
  - Bracing and physical therapy
- Surgical
- Decompression/neurolysis
- Grafting
- Nerve transfers

Surgical Technique

This procedure can be accomplished in a single anterior approach, or in two stages: first prone for shoulder reanimation, and then supine for musculocutaneous reanimation. We prefer the two-stage procedure, as it affords the easiest access to the distal spinal accessory nerve and offers advantages for axillary nerve reinnervation (Figures 87-3, 87-4, and 87-5).

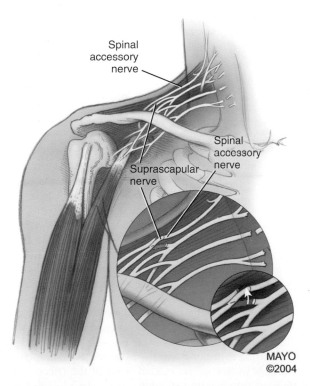

FIGURE 87-3   Transfer of the spinal accessory nerve to the suprascapular nerve. *(Reprinted with permission from the Mayo Foundation for Medical Education and Research. All rights reserved. From Spinner RJ, Shin AY. Green's Operative Hand Surgery. Elsevier; 2011.)*

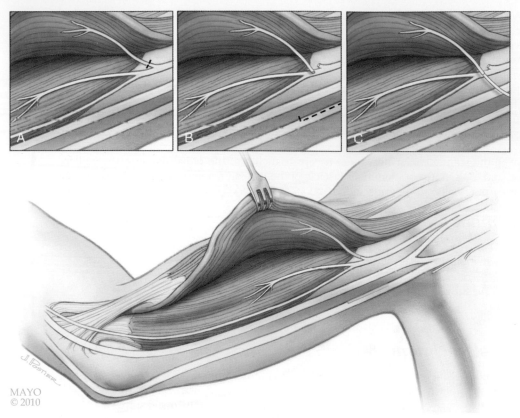

FIGURE 87-4 Ulnar fascicular transfer to the biceps motor branch (Oberlin's method). **(A)** The biceps motor branch is identified and carefully dissected from the musculocutaneous nerve. **(B)** The ulnar nerve undergoes internal neurolysis, and a nerve stimulator is used to choose an appropriately sized fascicle for stimulation of wrist flexion without stimulation of intrinsic hand function. **(C)** The ulnar nerve fascicle is divided and transferred under an operative microscope to the biceps motor branch. *(Reprinted with permission from the Mayo Foundation for Medical Education and Research. All rights reserved. From Spinner RJ, Shin AY.* Green's Operative Hand Surgery. *Elsevier; 2011.)*

Initially, the patient is intubated and placed on gel rolls with the right shoulder and arm supported. A 3 inch horizontal incision is made a finger breadth above the transverse spine of the scapula and centered halfway between the acromion and the spinous processes. As the skin is divided, the trapezius is exposed. A plane is developed between the horizontal fibers of the trapezius; the spinal accessory nerve can be identified on the underside of the trapezius muscle, approximately at the medial border of the scapula. A vessel loop is placed around the spinal accessory nerve and it is dissected as distally as possible, and then divided. Deep to the trapezius and above the suprascapular muscle, the superior border of the scapula is exposed and followed laterally until the suprascapular notch is identified with its associated vessels. The superior transverse scapular ligament is divided, facilitating identification of the suprascapular nerve. This nerve is dissected as proximally as possible and divided. The divided spinal accessory nerve is brought to the proximal divided end of the suprascapular nerve and microcoaptation is undertaken with a 9-0 nylon suture (Figure 87-6).

Next, an incision is made along the posterior deltoid border to the midhumeral level, centered over the triceps. The muscle fascia is exposed and divided, and a plane between the lateral and the long heads of the triceps is developed. At the depth of this interval the radial nerve can be identified running along the humerus. The branches to the triceps are separated and two long branches to the medial head of the triceps are identified. These are followed as distally as possible and divided. Next, the posterior deltoid is retracted, and the axillary nerve is identified deep within the quadrangular space. The cutaneous branch of the axillary nerve serves as an excellent guide to the axillary nerve. The main

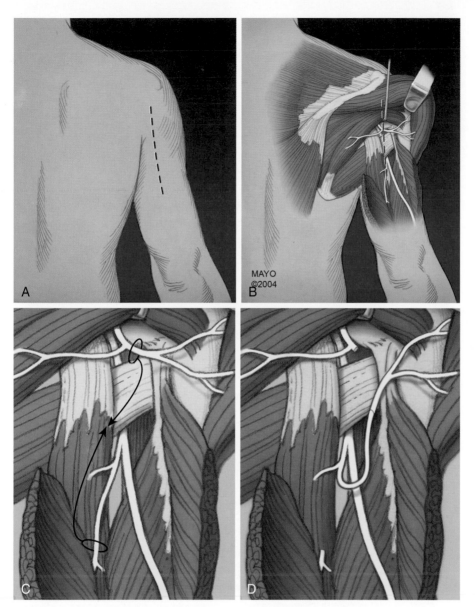

FIGURE 87-5 Transfer of the right triceps branch to the axillary nerve (Leechavengvongs' procedure). **(A)** Skin incision. **(B)** Identification of the axillary nerve in the quadrilateral space and the radial nerve and triceps branches in the triangular interval. **(C)** The long head triceps motor branch is selected and transferred to the anterior division of the axillary nerve. **(D)** Direct nerve repair without tension. *(Reprinted with permission from the Mayo Foundation for Medical Education and Research. All rights reserved. From Spinner RJ, Shin AY.* Green's Operative Hand Surgery. *Elsevier; 2011.)*

axillary, including both anterior and posterior divisions, is followed as proximally as possible and divided. The triceps branches are then brought to the stump of the axillary nerve and coaptated. Ideally, the sensory branch should be excluded from the repair.

In the second stage of the operation, the patient is placed in the supine position with the arm on an arm board. A linear incision is made from the distal axilla to the midhumerus, centered on the medial intermuscular septum. Typically, the median nerve can be identified just beneath the brachial fascia. A vessel loop is placed around the median nerve, and attention is directed to the proximal biceps. The musculocutaneous nerve is identified within a cleft of the proximal biceps near the humerus. A vessel loop is placed around the musculocutaneous nerve and dissected distally. At about one third of

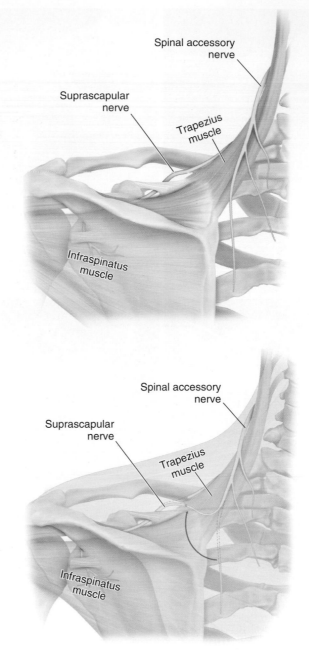

FIGURE 87-6 Nerve transfer of the spinal accessory nerve to the suprascapular nerve. *(Reprinted with permission Kim DH, Hudson AR, Kline DG. Atlas of Peripheral Nerve Surgery. Elsevier; 2013.)*

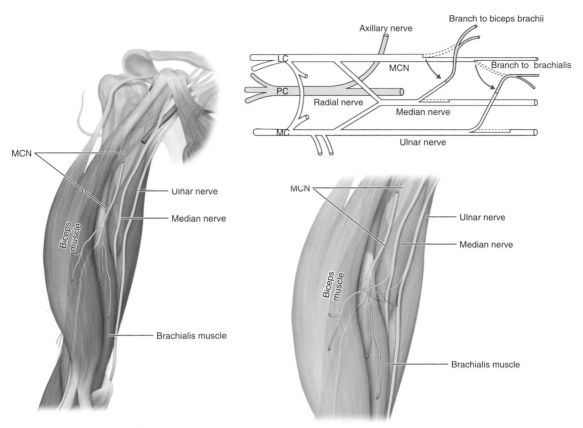

FIGURE 87-7   Nerve transfer of the median and ulnar nerves to musculocutaneous nerve branches. *LC,* lateral cord; *MC,* medial cord; *MCN,* musculocutaneous nerve; *PC,* posterior cord. *(Reprinted with permission Kim DH, Hudson AR, Kline DG. Atlas of Peripheral Nerve Surgery. Elsevier; 2013.)*

the distance to the elbow, a motor branch to the biceps usually deviates from the musculocutaneous nerve heading to the underside of the biceps muscle. This branch is separated from the main trunk of the musculocutaneous nerve and dissected from within the musculocutaneous branch as proximally as possible. The biceps motor branch is divided and brought immediately adjacent to the median nerve. At this location of the median nerve, the epineurium is opened and the nerve is separated into individual fascicles, generally at least four fascicles. These are each stimulated until one that innervates wrist flexion function is identified. This fascicle is then divided and coapted to the biceps branch of the musculocutaneous nerve (Figure 87-7).

Complication Avoidance and Management

- Median nerve finger flexion weakness
  - It is critical that the muscles innervated by the anterior interosseous nerve are preserved. If stimulation of the potential donor fascicle provided function to the flexor pollicis longus and flexor digitorum profundus, the surgeon must confirm that other fascicles that will be preserved also contain these same functions.
  - When C7 is involved in the injury, the innervation to the triceps may be compromised. It is important to assess this muscle with EMG prior to undertaking the triceps-to-axillary-nerve transfer. If the innervation is quite poor, alternative sources should be considered.

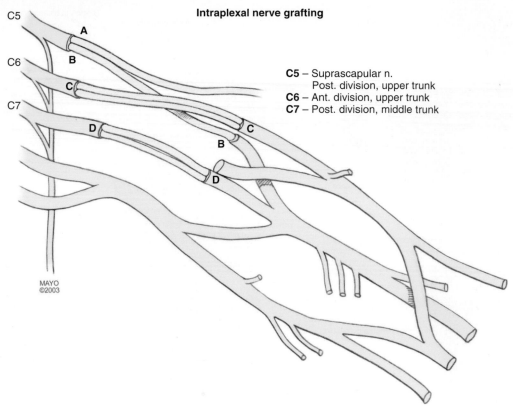

Intraplexal nerve grafting

C5

C6

C7

A

B

C

D

B

C

D

C5 – Suprascapular n.
        Post. division, upper trunk
C6 – Ant. division, upper trunk
C7 – Post. division, middle trunk

MAYO
©2003

FIGURE 87-8 Anatomic reconstruction of the brachial plexus is done whenever possible with intraplexal nerve grafts: C5 to shoulder targets, C6 to elbow flexors, and C7 to extensor muscles. *(Reprinted with permission from the Mayo Foundation for Medical Education and Research. All rights reserved. From Spinner RJ, Shin AY.* Green's Operative Hand Surgery. *Elsevier; 2011.)*

Alternative Procedures: Nerve Grafting

- Brachial plexus post ganglionic nerve grafting technique (Figure 87-8)
- When the trunks of the brachial plexus are injured, with continuity of the roots to the spinal cord, and the planned repair is within at most 6 months of the injury, grafting of the brachial plexus is an option.
- Grafting is typically performed to direct specific roots to specific functions, as shown in figure 87-8. Here, the C5 root is grafted for shoulder function, i.e., suprascapular nerve and posterior division of the upper trunk. The C6 root is grafted for elbow flexion, i.e., to the anterior division of the upper trunk. The C7 root is grafted to the middle trunk.

KEY PAPERS

Colbert SH, Mackinnon S. Posterior approach for double nerve transfer for restoration of shoulder function in upper brachial plexus palsy. *Hand (N Y)*. 2006;1(2):71-77. doi:10.1007/s11552-006-9004-4.

Estrella EP, Favila AS Jr. Nerve transfers for shoulder function for traumatic brachial plexus injuries. *J Reconstr Microsurg*. 2014;30(1):59-64. doi:10.1055/s-0033-1354737; [Epub 2013 Sep 9].

Ray WZ, Pet MA, Yee A, et al. Double fascicular nerve transfer to the biceps and brachialis muscles after brachial plexus injury: clinical outcomes in a series of 29 cases. *J Neurosurg*. 2011;114(6):1520-1528. doi:10.3171/2 011.1.JNS10810; [Epub 2011 Feb 25].

Shin AY, Spinner RJ, Steinmann SP, et al. Adult traumatic brachial plexus injuries. *J Am Acad Orthop Surg*. 2005;13(6):382-396.

Case 88

Parsonage-Turner Syndrome

Justin Brown, MD ● Mark A. Mahan, MD

Presentation

A 57-year-old right hand–dominant male undergoes a lumbar microdiskectomy for an S1 radiculopathy. The surgery is uneventful, but the following morning he complains of severe pain in his right shoulder and arm that developed overnight. He is treated with pain medication and discharged the following day with a referral to PT to address the shoulder pain. In PT the following week he is noted to have a winging scapula and significant weakness in his deltoid and biceps. He presents for a post-op checkup 2 weeks after surgery at which time his lumbar radiculopathy has resolved, but he is suffering from significant right shoulder and arm pain and weakness.

- PMH: otherwise unremarkable
- Exam:
  - Sensory exam intact, except for some paresthesias over the dome of the shoulder
  - Passive range of motion about the shoulder and elbow is full
  - Weakness – 2/5 in the right deltoid and 3/5 in the right biceps with notable scapular winging; distally full strength; very mild abduction weakness in the left deltoid, otherwise fully intact on that side
  - Reflexes – right biceps reflex is not elicitable, otherwise triceps and brachioradialis are intact bilaterally

Differential Diagnosis

- Idiopathic
  - Peripheral nerve vasculitis
  - Multifocal motor neuropathy
  - Brachial amyotrophic diplegia
  - Inflammatory or degenerative shoulder disease
  - Radiation plexopathy
- Trauma
  - Positioning-related brachial plexus traction
  - Positioning-related aggravation of prior shoulder pathology
  - Acute cervical disk herniation
  - Previously undiagnosed cervical foraminal stenosis exacerbated by positioning for intubation or surgery
  - Previously undiagnosed cervical central canal stenosis aggravated by positioning or blood pressure fluctuations during surgery (e.g., induction)

Initial Imaging

- Chest X-ray
- Shoulder X-ray
- MRI of cervical spine and brachial plexus (Figure 88-1)

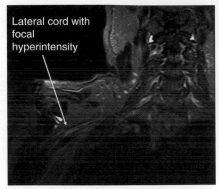

Lateral cord with focal hyperintensity

FIGURE 88-1   *(Printed with permission from the Department of Neurosurgery, University of Utah.)*

Imaging Description and Differential

- MRI of the cervical spine demonstrates some degenerative changes, but widely patent central canal and neural foramen at all levels.
- MRI of the brachial plexus shows thickened and hyperintense upper trunk on coronal STIR sequences. STIR imaging demonstrated hyperintensity of the lateral cord in association with severe denervation and atrophy of the biceps and brachialis. This MRI was obtained 9 months after the onset of symptoms. MRI in the acute period is frequently normal or minimally abnormal – such that detection is difficult to distinguish from background noise.

Further Workup

- Imaging
  - Chest and shoulder X-rays
- Electrodiagnostic studies
  - Electrodiagnostic: can be performed reliably after about 3 weeks. In this case fibrillations and positive sharp waves are seen in the serratus anterior, supra and infraspinatus, deltoid, biceps, and brachioradialis with decreased recruitment, particularly in the serratus anterior, infraspinatus, and deltoid.
- Consultants
  - PT
  - Neurology

Pathophysiology

Parsonage-Turner syndrome, or neuralgic amyotrophy, is typically characterized by severe neuropathic pain, followed by weakness and atrophy within hours to days. This syndrome is typically triggered by an antecedent viral infection (40%), although exercise and surgery have been found to be triggers in about 15% of cases each. Additional triggers may include childbirth, trauma, vaccinations, and even psychological stress.

The most typical symptoms are pain in the neck and shoulder, followed by an increase in intensity over a few hours that then persists. As the nadir of the pain begins to abate, the weakness and atrophy become more apparent. There are two additional pain types that follow: first, a neuritis-type nerve sensitivity that typically results in "shooting" or "shocking" sensations and second, a musculoskeletal mechanical pain from the subsequent muscle imbalance that results from ensuing weakness. Finally, depression of the shoulder girdle, as a result of this weakness, can result in traction on the brachial plexus, further exacerbating the neuritis symptoms.

The ensuing weakness can involve any component of the brachial plexus, but the upper plexus is most common. The majority of these, in addition to shoulder and biceps weakness, have notable involvement of the long thoracic nerve with scapular winging. Alternatively, the middle and lower plexus can also be the predominant distribution of weakness.

Additionally nonplexus distributions can occur and may include the anterior interosseous nerve, phrenic nerve, recurrent laryngeal nerve, or even the lumbosacral plexus. At least one third of all cases have some degree of bilateral involvement, though the less affected side is often not brought to clinical attention. Nerve distributions affected are rarely contained within a single nerve root or single peripheral nerve distribution, which can be helpful in arriving at the diagnosis. Sensory changes are typically mild and may amount to no more than paresthesias in the distribution most affected.

The diagnosis is usually primarily derived from the clinical history and confirmed by physical exam and electrodiagnostics. The pain syndrome followed by weakness is quite characteristic. Onset of pain is typically acute and severe without a corresponding inciting injury source to explain it. Evaluation of the shoulder complex typically reveals no mechanical impediment to full range of motion to explain such a pain syndrome. Finally the muscles affected involve multiple nerve sources. EMG can assist with determining this as examining a painful limb can sometimes provide less than ideal information. MRI, and particularly neurography sequences (T1- and T2-weighted spin ECHO sequences and STIR), can demonstrate hyperintensity and thickening in a region of the brachial plexus that corresponds with the distributions affected.

Initial management of pain typically includes long-acting NSAIDs and opioids. Lyrica, gabapentin, or amitriptyline are also useful adjuncts to this, particularly when the shooting pain begins. PT helps the patient correct postures that aggravate the pain and strengthen weakened muscles as the disease course abates. Shoulder harnesses may help avoid traction on the plexus from a weakened shoulder girdle.

The majority of patients demonstrate signs of recovery by 6 months from the onset of weakness. Complete paralysis of muscle groups (0/5) is relatively rare, accounting for <5% of all cases. When complete paralysis is present and persists beyond 6 months, or when severe weakness (MRC 1-2/5) does not show any evidence of improvement between 9 to 12 months, nerve transfers are considered.

Treatment Options

- Conservative measures
  - Pain control (NSAIDs, opioids, antidepressants)
  - PT
  - Bracing
  - Serial physical exams and electrodiagnostics to confirm recovery with time
- Surgical intervention
  - With severe weakness and no signs of recovery at 9 to 12 months
  - Nerve transfers
  - Tendon transfers

Complication Avoidance and Management

- Patients who do not receive proper therapy and pain control may have persisting pain even years after onset. Additionally, patients with severe weakness who do not undergo intervention by 12 months may have persistent disability for the rest of their lives. Finally, as surgery can be a triggering event appropriate counseling is important if surgical repair is advised, i.e., a risk of surgery for repair may be repeated as a neuritis episode. However, the risk associated with surgery is low and probably under 10% (lifetime risk of recurrent episode).

KEY PAPERS

Brown JM, et al. Post-cervical decompression Parsonage-Turner syndrome represents a subset of C5 palsy: six cases and a review of the literature. *Neurosurgery.* 2010;67(6):E1831-E1844.

Duman I, et al. Neuralgic amyotrophy, diagnosed with magnetic resonance neurography in acute stage: a case report and review of the literature. *Neurologist.* 2007;13(4):219-221.

Van Alfen N. The neuralgia amyotrophy consultation. *J Neurol.* 2007;254:695-704.

Van Alfen N, van Engelen BG. The clinical spectrum of neuralgic amyotrophy in 246 cases. *Brain.* 2006; 129:438-450.

Case 89

Radial Nerve Injury

Justin Brown, MD ● Gehaan D'Souza, MD ● Mark A. Mahan, MD

Presentation

A 14-year-old right hand–dominant girl is referred to the clinic 2 weeks after a fall from a horse where she sustained an open fracture of the humerus. Immediately after the fall, she was unable to extend the wrist and fingers and had numbness on the dorsal aspect of her hand. Upon initial arrival to the hospital, she was treated with open fracture reduction and internal fixation (ORIF), and tagging of the proximal and distal ends of a visibly torn radial nerve.

- PMH: otherwise unremarkable
- Exam:
  - Anesthesia – dorsal hand
  - Weakness – loss of extension of wrist, fingers, and thumb

Differential Diagnosis

- Idiopathic
  - Parsonage-Turner syndrome
- Trauma
  - Brachial plexus/posterior cord injury
  - Forearm compartment syndrome
  - C6–C7 nerve root injuries
- Iatrogenic
  - Surgical trauma (e.g., under the ORIF plating)
  - Positioning during surgery/casting or other pressure palsy

Initial Imaging

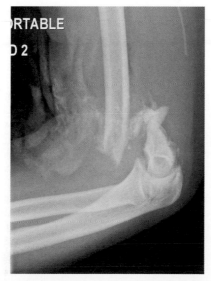

FIGURE 89-1 *(Printed with permission from the University of Utah.)*

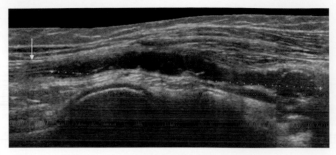

FIGURE 89-2

Imaging Description and Differential

- X-ray of humerus, shoulder, forearm (Figure 89-1)
- Electrodiagnostic evaluation can be performed reliably after about 3 weeks. When the nerve is visibly torn, electrodiagnostic studies are generally not necessary, except to potentially exclude proximal injuries not identified on physical exam.
- Ultrasound or MRI can be performed, especially for preoperative location of the proximal end of the lacerated nerve; otherwise no imaging is necessary.

Further Workup

- Laboratory
  - CBC, BMP
  - ESR, CRP
- Imaging
  - X-ray: include forearm, wrist, and hand
  - CT: evaluate for bony callus, misplaced screw, etc.
  - MRI: will have significant metal artifact, but may be able to visualize the nerve
- Consultants
  - Occupational therapy, possibly hand surgery

Pathophysiology

Radial nerve loss of function is seen in both open and closed injuries, including 22% of humeral shaft fractures. A functional radial nerve is essential for a functional hand, including wrist and finger extension, which provides for effective hand opening. In the absence of this, the hand is rendered ineffective for most activities. Isolated radial nerve injury additionally leads to the loss of power grip, due to the inability to position the wrist in extension.

The type of fracture and extent of displacement are the key factors affecting the occurrence of radial nerve palsy at the time of trauma. The Holstein-Lewis fracture, at the distal third of the humerus, is a fracture pattern that may entrap the nerve between the bone fragments. Alternatively, some studies have found that midshaft fractures, where there is no muscle interposed between the radial nerve and the humerus, have the highest neurologic injury rate.

Fixation of a humeral fracture may also be fraught with risks. Nerves have been entrapped under plates and bicortical screws have been found to pierce the nerve after traversing bone in some cases. Finally, delayed development of large bony calluses can result in pressure on the nerve. This would typically appear as delayed neuropathy, and not acute palsy.

If the nerve appears intact, it can be followed with serial EMG studies focusing on the brachioradialis. If there are no motor unit potentials in the brachioradialis muscle by 6 months, the axon front has failed to advance and surgery should be undertaken.

Treatment Options

- Surgery
  - Primary repair of nerve injury using nerve graft
  - Nerve transfer
  - Tendon transfer

Surgical Technique

The patient's prior antecubital incision is reopened. The skin and subcutaneous tissue are dissected free from the deep fascia. Proximal to the elbow, the radial nerve can be found between the brachialis and the triceps; proximal to the so-called mobile wad, which is the humeral insertion of the brachioradialis, extensor carpi radialis longus, and the common extensor tendon, including extensor carpi radialis brevis, extensor digitorum communis, and others.

The nerve is identified and then carefully neurolysed from the surrounding scar tissue, bone, and hardware (Figure 89-3). It is critical to go as far proximally and distally as necessary to identify healthy-appearing nerve. Injured nerve is typically very firm to the touch and healthy nerve is soft and mobile when rolled between the fingers.

Once the decision to graft is made, a nerve graft is harvested (Figure 89-4). The sural nerve is typically used, although local nerves such as the posterior antebrachial cutaneous nerve can also be used. The hardest part of the scarred nerve is resected and each nerve end is trimmed further using a fresh blade until fascicular structure is identified. Vigorous arterial bleeding is usually encountered once the scarred segment has been removed. Specimens can be sent for pathological analysis to assess the architecture if there is question. Once healthy-appearing nerve is prepared at both ends, the graft is interposed and sutured into position using 9-0 nylon sutures. Enough cables should be used to cover the surface area of the ends being sutured to. The length of the nerve should be selected to allow elbow extension with minimal tension on the nerve repair sites. Additionally, nerve tubes can be used to cuff the repair sites and fibrin glue to reinforce the sites of repair (Figure 89-5).

The wound is closed, and the arm is placed in a splint and immobilized for 2–3 weeks to avoid disrupting the repair with extreme movement. A variable angle elbow locked

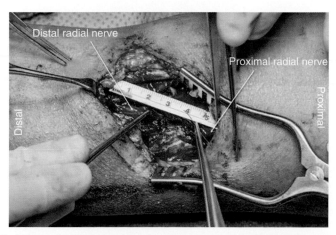

FIGURE 89-3 Radial nerve in the antecubital fossa following supracondylar fracture 2 weeks prior. The previously tagged ends of the lacerated radial nerve are easily identified by the Prolene (blue) sutures. Thorough neurolysis of each stump is performed to allow maximal mobilization and, consequently, minimal graft length. Tension is placed on each of the proximal and distal stumps and the requisite length of the nerve graft is estimated with the elbow in extension. The amount of proximal and distal stump to be resected to achieve normal nerve is estimated by palpation. In this case, 1 cm of proximal nerve stump was resected and 0.5 cm of distal nerve stump was resected. With the 3 cm gap, a 4.5 cm cabled graft was prepared. *(Printed with permission from the University of Utah.)*

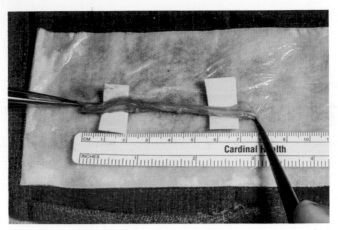

FIGURE 89-4   Preparation of a cabled sural graft. Approximately 36 cm of sural nerve is harvested through a series of four serial incisions along the course of the sural nerve. The nerve is then folded in half twice, to achieve a four cable graft. Fibrin glue is then placed at two locations, approximately 4.5 cm apart. Using yellow plastic, the four cables are glued together to facilitate suture repair. *(Printed with permission from the University of Utah.)*

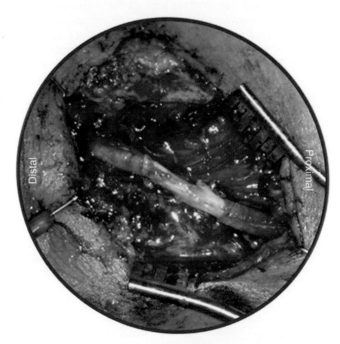

FIGURE 89-5   View of the completed graft from the operating microscope. The 4.5 cm four-cable sural graft was sewn to the trimmed ends of the proximal and distal stumps with 9-0 nylon sutures. Once sutured, nerve conduits are placed on both proximal and distal coaptation sites with epineurial sutures. The addition of the collagen tube is designed to reduce the "wandering" of regenerating axons to the adjacent musculature, and to provide additional buttress to nerve tension along the repair sites. *(Printed with permission from the University of Utah.)*

brace is preferred, allowing immediate mobilization – generally allows progressive extension once the nerve has had adequate time to heal across the coaptation sites.

Alternative Procedures

- Excessive scarring and difficult proximal dissection
  - In some cases of long segment radial nerve injuries, we have found it difficult to access a healthy proximal stump without further injuring the healthy triceps branches.

This also indicates that the distance of regeneration is quite long. In patients with long segment injuries, or in patients who have symptoms well past 6 months after injury, we have often utilized nerve transfers to restore function. Branches of the median nerve within the forearm are used to reinnervate extensor carpi radialis brevis and the posterior interosseous nerve. This approach typically is used in previously undisrupted tissue when the donor nerves are known to be perfectly healthy. Distal nerve transfers shorten the distance of regeneration and produce a more rapid result, but may also require more occupational therapy to teach the patient how to activate the reinnervated muscles.

- Radial nerve palsy
  - Tendon transfers are well established for radial nerve palsy. If there is inadequate recovery after 18 months following nerve repair, tendon transfers should be considered. Typically, the pronator teres is used for wrist extension, the palmaris longus for thumb extension (extensor pollicis longus), and the flexor carpi radialis for finger extension.

Complication Avoidance and Management

- Confirmation of bone healing is important when considering removal of hardware. Use of an extension lock-out brace can avoid excessive tension on nerve grafting or repair. Distal nerve transfers can be considered for failures of nerve grafting procedures. Nerve transfers have to be carefully considered to avoid denervation of tendon transfer donors.

KEY PAPERS

Brown JM, Tung TH, Mackinnon SE. Median to radial nerve transfer to restore wrist and finger extension: technical nuances. *Neurosurgery*. 2010;66(3 suppl Operative):75-83, discussion 83.

Korompilias AV, Lykissas MG, Kostas-Agantis IP. Approach to radial nerve palsy caused by humerus shaft fracture. Is primary exploration necessary? *Injury*. 2013;44:323-326, pii: S0020-1383(13)00016-8. doi:10.1016/j.injury.2013.01.004.

Seiler JG 3rd, Desai MJ, Payne SH. Tendon transfers for radial, median, and ulnar nerve palsy. *J Am Acad Orthop Surg*. 2013;21(11):675-684. doi:10.5435/JAAOS-21-11-675.

Shao YC, Harwood P, Grots MRW, et al. Radial nerve palsy associated with fractures of the shaft of the humerus: a systematic review. *J Bone Joint Surg Br*. 2005;87(12):1647-1652.

Wang X, Zhang P, Zhou Y, et al. Secondary radial never palsy after internal fixation of humeral shaft fractures. *Eur J Orthop Surg Traumatol*. 2014;24(3):331-333. doi:10.1007/s00590-013-1197-y.

Case 90

Ulnar Nerve Injury

Justin Brown, MD ● Mark A. Mahan, MD

Presentation

A 42-year-old right hand–dominant male is referred to the clinic 6 weeks after an altercation in which he suffered multiple stab wounds, including one to his medial right arm. Most of the wounds were superficial, and when originally seen he was treated with suture closure and local dressings for the stab incisions. He noted new numbness and discoordination of his hand, which began at that time and has persisted to the present.

- PMH: otherwise unremarkable
- Exam:
  - Anesthesia – dorsal and volar aspect of the palm, half of the fourth digit, and the entire fifth digit
  - Weakness – wasting of the intrinsic muscles of the hand, clawing of the last two digits and radial deviation of wrist flexion (Figure 90-1)

Differential Diagnosis

- Idiopathic
  - Syringomyelia
  - Spinal cord tumor
  - C8 radiculopathy
  - ALS
  - Cubital tunnel syndrome
  - Thoracic outlet syndrome
  - Pancoast tumor
  - Parsonage-Turner syndrome
- Trauma
  - Brachial plexus/lower trunk injury
  - C8 nerve root injuries

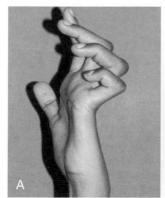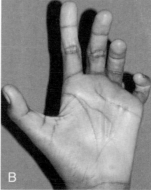

FIGURE 90-1   Preoperative photographs of a mobile claw deformity of the left hand of 2 years in duration. **(A)** Open hand position and **(B)** palmar view. *(Reprinted with permission from* Journal of Hand Surgery. Rath Santosh MS. Published February 1, 2008. Volume 33, Issue 2. Pages 232240. © 2008.)

Initial Imaging

- MRI or ultrasound

Imaging Description and Differential

- Ultrasound demonstrates loss of continuity of the ulnar nerve at the mid humeral level.

Further Workup

- Laboratory
  - CBC, BMP
  - ESR, CRP
- Electrodiagnostic studies
- Electrodiagnostic: reliable after about 3 weeks
  - In this case NCVs demonstrate no measurable conduction below the elbow; good innervation with normal motor unit potentials in median and radial distributions; fibrillations and positive sharp waves with no motor unit potentials in the ulnar-innervated muscles.
- Imaging
  - X-ray of humerus to look for metal fragments prior to MRI
- Consultants
  - Occupational therapy, possibly hand surgery

Pathophysiology

Ulnar paralysis can be severely disabling, resulting in a loss of fine motor skills, difficulty with proper opening of the hand, loss of power grip (reduction in grip strength by up to 80%), and a sensory deficit in the medial aspect of the hand including the last two fingers. The claw hand deformity includes hyperextension of the fourth and fifth MCP joint as a result of a loss of lumbrical (flexion at MCP) innervation, and flexion of the fourth and fifth PIP and DIP from a loss of PIP and DIP extension by lumbricals and interossei.

Repair of a high ulnar nerve lesion should be performed in a timely fashion, but even in the best circumstances it typically does not restore useful hand intrinsic function. Tendon transfers are available to improve intrinsic balance in the hand and augment power grip, but these tend to be less efficacious than those available for median and radial nerve injuries.

Negative prognostic factors in the likelihood of successful recovery following nerve injury include advanced age, delay in repair, proximal site of injury, and the ulnar nerve being the injured nerve. Primary repair typically produces the most effective results if the fascicles are aligned properly. Grafts >5 cm are associated with poorer results than those shorter.

Once it is clear that the nerve is severed and will require repair, there should be no further delay in bringing this patient into the operating room for repair.

Treatment Options

- Surgery
  - Primary repair of nerve injury
  - Nerve transfer
  - Tendon transfer

Surgical Technique

The patient is positioned supine with arm outstretched on an arm table. Tourniquet may be used based on surgeon preference. Incision is planned based on the site of the stab wound and the findings on ultrasound. Incision is made longitudinally in the interval between the biceps and triceps, medially. Skin and subcutaneous tissues are cleared from the brachial fascia and the fascia is then divided. Typically, the medial antebrachial cutaneous nerve is encountered first, followed by the median nerve. Posterior to these and often inferior to the brachial vein, the ulnar nerve can be identified. Use of a hand-held stimulator can help identify the uninjured nerves. Once the ulnar nerve ends are identified, the ends are trimmed and the nerves are mobilized both proximally and distally to achieve direct repair if possible (Figures 90-2 and 90-3). If excessive traction has apparently precluded direct repair, an ulnar nerve transposition should be undertaken to achieve additional length. Once ends are able to be brought directly together, the trimmed ends

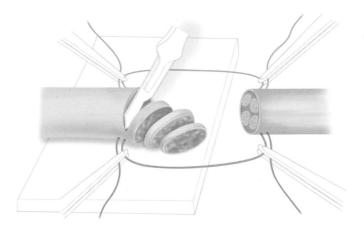

FIGURE 90-2 Nerve stumps are sectioned back to healthy fascicular tissue. Preplaced sutures are used to hold the stumps in place as they are trimmed on a firm surface, such as a moistened tongue blade or sterile wooden block. *(Reprinted with permission from Kim DH, Hudson AR, Kline DG. Atlas of Peripheral Nerve Surgery. 2nd ed. Elsevier; 2013.)*

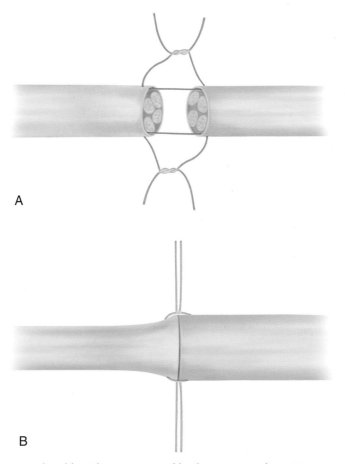

FIGURE 90-3 **(A)** Preplaced lateral sutures are tied by the surgeon and surgeon's assistant. **(B)** Lateral sutures are tied and placed on mild traction to prepare the topside for suture. *(Reprinted with permission from Kim DH, Hudson AR, Kline DG. Atlas of Peripheral Nerve Surgery. 2nd ed. Elsevier; 2013.)*

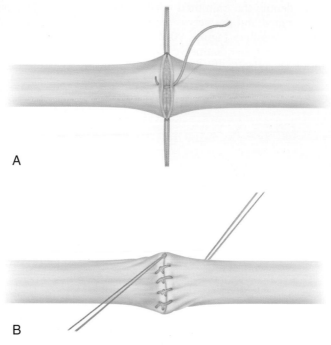

FIGURE 90-4 **(A)** An epineurial suture is placed between tied lateral sutures. **(B)** After placement of a series of epineurial sutures on the topside, the lateral sutures are inverted so that the backside of the repair site is exposed. *(Reprinted with permission from Kim DH, Hudson AR, Kline DG. Atlas of Peripheral Nerve Surgery. 2nd ed. Elsevier; 2013.)*

are carefully examined under magnification to identify the fascicular pattern. Ideally the pattern is matched and the nerve is repaired in its anatomical configuration using four epineurial sutures (9-0 nylon), which can be wrapped in a nerve conduit if the surgeon so chooses.

Complication Avoidance and Management

- Late presentation
  - Because recovery of intrinsic hand function is quite difficult to achieve in high ulnar nerve injuries, it is often valuable to augment reinnervation of the hand intrinsic muscles using a nerve transfer. Typically, the median nerve branch to the pronator quadratus is used as the donor nerve. An extended Guyon's canal incision can be used to expose the ulnar nerve and separate motor and sensory nerve components. These components are frequently distinct into the proximal third of the forearm. By following the motor branch proximally, the nerve to the pronator quadratus muscle can be coapted directly to the motor component of the ulnar nerve at this level (Figure 90-4).
- Insufficient grasp recovery
  - If nerve surgery fails to completely correct the claw deformity and recover reasonable grasp, tendon transfers should be considered.

KEY PAPERS

Brown JM, et al. Distal median to ulnar nerve transfers to restore ulnar motor and sensory function within the hand: technical nuances. *Neurosurg.* 2009;65(5):966-977.

Gottschalk HP, et al. Late reconstruction of ulnar nerve palsy. *Orthop Clin North Am.* 2012;43(4):495-507.

Ruijs ACJ, et al. Median and ulnar nerve injuries: a meta-analysis of predictors of motor and sensory recovery after modern microsurgical nerve repair. *Plast Reconstr Surg.* 2005;116(2):484-494.

Case 91

Median Nerve Injury

Mark A. Mahan, MD ● Justin Brown, MD

Presentation

An obese 62-year-old right hand–dominant woman presents to the emergency room with multiple gunshot wounds to the neck, shoulder, and left arm. Her wounds are dressed, and she is referred to the clinic 3 weeks later with complaints of left hand numbness and weakness.

- PMH: otherwise unremarkable
- Exam:
  - Hand is mildly cyanotic and cooler compared with the contralateral side.
  - Complete anesthesia on radial palm and first, second, third, and radial half of the fourth digit
  - Weakness
    - Loss of flexion of thumb and index, with relative weakness of third finger flexion
    - Thenar atrophy with weakness in thumb palmar abduction
    - Weak pronation of the forearm against resistance with the elbow flexed (Figure 91-1)

Differential Diagnosis

- Trauma
  - C8 nerve root injury
  - Medial cord injury
  - Direct transection or laceration
  - Compartment syndrome/ischemic injury to the nerve
  - Blast (concussive) injury to the nerve

Initial Imaging

- X-ray (to assess for bony injuries and bullet fragments)
- Ultrasound (to assess the nerves of the arm and forearm)

Imaging Description and Differential

- Ultrasound
  - The median nerve in the medial intramuscular region, at the level of the mid humerus, has normal caliber and a preserved fascicular appearance. As we approach the antecubital fossa, the nerve becomes hypoechoic and the fascicular appearance less distinct. Just beyond the antecubital fossa, the nerve appears to end in a region of hyperechoic scar tissue. This may represent a terminal neuroma. Similarly, working proximally from the wrist, the nerve has normal caliber but becomes indistinct as we approach the proximal forearm.

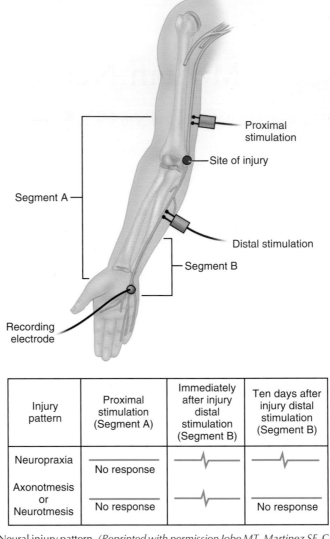

Injury pattern	Proximal stimulation (Segment A)	Immediately after injury distal stimulation (Segment B)	Ten days after injury distal stimulation (Segment B)
Neuropraxia	No response	⟋⟍	⟋⟍
Axonotmesis or Neurotmesis	No response	⟋⟍	No response

FIGURE 91-1 Neural injury pattern. *(Reprinted with permission Jobe MT, Martinez SF. Campbell's Operative Orthopaedics. 6th ed. Elsevier; 2013.)*

- Differential
  - Direct transection, which requires early reconstruction, versus concussive injury with nerve continuity, which is initially managed with serial exam to assess for spontaneous recovery

Further Workup

- Neurophysiology
  - EMG/NCS
- Imaging
  - MRI is useful for delineating the pattern of denervation and can frequently localize the site of injury and assess the continuity of the nerve; if metal fragments are present, it cannot be utilized.
- Consultants
  - Physical therapy, occupational therapy, and possibly hand surgery (if tendon transfers are considered)

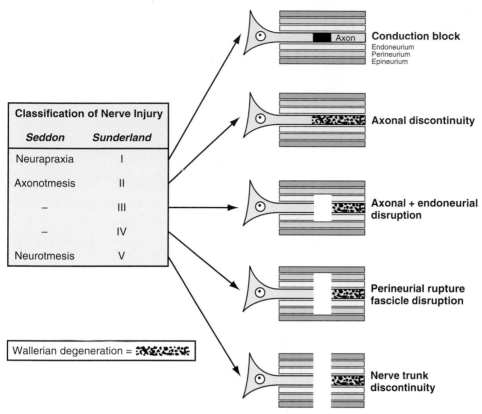

FIGURE 91-2 Seddon and Sunderland classifications of nerve injuries. *(Reprinted with permission from Ellenbogen RG, Abdulrauf SI, Sekhar LN. Principles of Neurological Surgery. 3rd ed. Elsevier; 2012.)*

Pathophysiology

Gunshot wounds to the extremities can result in nerve injury via direct or indirect injuries. An indirect injury is a result of the temporary cavity and compression of the nerve at the time that the missile traverses the limb (Figure 91-2). Indirect injuries are frequently neurapraxic, that is, axons are predominantly preserved while myelination is lost. Such injuries benefit from watchful waiting while remyelination ensues. If ischemia is the source of the conduction block, removing the constriction that is limiting blood flow can sometimes provide rapid reversal of symptoms. When Schwann cells are damaged, the time to recovery depends on the severity of the damage. Mild damage can recover in days to weeks. A larger segment of lost Schwann cells can take 3 to 4 months to recover as those cells regenerate and mature in their ability to properly insulate a segment of the nerve (Figure 91-3).

Alternatively, if the missile passed near the nerve or there was high-energy impact, axonotmesis (injury to the axons) may occur. This is hallmarked by evidence of denervation on EMG and requires a greater length of time for recovery (commonly 1 mm per day or 1 inch per month). Recovery after axonotmesis is variable and is best assessed by serial EMG.

When a nerve is directly lacerated by a missile fragment, spontaneous recovery is not possible because of the recoil of severed ends away from each other.

Delayed treatment of a compartment syndrome frequently results in ischemic injury to the nerve and muscle. This is generally an irreversible injury with loss of both the muscle and the nerve. Secondary neuropathic pain frequently occurs.

Treatment Options

Sharp transections (knife) are repaired in <3 days. Blunt transections (propeller blade) are treated in 3 weeks, after neuroma is allowed to form, allowing discernment of healthy

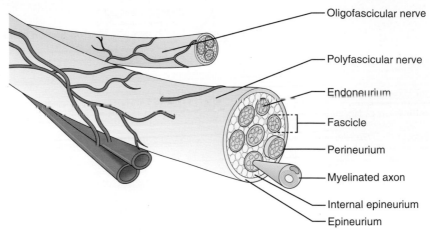

FIGURE 91-3 Microscopic anatomy of the peripheral nerve. *(Reprinted with permission from Ellenbogen RG, Abdulrauf SI, Sekhar LN.* Principles of Neurological Surgery. *3rd ed. Elsevier; 2012.)*

fascicular ends. Blunt injuries (GSW, stretch, trauma) are treated after 3 to 6 months if there is failure to improve with clinical and nerve conduction studies.

- Surgery
  - Nerve grafting
  - Nerve transfers
  - Tendon transfers
  - A combination of these

Surgical Technique

The patient is placed in a supine position with the arm abducted on an arm board. The shoulder is abducted and externally rotated. The incision is made 2–3 inches above the medial epicondyle, over the medial intermuscular septum. The incision moves volar distally, utilizing a Bruner's type Z-plasty incision across the antecubital fossa, and then a curvilinear path across the proximal half of the volar forearm. The incision is opened proximally and the brachial fascia is divided. First, the medial antebrachial cutaneous nerve is identified superficially; the median nerve is typically just beneath the medial antebrachial cutaneous nerve. A nerve stimulator can be used to confirm identity. In this case, the median nerve may provide only weak pronation. The nerve is then traced into the forearm. As we move distally, the nerve becomes encased in increasingly thick scar tissue. At the level of the distal aspect of the brachialis muscle belly, the nerve is found to end in scar tissue (Figure 91-4).

Next, the forearm incision is entered and the fascia of the forearm is divided, including the lacertus fibrosis proximally. After identifying the radial vessels and moving to the radial side of these, the insertion of the pronator teres onto the radius is identified. This is cut in a step lengthening–type incision for later reapproximation. Once cut, the entire flexor–pronator mass can be retracted, providing a view of the median nerve. Sometimes it is valuable to cut the leading edge of the flexor digitorum superficialis muscle to improve the view. The healthy distal end of the median nerve is identified in unscarred tissue within the forearm and a vessel loop is placed around it. It is then carefully followed proximally until the divided end is identified.

The two divided ends are about 2 inches from one another. The ends are cleared of adherent tissue, and then a sharp No. 15 blade is used to begin to trim the ends. This is done in 2 mm segments until we are able to visualize "pouting" fascicles instead of scar tissue. Once this healthy nerve is encountered, attention is turned to the harvest of a nerve graft.

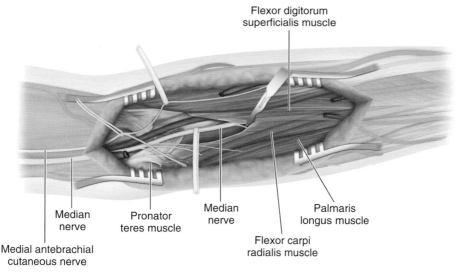

Flexor digitorum
superficialis muscle

Median
nerve

Pronator
teres muscle

Median
nerve

Palmaris
longus muscle

Medial antebrachial
cutaneous nerve

Flexor carpi
radialis muscle

FIGURE 91-4 After the surgeon incises the bicipital aponeurosis, the edge of the pronator is incised. Metzenbaum scissors are placed atop, or superficial to, the nerve and are gradually edged distally as the scalpel divides the overlying muscle and fascia. *(Reprinted with permission from Kim DH, Hudson AR, Kline DG.* Atlas of Peripheral Nerve Surgery. *2nd ed. Elsevier; 2013.)*

The sural nerve is most frequently chosen. The leg is flexed, placing the foot on a sandbag to maintain the knee flexion. The sural nerve is located via a longitudinal incision in the valley between the lateral malleolus and the achilles tendon, where it is often accompanied by the lesser saphenous vein. Traction is placed on the nerve until it can be palpated in the mid calf and then a second longitudinal incision is made. In this manner, the nerve is followed to the popliteal fossa using three to four noncontiguous incisions. Graft lengths of 30–40 cm are typically provided (Figure 91-5). Alternatively, a single longitudinal incision can be made down the midline of the calf for ease of harvest. Another alternative is to use the medial antebrachial cutaneous nerve graft, which would be harvested by taking the medial arm incision proximally to the level of the axilla. About 20–25 cm of graft can be harvested this way.

After trimming the proximal and distal stumps, the intervening defect is measured. A 7 cm gap is measured and the 30 cm graft is therefore divided into four equal-length segments. These segments are reversed in their orientation so that the formerly distal end is inserted proximally. Using 9-0 nylon sutures under the microscope, one to two sutures are placed in each graft strand to the epineurium of the median nerve to cover the face of the cut end (Figure 91-6); this is done at both ends. Redundancy in the grafts is intentional. Fibrin glue can be used to reinforce the repair. The arm is then closed with 3-0 Vicryl sutures in the dermal layer and a running 4-0 Monocryl subcuticular. The arm is placed in a splint, keeping the elbow bent at 90 degrees for 3 weeks, followed by gentle mobilization by occupational therapy over the next few weeks.

Complication Avoidance and Management

- Neuroma pain
  - During harvest of the sural nerve, it is critical that the proximal cut end be deep within the leg and far from the cut skin edge.
- Damage to repair
  - A secure repair, redundant graft, and limitation of activity all aid in avoiding pulling these delicate repairs apart and compromising the results of the operation.
- Incomplete recovery
  - If recovery is incomplete, tendon transfer options should be considered at 18 to 24 months from the time of repair.

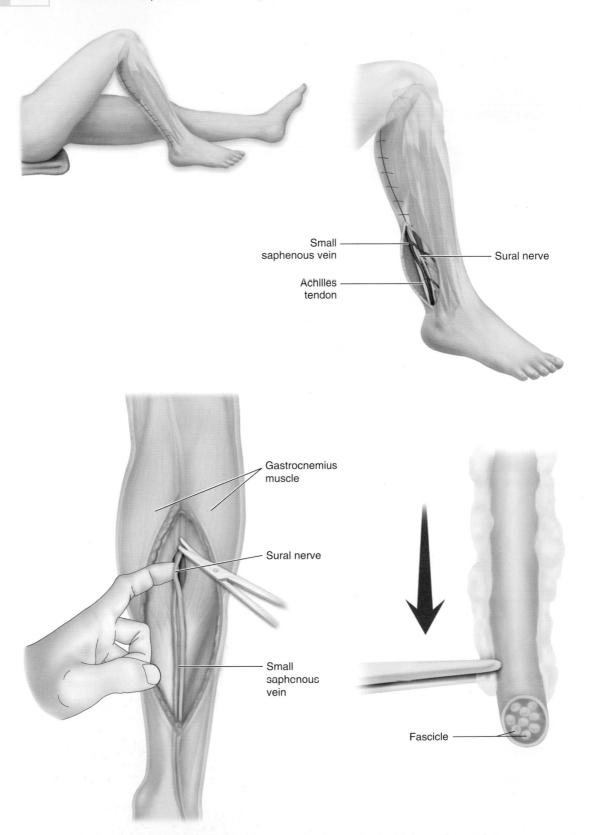

FIGURE 91-5 **(A)** Incision tracing and anatomical structures closely associated with the sural nerve that are encountered during conventional harvest of the nerve. **(B)** Pictorial depiction of anatomical structures encountered during conventional sural nerve harvest. *(Reprinted with permission from Kim DH, Hudson AR, Kline DG. Atlas of Peripheral Nerve Surgery. 2nd ed. Elsevier; 2013.)*

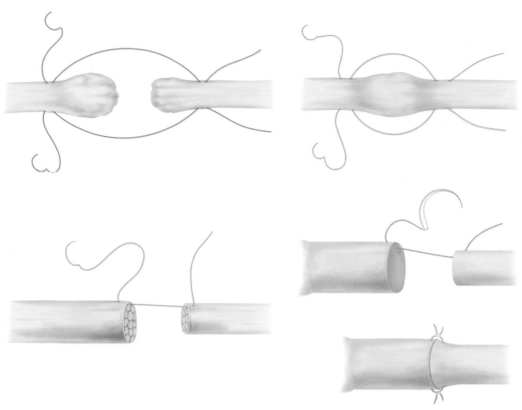

FIGURE 91-6 Epineurial suture technique. *(Reprinted with permission from Kim DH, Hudson AR, Kline DG. Atlas of Peripheral Nerve Surgery. 2nd ed. Elsevier; 2013.)*

KEY PAPERS

Colbert SH, Mackinnon SE. Nerve transfers for brachial plexus reconstruction. *Hand Clin.* 2008;24(4): 341-361.

Hsiao EC, Fox IK, Tung TH, et al. Motor nerve transfers to restore extrinsic median nerve function: case report. *Hand (N Y).* 2009;4(1):92-97.

Spinner RJ. Median nerve. In: Kim D, Midha R, Murovic JA, et al., eds. *Kline and Hudson's Nerve Injuries: Operative Results for Major Nerve Injuries, Entrapments and Tumors.* Philadelphia: Saunders; 2007.

Section VIII Neurology

Case 92

Multiple Sclerosis

Audrey Kohar, DO ● Neal Prakash, MD, PhD

Presentation

A 50-year-old female complains of "flashes" in her left eye that started 3 months ago. A few months later the patient has progressively worsening symptoms and starts to slur her speech. Within a few weeks she has developed a right facial droop, which acutely progressed to left-sided blindness, right-sided hemiplegia, sensory loss, and speech difficulties. The patient denies headaches, dysphagia, coughing, and seizures.

- PMH: unremarkable
- Exam:
  - HR ranges from 70 to 80 bpm; respiration 18; BP ranges from 100–150/50–60
  - No carotid bruits
  - No edema or cyanosis in UE/LE bilaterally
  - No numbness or tingling of extremities
  - Alert and oriented; extraoculomotor movements intact
  - Right-sided visual field defect
  - Expressive and receptive aphasia; unable to follow commands; able to respond to questions with yes/no answers
  - Right facial droop
  - Tongue and uvula midline
  - Right-sided motor strength UE/LE both 0/5, compared with 5/5 on left side
  - UE/LE DTRs +3 on right and +2 on left
  - Intact on finger to nose testing
- LP:
  - White count 3; protein 30; glucose 61; Lyme disease antibody (-); VDRL (-); oligoclonal bands/IgG (+); and NMO antibody (-)

Differential Diagnosis

- Neoplastic
  - Metastasis (h/o cancer)
  - Paraneoplastic encephalomyelopathies
  - Compressive spinal cord lesions
- Vascular
  - Spinal hematoma
- Infectious
  - HIV
  - Lyme neuroborreliosis
  - Neurosyphilis
  - Progressive multifocal leukoencephalopathy
  - Tropical spastic paraparesis
  - Sarcoidosis

- Autoimmune
  - Behcet's disease
  - Granulomatosis angiitis
  - Devic's disease
  - Sjögren's syndrome
  - SLE
  - Disseminated encephalomyelitis (acute)
  - Wegener's
- Other
  - Arnold-Chiari malformation
  - Vitamin B_{12} deficiency
  - Adrenoleukodystrophy
  - Adult metachromatic leukodystrophy
  - Lymphomatoid granulomatosis
  - Cerebral autosomal dominant arteriopathy with subcortical infarcts and leukoencephalopathy (CADASIL)
  - Chronic lymphocytic inflammation with pontine perivascular enhancement responsive to steroids (CLIPPERS)

Initial Imaging

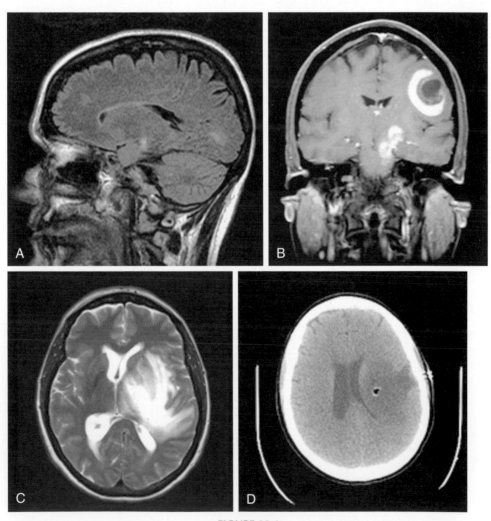

FIGURE 92-1

Imaging Description and Differential

- Figure 92-1A: MRI T2 FLAIR sagittal reflected a nonenhancing mass involving the motor cortex in the left facial area; a development from the small nonenhancing lesion involving the subcortical left parietal lobe on initial brain MRI
- Figure 92-1B: MRI T1 coronal reflected a ring-enhancing lesion in the left parietal lobe and enhancing the left mid brain extending to the posterior basal ganglia
- Figure 92-1C: MRI T2 axial showing minimally enhancing lesion that has increased in size; located in the left frontal temporal region with mild dural involvement in the left anterior temporal lobe; edema extending into the left thalamus, brainstem, and cerebellar vermis is strongly suggestive of a primary brain malignancy; mild periventricular edema present; no evidence of hydrocephalus or satellite lesions; bulk of the abnormality is nonenhancing
- Figure 92-1D: CT brain without contrast; postoperative change status post biopsy of posterior left frontal lobe lesion; abnormally decreased density in the left, from the posterior frontal lobe, extending to the left cerebral peduncle and pons, which is consistent with extensive tumor
- Differential: lesion in the left parietal lobe is not typical in terms of location for an MS plaque and the radiograph was initially strongly suggestive of a primary brain tumor. There was noted to be only slight edema around the left parietal lobe, which may be more associated with multiple sclerosis than a tumor.

Further Workup

- Laboratory
  - CSF analysis for presence of two or more oligoclonal IgG bands (positive predictive value 97%) – testing must run in parallel with sampling of serum obtained within 72 hours of lumbar puncture (preferred method of testing is isoelectric focusing on agarose gels, followed by immunodetection by blotting or fixation). Bands and IgG will be abnormal in CSF whereas they will be normal in serum.
  - CSF analysis for presence of neurofilament protein subunits may indicate acute axonal damage.
  - CSF protein <100 and WBC <5.
  - Serum immune biomarkers may help in diagnosis:
    - Anti-myelin oligodendrocytic protein and anti-myelin basic protein may predict MS.
    - Antibodies targeting alpha-glucose–based antigens predict MS progression to a more severe disease phenotype.
    - B-cell chemoattractant chemokine, CXCL13, may serve as a prognostic marker.
    - Other markers include osteopontin, TNF-α, various cytokines, chemokines, and ab-crystalin.
- Histology
  - Perivenular inflammatory lesions (consisting of mononuclear infiltrations) are evident in the earlier phases of the disease and result in demyelinating plaques and astrocyte proliferation with resultant gliosis (pathological hallmark of MS).
- Imaging
  - MRI for definite diagnosis of MS based on revised 2010 McDonald criteria (considered to have increased sensitivity without compromising specificity): evidence of dissemination pathology in time and space (DIT/DIS)
    - DIS could be met by one or more T2 lesions in at least two of the following four locations: spinal cord, infratentorial, periventricular, or juxtacortical, with no requirement for Gd-enhancing lesions; or await second clinical attack implicating a different CNS site. DIT could be met by simultaneous presence of asymptomatic T2 or Gd-enhancing lesions at any time; or a new T2 and/or Gd-enhancing lesion on any follow-up MRI at any time.
    - Lesions in the brain stem or spine do not count. Spinal cord lesions show minimal swelling.
    - Tumefactive usually display incomplete ring enahancement, the "C" sign, as in figure 92-1 B.

Pathophysiology

MS is a chronic disease of the central nervous system characterized by a loss of motor and sensory function. It is more prevalent in females. MS is caused by immune-mediated inflammation, demyelination, and subsequent axonal damage. Signs and symptoms of MS include: multiple disseminated MR lesions that can enhance, optic neuritis (decreased acuity), internuclear ophthalmoplegia (inability to adduct one eye), bladder spasticity, parathesias, spastic paraparesis and hyperreflexia, Lhermitte's, and euphoria (Labelle indifference). MS can also be a cause of trigeminal neuralgia. If so, facial sensation is decreased and often bilateral in contrast to the typical disease.

MS is propagated by an autoimmune cascade, involving the activation of CD4+ T-helper type 1 (Th1) cells that target myelin self-antigens. The activated immune cells secrete cytokines, such as IL-2, IFN-γ, and TNF-α; chemokines; and matrix metalloproteinases. This results in adherence of the activated immune cells to the endothelium, which in turn facilitates the migration of those immune cells across the blood-brain barrier. The autoimmune cascade also involves Th17 cells that target myelin self-antigens.

Once the migration occurs, the T-cells are reactivated by resident antigen-presenting cells, such as microglia, or by invading dendritic cells that present the local CNS antigens. This results in the recruitment of B-cells, myeloid cells, NK cells, cytokines, chemokines, and matrix metalloproteinases, and leads to the activation of resident microglia and astrocytes. MHC II restricted CD8+ cytotoxic T-cells recognizing myelin proteins create more damage to the myelin, oligodendrocytes, and axons. The B-cells continue to add injury by acting as antigen-presenting cells, thereby secreting cytokines and regulating T-cells. Impaired ability to combat the destruction is due to dysfunctional subsets of regulatory T-cells (T_{reg} cells).

Tumefactive MS has been defined as at least one large (>2 cm) acute demyelinating lesion with accompanying edema, mass effect, and ring enhancement.

Treatment Options

- Medical
  - Acute treatment: 3–7-day course of IV methylprednisolone (500–1000 mg daily, with or without a short prednisone taper)
  - 10 monotherapy options for long-term treatment (treatment is personalized to each patient due to varied benefit-risk profiles characteristic of each drug)
    - Interferon beta and glatiramer acetate (20 mg daily)
    - Fingolimod (daily – contraindicated in patients with cardiovascular pathology), teriflunomide (daily – teratogenic), dimethyl fumarate (BID) approved for relapsing MS
    - Alemtuzumab
    - Ocrelizumab
    - Laquinimod
    - Daclizumab
    - Mitoxantrone for rapidly worsening relapsing MS
    - Natalizumab (risk of progressive multifocal leukoencephalopathy); reserved for use in patients with "breakthrough" disease activity on one or more of the first-line disease-modifying therapies
- Interventional
  - Plasma exchange may be beneficial in patients with acute CNS inflammatory demyelinating disease who do not respond to glucocorticoid therapy for acute MS.
- Surgical
  - Biopsy is not typically indicated. However, GBMs can develop in the setting of MS. Therefore, biopsy progressive lesions in the setting of negative bands that were previously positive.

Surgical Technique

Stereotactic brain biopsy was performed on this patient due to initial suspicions of glioma.

Prior to the procedure, the patient is taken for either an MRI or CT scan while intubated and sedated. The brain scans will generate the images required to visualize the probe's trajectory prior to the procedure. After proper draping and preparation, a small incision is made in the scalp and the biopsy needle is carefully advanced along the chosen trajectory to the chosen depth. In general, a minimum of three small "core samples" are taken and sent to the OR pathologist for intraoperative confirmation that the tissue samples are indeed abnormal.

Complication Avoidance and Management

- Most MS patients experience recurrent episodes of neurological impairment, but 60%–80% have disease states that become chronic and progressive, resulting in cumulative motor disability and cognitive deficits.
- Brain biopsy has complications that are not limited to a 1% risk of significant cerebral hemorrhage, infection, bleeding, hematoma, seizures, and even death.

KEY PAPERS

Karussis D. The diagnosis of multiple sclerosis and the various related demyelinating syndromes: a critical review. *J Autoimm* (Department of Neurology, Multiple Sclerosis Center and Laboratory of Neuroimmunology). 2014; 48–49:134-142.

Milo R, Miller A. Revised diagnostic criteria of multiple sclerosis. *Autoimm Rev.* 2014;13(4–5):518-524.

Wingerchuk D, Weinshenker B. Acute disseminated encephalomyelitis, transverse myelitis, and neuromyelitis optica. *Continuum (Minneap Minn).* 2013;19(4):944-967.

Wingerchuk DM, Carter J. Multiple sclerosis: current and emerging disease-modifying therapies and treatment strategies. *Mayo Clin Proc.* 2014;89(2):225-240.

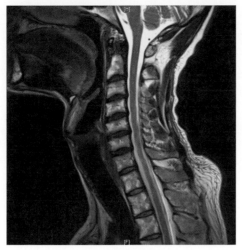

FIGURE 93-4

TABLE 93-1		
AWAJI-SHIMA CRITERIA: CLINICAL OR ELECTROPHYSIOLOGICAL PRESENCE		
Definite ALS	**Probable ALS**	**Possible ALS**
UMN+LMN signs in the bulbar region and 2+ spinal regions or UMN+LMN signs in 3 spinal regions	UMN+LMN signs in 2+ spinal regions, and some UMN signs rostral to the LMN signs	UMN+LMN dysfunction in only 1 region, or UMN in 2+ or more regions, or LMN rostral to UMN signs

UMN = upper motor neuron; LMN = lower motor neuron

Electrodiagnostic Studies

EMG is key for diagnosis. The old El Escorial criteria for diagnosis of ALS has been revised into the Awaji-Shima criteria. It elicits more accurately both UMN and LMN signs and symptoms (Table 93-1) Conduction velocities in the left arm and leg are essentially normal. Left median CMAP is low in amplitude. Needle electromyography demonstrates subacute denervation with spontaneous activity and axonal remodeling in multiple muscles of both arms and thoracic paraspinalis muscle (Table 93-2).

Differential Diagnosis

- Cervical
  - Myeloradiculopathy (prominent neck pain with sphincter involvement)
  - Hirayama's disease
- Endocrine
  - Basedow's disease (autoimmune hyperthyroidism – weakness, wasting, fasciculation)
  - Hyperparathyroidism
- Inflammatory
  - Inclusion body myositis (predilection for quadriceps and medial forearms; CK >1000 IU/L; muscle biopsy demonstrates rimmed vacuoles)
  - Polymyositis
- Autoimmune disorder
  - Multifocal motor neuropathy with conduction block (lack of atrophy; anti-GM1 antibody)
  - Myasthenic syndrome
  - Stiff person syndrome (glutamic acid decarboxylase, anti-amphiphysin antibody)

TABLE 93-2

ELECTRODIAGNOSTIC AWAJI-SHIMA CRITERIA NERVE

A

Nerve	Latency (msec)	Ampl	Velocity (m/s)
L Median m.	4.1	4.2	49
L Median s.	2.1	20.0	58
L Ulnar motor	3.3	5.8	51
L Musculocut	6.4	3.3	53
L Tibial	6.5	7.2	44

B

EMG	FIB/PSW	Fascic	Recruit
Lt FDI	+1	0	↓
Lt ABP	+1	0	↓
Lt Biceps	+2	+2	↓↓
Lt Triceps	+2	+1	↓↓
Lt Infraspin	+1	0	↓
Rt FDI	+1	0	↓
Rt Biceps	+2	+2	↓↓
Rt Triceps	+2	+1	↓↓
Rt Deltoids	+2	+1	↓↓
Lt TA	0	0	NI
Lt MG	0	0	NI
Lt Glut	0	0	NI
Lt T6 PS	+2	0	
Lt Tongue	0	0	

- Hereditary
  - Kennedy's disease (spinal and bulbar muscular atrophy; expansion of CAG repeat in the androgen receptor gene)
  - Late onset hexosaminidase deficiency (white cell enzyme; usually younger than 30 years)
- Others
  - Postpoliomyelitis syndrome
  - Benign cramp fasciculation syndrome

Further Workup

- Laboratory
  - SPEP, CK, ESR, TSH
  - Anti-GM1 ganglioside antibodies (present in 50% of MMN cases)
  - Anti-MuSK/AChR antibodies
  - LP: if protein >75 mg/dL, consider monoclonal paraproteinemia
- DNA analysis in appropriate setting
  - SOD1 gene mutation
  - Androgen receptor mutation (Kennedy's disease)
  - Spastin (progressive UMN disease)
  - Dynactin gene mutation (familial LMN disease)
- Additional imaging
  - CT of the chest and abdomen, with contrast
  - Mammography
- Consultants
  - Neurology/neuromuscular subspecialist (EMG/NCS)
  - Pulmonology
  - Physiatrist
  - Speech/occupational therapy

Pathophysiology

ALS is a progressive neurodegenerative-neurogenetic disorder that affects the motor neurons. The spectrum of clinical heterogeneity falls into six main categories: progressive bulbar palsy, classic or Charcot ALS with upper motor neuron (UMN) and lower motor neuron (LMN) symptoms, progressive spinal muscular atrophy (LMN form), primary lateral sclerosis (UMN variant), brachial amyotrophic diplegia (man-in-the-barrel syndrome), and flail leg syndrome. The median survival ascends from 36 months for the bulbar phenotype to 65 months for flail leg syndrome.

Classic presentation is that of lower extremity spasticity (upper motor neuron death) and atrophy and fasciculations in the upper extremities. Other signs and symptoms include clumsiness, foot drop, atrophy of intrinsic hand muscles, especially preferential wasting of the first dorsal interosseous and abductor pollicis brevis ("split hand" sign), preserved sensation, and hyperreflexia (especially lower extremities). Bulbar onset occurs in 20%, manifesting as dysarthria and impaired tongue movement. Brachial amyotrophic diplegia (segmental proximal spinal muscular atrophy), as in this patient, corresponds with asymmetrical weakness and wasting isolated to the upper extremities, without UMN or bulbar involvement. ALS can often be mistaken for cervical spondylitic myelopathy but there is no neck pain, no sensory changes, and fasciculations are classically present.

Family history is often positive; however, no clear genetic or environmental causes have been identified. Microglial cells are activated early in the disease via signal transducer and activator of transcription-3 (STAT3) and upregulation of TLR4 (Toll-like receptor 4). Mitochondrial dysfunction, oxidative stress, dimerization of neuronal calcium sensor protein visinin-like protein 1 (VILIP-1), glutamate excitotoxicity, toxic misfolding and aggregation of SOD1, inflammation and apoptosis due to imbalance of Bcl-2 oncoproteins, and overexpression of caspases have been implicated in the pathogenesis of ALS. Five to 10% of people with motor neuron disease have a familial form, and 20% of these patients have 1 of 100 mutations in the gene for copper/zinc superoxide dismutase (SOD1), most being point missense mutations. Furthermore, carriers of SOD1 gene mutations do not develop denervation until the onset of clinical symptoms. D90A mutation is linked to a slowly progressive type of ALS.

Treatment Options

- Medical management
  - Riluzole: 50 mg every 12 hours, taken at least 1 hour before, or 2 hours after, a meal; effect is modest, with survival prolonged by no more than 4 months
- Supportive
  - Percutaneous endoscopic gastrostomy placement
  - Endotracheal/ventilator support
  - Muscle biopsy if other medical conditions seem plausible
  - Palliative/end-of-life/hospice care
- Surgery
  - Do not operate

KEY PAPERS

Leigh PN, Abrahams S, Al-Chalabi A, et al. The management of motor neurone disease. *J Neurol Neurosurg Psychiatry*. 2003;74(suppl IV):iv32-iv47.
Oliveira ASB, Pereira RDB. Amyotrophic lateral sclerosis (ALS). Three letters that change the people's life forever. *Arq Neuropsiquiatr*. 2009;67(3–A):750-782.

Case 94

Guillain-Barré Syndrome

Ramsis Benjamin, MD

Presentation

A 63-year-old manager of apartment complexes was diagnosed a year prior with T-pro-lymphocytic leukemia, negative for the CD30 and ALK1 markers. He began to experience pins-and-needles sensation in his toes, feet, fingers, and hands approximately 4 weeks after having completed his second cycle of nelarabine. Within 6 days, the numbness ascended to his lower abdomen. He felt clumsy, had difficulty driving, nearly fell on multiple occasions, and was unable to pinch with his fingers. He has dropped his cell phone repeatedly. There has been no cough, dyspnea, fever, chills, tinnitus, or vertigo.

- PMH:
  - Coccidioides immitis in the left eye 5 years prior
  - *Clostridium difficile* colitis
- Exam:
  - HR ranges between 63 and 95 bpm; respirations 18; and BP stable
  - Applying bilateral ocular pressure for 25 sec produces bradycardia (< 50 bpm)
  - Sensation is normal to elementary testing
  - Hand pincers, hip flexion, and leg extension 4-/5 in strength; dorsiflexion 3+/5 b/l
  - DTR 1+/4 biceps; unobtainable brachioradialis, patellae, and achilles; toes equivocal
  - Requires a walker for stability
- CSF
  - WBC = 0/μL; RBC = 1/μL; protein = 100 mg/dL; glucose 94 mg/dL; negative cytology/cultures

Initial Imaging

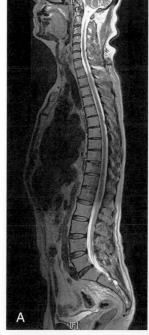
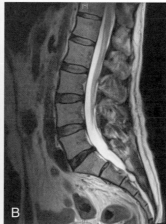

FIGURE 94-1

Diagnostic Tests

- Thoracic spine MRI demonstrates a 3 mm posterior extrusion at T2-T3, extending over a cephalocaudal distance of 1 cm, with a borderline central canal stenosis and mild impingement on the anterior thoracic cord.
- Lumbar spine MRI shows mild loss in height at L5-S1 disc with a 2 mm posterior protrusion minimally impressing the thecal sac; no central canal stenosis or nerve root impingement is noted.
- Cervical spine is unremarkable.

Electrodiagnostic Study

- EMG/NCS: demyelinating > axonal motor-sensory polyneuropathy, + dispersion, and no denervation
- Needle exam (Figure 94-2, Table 94-1, Figure 94-3, and Figure 94-4)

Differential Diagnosis

- Autoimmune disorder
  - Miller-Fisher syndrome (anti-GQ1b and GT1a)
  - Vasculitic neuropathy (Sjögren's syndrome)
  - Myasthenic syndrome
- Other
  - Chemotherapy-induced toxic neuromyopathy
  - Acute intermittent porphyria (in patients with predominantly axonal neuropathy)
  - Periodic paralysis (in those without sensory complaints)

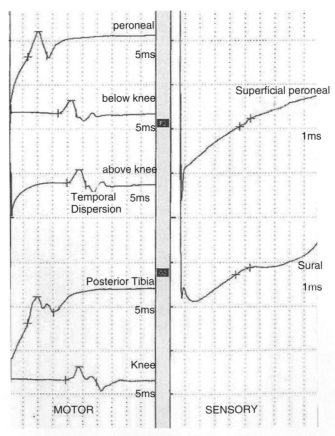

FIGURE 94-2 Motor sensory.

TABLE 94-1

EMG RESULTS

Nerve	Latency (msec)	Ampl	Velocity (m/s)
Median m.	5.1	6.2	42
Ulnar m.	3.5	7.8	46
Median s.	2.5	18.0	40
Ulnar s.	2.7	3.0	30
Tibial	6.5	1.2	34
Peroneal	6.7	1.2	32
Sural	4.4	4.0	32

F Waves	(msec)		
Rt Median n.	35.4		
Rt Ulnar n.	36.2		
Rt Tibial n.	77.1		
Lt Tibial n.	NR		
B/L Peroneal n.	NR		

Muscle EMG	Ampl	Polyphasic Potentials	Recruitment
Rt VM	NI	None	↓
Rt TA	Giant	+1	Doublets
Rt MG	NI	None	Discrete
Rt TP	NI	+1	↓

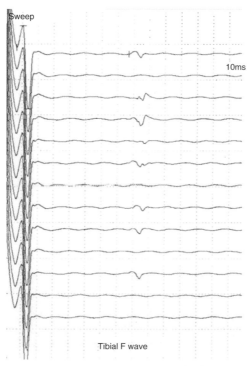

Sweep

10ms

Tibial F wave

FIGURE 94-3   GBS F wave tibial.

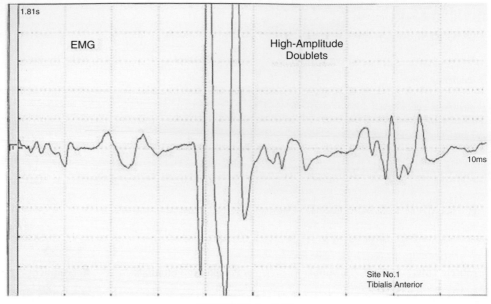

FIGURE 94-4 EMG.

- Acute transverse myelopathy
- Diphtheria (ascending paralysis in 33% and descending paralysis in 27%)
- Acute anterior poliomyelitis
- Tick paralysis
- Botulism (descending paralysis)
- Paraneoplastic syndrome
  - Anti-Hu antibody syndrome

Further Workup

(For Guillain-Barré syndrome [GBS])

- Laboratory
  - ESR <50 mm/hr
  - CPK may be mildly elevated (with radicular symptoms)
  - AST/ALT elevated in 10%
  - Anti-ganglioside antibodies: GQ1b, GT1b, GM1, GalNac-GD1a
  - Stool cultures if GI complaints (Campylobacter)
- EMG/NCS
  - If tested within 7 days
  - Abnormal H reflex (95%)
  - Low amplitude/prolonged F-waves (85%)
  - Within 3 weeks: demyelination
  - Distal latencies prolonged by >150% UNL
  - Temporal dispersion of CMAP
  - Slow conduction velocity
- CSF
  - Protein-cytological dissociation in 80% by the second week: protein 55–1000 and less than 10 WBC
  - Oligoclonal bands (positive in 10%–30%)
- Additional imaging
  - Chest X-ray
  - MRI lumbar spine with contrast shows diffuse nerve root enhancement in 95% of cases

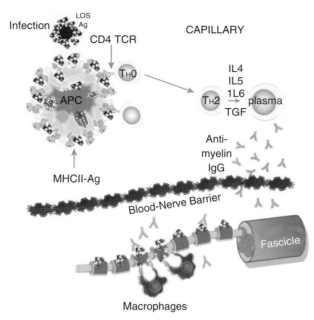

FIGURE 94-5 GBS–BNB AB macrophage.

- Consultants
  - Neurology
  - Hospital intensivist/pulmonology

Pathophysiology

GBS is a heterogeneous condition. Its most common form includes acute inflammatory demyelinating polyneuropathy (AIDP). The disease may also manifest as acute axonal neuropathy, Miller-Fisher syndrome (triad of ataxia, areflexia, and ophthalmoparesis), and as acute motor sensory axonal neuropathy (AMSAN). Clinically, patients exhibit symmetric ascending paralysis in the distal and proximal leg muscles, associated with radiating lumbar pain. There is frequent subjective paresthesia without objective findings. Areflexia and autonomic dysfunction are often evident. Approximately one third will develop vital capacity, <1 L, requiring intubation.

A genetic risk factor is FcγRIIa-H131 allele homozygosity. A misdirected humoral immune response, with immunoglobulins against tubulin, gangliosides, heparan sulfate, glycolipids, gliomedin, and neurofascin-186 (in axonal variation), is believed to be the pathological basis of the disease (Figure 94-5).

Peptide antigens (derived from lipooligosaccharides [LOS] of a pathogen) are displayed on the antigen-presenting cells (APC) in association with MHC II receptors. The T-cell zone of secondary lymphoid organs is where APCs migrate and T-cells are activated. Autoantibodies are produced by plasma cells, pass the blood-nerve barrier, and cross-react with autoantigens expressed on Schwann cells (molecular mimicry), forming a membrane attack complex. Microglial cells expressing Fc and complement receptors, and CD4+ helper T-lymphocytes, release proinflammatory cytokines such as IFNγ, TNF-α, and nitric oxide, causing demyelination, and if severe, subsequent axonal degeneration.

This particular patient was given 5 days of IVIG (total 2 g/kg). The sensory complaints stabilized and he was able to walk independently after several months. Given the normal CSF protein concentration and AMSAN, it was assumed, however, that the patient had developed GBS-like disorder as a result of nelarabine.

Potential Antecedent Etiologies

- *Campylobacter jejuni* (~6.5%)
- CMV (~2%)

- EBV (~1%)
- Mycoplasma pneumonia (~2%, antibodies to galactocerebroside)
- Haemophilus influenza
- Human immunodeficiency virus
- Post vaccine
- About 30% of patients with GBS have no history of antecedent infection.

Treatment Options

- Medical management
  - IVIG = 0.4 g/kg a day, for 5 days (total of 2 g/kg); initial rate of infusion is 40–60 mL/hr for 30 min and increased to 120–150 mL/hr as tolerated; vitals are checked every 15 min during the first 60 min.
  - Alternative 2-day regimen: on the first day a test dose of 0.2 g/kg is infused. If tolerated, the remaining 0.8 g/kg is infused; next day, 1 g/kg is infused in divided doses.
  - Alternative 3-day regimen: 0.4 g/kg the first day, then 0.8 g/kg the following 2 days
  - For plasmapheresis (used for severe cases), a Shiley catheter is required; continuous flow plasmapheresis machine is preferable, with 5% salt-poor albumin replacement fluid; standard therapy is five exchanges over 8–10 days, to a total of 250 mL/kg.
  - For both IVIG and plasmapheresis, it is important to check serum IG levels; low levels of IgA may place the patient at potential risk for anaphylaxis.
  - In GBS with identified antibodies against GM1, GM1b, or GalNAc-GD1a gangliosides, IVIG is more effective. Steroids are ineffective.
- Supportive
  - Elective intubation is needed when a patient's forced vital capacity (VC) drops to <12–15 mL/kg, especially with rapid decline, and/or with a negative inspiratory force (NIF) <25 cmH$_2$O, or PaO2 < 80 mmHg.
  - Intubate patients with bulbar symptoms having a VC of 15–18 mL/kg.
  - Antihypertensive medications should be avoided as a result of autonomic dysregulation.
  - Heparin, 5000 units for prophylaxis DVT
- Surgery
  - Surgery is avoided. Biopsy is not advised. If patients have other causes of myelopathy (i.e. severe cervical stenosis) then consider allowing recuperation from GBS first.

KEY PAPERS

Hughes RA, Cornblath DR. Guillain-Barré syndrome. *Lancet*. 2005;366(9497):1653-1666.

Reilly KM, Kisor DF. Profile of nelarabine: use in the treatment of T-cell acute lymphoblastic leukemia. *Onco Targets Ther*. 2009;2:219-228.

Vucic S, Kiernan MC, Cornblath DR. Guillain-Barré syndrome: an update. *J Clin Neurosci*. 2009;16:733-741.

Case 95

Devic's Syndrome

Audrey Kohar, DO ● Noriko Salamon, MD ●
Neal Prakash, MD, PhD

Presentation

A 45-year-old thin female with a recent history of intermittent bilateral eye pain and blurry vision presents with acute left eye blindness and weakness in the bilateral legs. The patient had no lesions on brain MRI, was refractory to conservative measures, and eventually developed progressive difficulty with ambulation.

- PMH: otherwise unremarkable
- Exam:
  - Tender to palpation at thoracolumbar midline spine
  - Normal UE exam
  - LE 3/5 weakness at adductor, obturator, and quadriceps
  - Sensory level at L1-L3 and decreased temperature sensation
  - Weak rectal tone

Differential Diagnosis

- Neoplastic
  - Metastasis (h/o cancer)
  - Spinal cord tumor
- Vascular
  - AVM (more chronic course, often with stepwise progression)
- Infectious
  - Spinal abscess (h/o IVDA and manifestations of infection)
  - EBV and varicella
  - HIV
  - TB
- Autoimmune
  - MS
  - SLE
  - Sjögren's syndrome
  - P-ANCA autoantibodies
  - Anticardiolipin
- Other
  - Transverse myelopathy or optic neuritis (acute onset)
  - Vitamin B_{12} deficiency (h/o alcoholism)
  - Folate deficiency
  - Radiation myelopathy
  - Disseminated encephalomyelitis (acute)

Initial Imaging

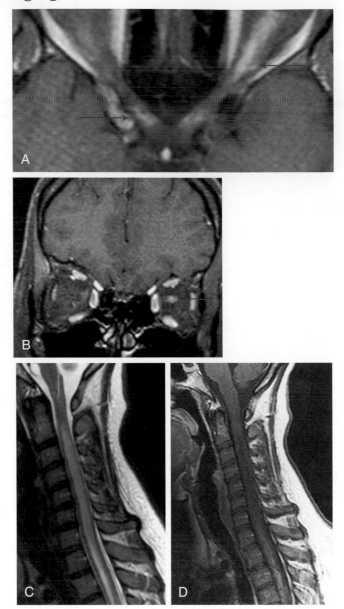

FIGURE 95-1

Imaging Description

- Figure 95-1A: optic nerves shown are hyperintense on T2, consistent with optic neuritis.
- Figure 95-1B: spinal cord lesions appears hyperintense on T2 and (Figure 95-1C) hypointense on T1-weighted images. (Gadolinium is enhanced when structures are inflamed [more indicative of acute phase].)

Further Workup

- Laboratory
  - Routine labs
  - ESR, CRP

- NMO-IgG, anti-AQP4 (strong predictor of future relapses)
  - CSF analysis
- Imaging
  - CT for evaluation of spine, brain, and optic nerves
  - MRI with contrast to evaluate optic nerve and spinal cord lesions
  - MRI to also evaluate brainstem, hypothalamus, and periventricular white matter (may be present in late courses)
- Consultants
  - Medical oncology
  - Neurology

Pathophysiology

Devic's syndrome is an immune-mediated disorder similar to MS. It is characterized by the presence of NMO-IgG, a serum autoantibody against the water channel protein aquaporin-4 (AQP4). AQP4 is a transmembrane protein that regulates the flow of water in cells. AQP4 is also expressed by CNS astrocytes and astrocytic processes surrounding small blood vessels at the glia limitans. NMO autoantibodies concentrate in AQP4 areas, resulting in a binding reaction on the astrocytic foot processes. Complement is then activated, leading to polymorphonuclear cell mobilization (neutrophils and eosinophils), resulting in inflammation and tissue swelling. Loss of AQP4 and glial fibrillary acidic protein, with relatively preserved myelin, is the pathological hallmark of active NMO lesions.

Recent studies also indicate that Th17 (interleukin 17 producing T-cells) cells specific to AQP4 may be the cause of the breakdown of the blood-brain barrier (BBB). The disruption of the BBB enables access of AQP4 antibodies and polymorphonuclear cells to the lesion sites, resulting in an upregulation of autoantibodies against the antigens on the surface of the myelin sheath or oligodendrocytes. This leads to demyelination. It is currently unknown why the antibodies only react with self-antigens on the optic nerve or spinal cord.

This disease has a predilection for middle-aged, non-Caucasian females. Diagnosis requires the presence of optic neuritis and acute myelitis and two of three supporting criteria: contiguous spinal cord MRI lesion extending over ≤3 vertebral segments, brain MRI not meeting the diagnostic criteria for multiple sclerosis, and seropositive NMO-IgG.

Treatment Options

- Medical
  - Short course IV corticosteroids are indicated for cord compression (1000 mg daily for 5 days)
  - Extended oral prednisone to follow after IV corticosteroids (taper at 60–100 mg per day)
- Interventional
  - Plasmapheresis to remove NMO-IgG and Th17 (QOD 1.5 × plasma volume exchange)
  - Immunotherapeutic agents targeting T- and B-cells (azathioprine, mycophenolate, rituximab, eculizumab, cyclosporine, mitoxantrone, methotrexate, and tocilizumab [anti-interleukin 6])
- Consults
  - Medical oncology
  - Neurosurgery for progressive symptomatic lesions refractory to treatment

Surgical Technique

There is typically no role for neurosurgery in Devic's. However, lesions that do not respond to therapy may require biopsy to confirm the diagnosis. A percutaneous technique is described below. Once a safe path to the target lesion has been chosen, the entry site on the skin's surface is marked with indelible ink marker. The region of interest is then prepped and draped in a sterile fashion. A 1 cm wheal is raised at the skin entry site with a 25 gauge needle and local anesthetic agent. A No. 11 blade scalpel is used to make a dermatotomy incision at the skin entry site. A stylet-bearing thin needle is then advanced with image guidance to administer local anesthetic to the deeper soft tissue. If vertebra is entered, infiltration of the anesthetic agent into periosteum is helpful in decreasing discomfort.

The position of the needle tip relative to the lesion is adjusted and confirmed by means of image guidance. When the needle tip is in satisfactory position, the needle hub is removed and the needle then serves as a stiff guidewire. A guiding cannula is inserted over the hubless needle and advanced to the desired level under image guidance. Aspiration or core needles are then passed through this guiding cannula to obtain specimens.

Complication Avoidance and Management

- Demyelination can cause respiratory arrest or difficulties and may require the use of artificial ventilation; respiratory complications are the most common cause of death for patients with Devic's syndrome
- Complications of spinal cord biopsy can entail active hemorrhage, hematoma, vascular injury, neural injury (results in transient or permanent paralysis), pneumothorax, and infection. Incidence of reported complications in percutaneous skeletal biopsy is low and estimated to be <0.2%.

KEY PAPERS

Bienia B, Balabanov R. Immunotherapy of neuromyelitis optica. *Autoimmune Dis.* 2013;2013:Article ID 741490, 7 pages, doi:10.1155/2013/741490.

Cohen-Gadol AA, et al. Spinal cord biopsy: a review of 38 cases. *Neurosurgery.* 2003;52(4):806-815, discussion 815-816.

Orlando Ortiz A, et al. Image-guided percutaneous spine biopsy. *Image Guided Interventions.* 2010; doi:10.1007/978-1-4419-0352-5_5.

Sato DK, et al. Aquaporin-4 antibody-positive myelitis initially biopsied for suspected spinal cord tumors: diagnostic considerations. *Mult Scler.* 2014;20:621. doi:10.1177/1352458513505350.

Case 96

Human Immunodeficiency Virus

Ramsis Benjamin, MD

Presentation

A 36-year-old woman, married with five children, presents with 1 month of fatigue, malaise, 10 pounds of weight loss, and swollen glands. She has had a left frontotemporal pressure headache for 1 week, associated with word impairment and progressive lethargy.

- PMH:
  - Para 0125 and gravida 8
  - Migraines with visual auras
  - Contact with multiple stray cats
- Exam:
  - Dysarthria with dysnomia
  - Sensation normal to elementary testing
  - Right hand grasp, leg extension, hip flexion 4-/5 in strength
  - DTR 2+/4 right biceps; patellae, achilles; up going right toe
  - Electrolytes within normal limits; peripheral WBC 3.8/mm^3; mononucleosis negative

Initial Imaging

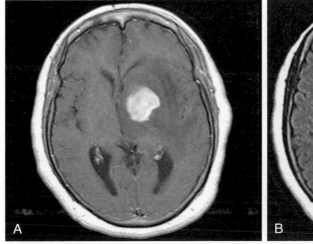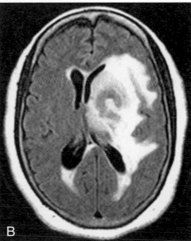

FIGURE 96-1

Imaging Description

- MRI of the brain – axial T1-weighted images with gadolinium contrast and T2/FLAIR. A homogenous enhancing lesion in the left basal ganglia is shown, with extensive vasogenic edema, mass effect, and left to right 8 mm shift.

Diagnostic Workup
CSF

- WBC <1; RBC 0; protein 76 mg/dL; glucose 65 mg/dL; and negative cytology

Brain Biopsy

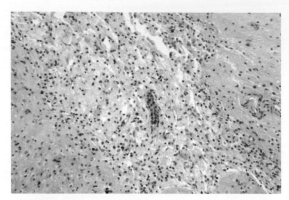

FIGURE 96-2   Lymphoma cells invading brain tissue.

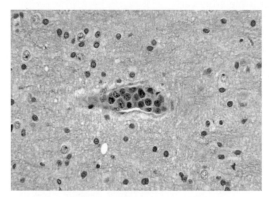

FIGURE 96-3   Accumulation of malignant cells within the vascular structure.

Differential Diagnosis (Box 96-1)

- Primary and secondary brain tumors
  - Astrocytoma/glioblastoma
  - Metastatic breast and lung cancer
  - Primary CNS lymphoma
- Infections
  - Abscess
  - Tuberculoma
- Other
  - Tumefactive multiple sclerosis
  - Stroke

Further Workup

- Laboratory
  - Serum human immunodeficiency virus (HIV)-1, toxoplasma serum titer
- Imaging
  - CT chest/abdomen/pelvis

BOX 96-1	Neurologic Complications in HIV/AIDS (Each with a Prevalence of <5%)
Toxoplasmosis	
PML	
Central nervous system lymphoma	
Cryptococcal meningitis	
Myopathy	
Neurologic cytomegalovirus	
Neurosyphilis	
Stroke	

- CSF (abnormal in 45%)
  - Cryptococcal/toxoplasma antigen titers
  - VDRL, PML, flow cytometry; cell cytology
  - Stains and cultures for acid-fast bacteria (glucose <35 mg/dL)
- Biopsy – indication:
  - For a definitive diagnosis of intracranial solitary mass
  - Negative antitoxoplasma serology
  - Failure of empiric treatment for toxoplasmosis
  - CD4+ cells >200/mm^3
- Consultants
  - Infectious disease
  - Radiation oncology (CNS lymphoma)

Epidemiology

HIV is a lentivirus that infects helper T-cells and monocytes. It belongs to Group III of the Baltimore Classification System double stranded RNA viruses. The "4 × 40" rule refers to a worldwide infection of 40 million people, 40% of whom are younger than 40 years, and seroconversion that occurs after 4 weeks. HIV transmission by male-to-male sexual contact is climbing in the United States, from 55% in 2008 to 62% in 2011 and 85% of women contract HIV-1 heterosexually.

HIV can involve the entire neuraxis (central and peripheral). In developed countries with access to antiretroviral therapy, peripheral neuropathy and HIV-associated neurocognitive disorder (HAND) account for the majority of neurological illnesses. Elsewhere, opportunistic infections (cryptococcal meningitis, neurotuberculosis, toxoplasmosis, and neurosyphilis) carry a higher prevalence.

Pathophysiology

Embedded throughout the viral envelope are nearly 72 copies of a complex protein known as Env, comprised of glycoprotein 120 (gp120) that is anchored by gp41. With its six regulatory genes (tat, rev, nef, vif, vpr, and vpu), HIV-1 can infect and replicate within a host cell, and infected monocytes can traverse the blood-brain barrier. Cell-to-cell fusion involving microglial cells that express CD4 and HIV coreceptors results in the formation of multinucleated giant cells within the brain, a hallmark of AIDS dementia complex. Gp120 may also induce apoptotic cell death in neurons via the activation of p38 mitogen-activated protein kinase (MAPK) (Figure 96-4).

CD4 glycoprotein and its coreceptor CXCR4 (or CCR5) are the primary receptors used by HIV to gain entry into helper T-cells or monocytes by binding to the gp120 protein of HIV. Once fused within the host cell membrane, HIV proteins and nucleic acids enter the cell. Reverse transcriptase (RT) creates double-stranded DNA using viral RNA as a template and host tRNA as primers. The viral DNA is integrated into the host DNA. New virus particles assemble at the cell's surface.

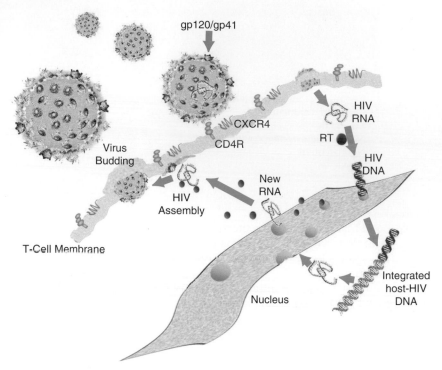

FIGURE 96-4 Pathophysiology of HIV.

Differential Diagnosis

The most common focal lesions in patients with HIV-1 and low CD4+ count (<200 cells/mm³) are lymphoma, PML, cryptococcal meningocerebritis, and toxoplasmosis.

- CNS lymphoma
  - Typically a diffuse large B-cell non-Hodgkin's lymphoma
  - Signs and symptoms are confusion, lethargy, and personality changes, usually with focal deficits; similar to toxoplasmosis.
  - Usually solitary or a few enhancing lesions associated with marked edema and mass effect; common locations are in the periventricular white matter and in the deep gray matter
  - Definitive diagnosis: brain biopsy or positive CSF cytology (occurs in ~20% of cases)
- Toxoplasmosis
  - The most common cause of intracerebral mass lesions.
  - Initial glandular symptoms herald confusion, headache, change in personality, generalized or focal seizures, and hemiparesis.
  - Radiologic appearance varies: typically, many ring-enhancing lesions with marked surrounding edema.
  - CSF sampling in toxoplasmosis can be normal, or show a mononuclear pleocytosis and elevated protein.
  - Serology is positive in 85% of cases.
  - Stereotactic biopsy is sometimes required.
- PML
  - Caused by John Cunningham/Jamestown Canyon (JC) virus, a ubiquitous polyoma virus
  - Subacute or chronic progressive symptoms of speech and visual impediment, hemiparesis, and gait abnormalities. Encephalopathy can occur with fulminate disease; seizures are uncommon.
  - Nonspecific mild pleocytosis and/or protein elevation in CSF is usually the norm; CSF PCR detection of JC virus DNA.

- Imaging studies show asymmetric, posterior, hypointense, nonenhancing lesions with minimum edema on T1-weighted in the subcortical U-fibers, sparing the periventricular white matter.
- Cryptococcus
  - Multiple non-enhancing (enhances in immunocompetent) basal ganglia lesions

Treatment Options

- Medical management
  - HIV-1
    - Protease inhibitors (PIs): nelfinavir, ritonavir, indinavir, saquinavir, and amprenavir
    - Nucleoside reverse transcriptase inhibitors (NRTIs): zidovudine (AZT and retrovir), didanosine (ddI and videx), zalcitabine (ddC and hivid), stavudine (d4T and Zerit), and lamivudine (3TC and epivir)
    - Nonnucleoside reverse transcriptase inhibitors (NNRTIs): nevirapine, delavirdine, efavirenz, HBY 097, and MKC 442
    - Nucleotides: adefovir and b-p PMPA
  - Toxoplasmosis
    - Initial approach: 10- to 14-day trial of pyrimethamine and folinic acid, and either sulphadiazine or clindamycin
    - If lesions improve, continue treatment for a total of 6 weeks, followed by co-trimoxazole.
    - Avoid steroids if possible so as not to mask the diagnosis of primary CNS lymphoma.
    - Antiretroviral therapy is initiated 2 weeks after the acute phase.
  - CNS lymphoma
    - 4000–5000 cGy whole brain radiation over 3 weeks
    - Tumor is radiosensitive, but has high recurrence rate.
    - Dexamethasone: lympholytic and anti-vasogenic
    - A trial of rituximab +/− methotrexate
    - Possible autologous stem cell transplant
  - PML
    - Standard of care: HAART
    - Cidofovir, cytosine arabinoside, interferon-α have proven ineffective against PML.
    - Worsening of PML from HAART has occurred due to immune reconstitution inflammatory syndrome (IRIS).
  - Cryptococcus
    - Amphotericin
- Preventive
  - Truvada (emtricitabine-tenofovir) prevents HIV-1 infection.
- Supportive
  - Patients generally live an almost normal life while taking antiretroviral medications, and withholding treatment causes recurrence of symptoms within 2 weeks.

KEY PAPERS

Hogan C, Wilkins E. Neurological complications in HIV. *Clin Med (Northfield Il)*. 2011;11(6):571-575.

Kranick SM, Nath A. Neurologic complications of HIV-1 infection and its treatment in the era of antiretroviral therapy. *Continuum Lifelong Learning Neurol*. 2012;18(6):1319-1337.

Manji H, Miller R. The neurology of HIV infection. *J Neurol Neurosurg Psychiatry*. 2004;75(suppl I):i29-i35.

Case 97

Status Epilepticus

Neal Prakash, MD, PhD

Presentation

A 47-year-old right-handed male nonsmoker who was diagnosed with stage IV adenocarcinoma of the lung with brain metastases is now having symptoms of progressive clumsiness with the right hand and frontal headaches.

He underwent a left frontoparietal craniotomy for gross total resection of a premotor left frontal tumor and a separate medial left frontal mass, located in the motor cortex and subcortical white matter using intraoperative SSEP, motor-evoked potentials, and direct cortical stimulation for motor mapping.

He was prescribed levetiracetam, 500 mg preoperatively; however, he was noted to have had a right upper extremity focal motor seizure intraoperatively. Postoperatively, he experienced right upper extremity weakness with multiple intermittent right upper extremity and head tremors. Intravenous boluses of lorazepam were given after each episode, which resulted in mild sedation, and levetiracetam was increased to 1500 mg intravenously every 12 hours over the next 24 hours. Despite these therapies, as you are rounding several days after surgery the nurses inform you that he is having a generalized seizure which has lasted over 5 minutes. You control your panic and …

• PMH: type 2 diabetes mellitus and taking oral medications; hypercholesterolemia

Differential Diagnosis

Seizures caused by hemorrhage, meningitis, electrolyte abnormalities, inadequate therapy

Initial Imaging

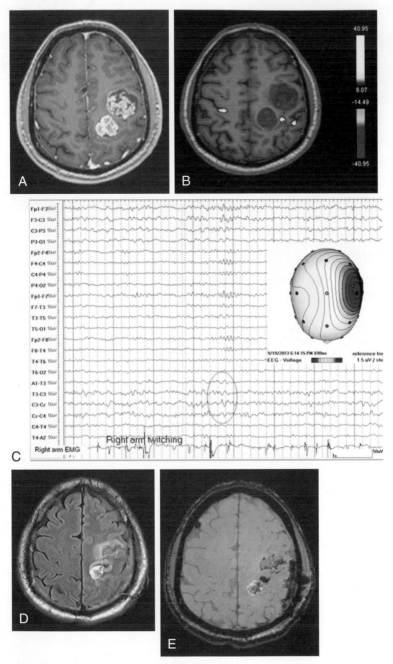

FIGURE 97-1

Imaging Description

- Preoperative MRI (Figure 97-1A) and functional MRI (Figure 97-1B) show: (1) two large enhancing lesions in the left posterior frontal and left parietal lobes. No significant mass effect is demonstrated and minimal surrounding vasogenic edema is present; (2) small lesions consistent with metastases in the inferior right frontal lobe and right cerebellum; (3) functional MRI showing activity consistent with motor activity just posterior to the more anterior lesion and extending directly up to the more posterior lesion, suggesting this lesion may involve the motor strip.
- Ictal EEG (Figure 97-1C) shows bursts of left central sharp waves and rhythmic theta activity during right hand and arm 3–4 Hz twitching episodes.

- Postoperative MRI images (Figure 97-1 D and E) show: (1) post resection left posterior frontal and left parietal metastases; (2) moderate hemorrhage within the left parietal metastasis; (3) subdural fluid collection beneath the craniotomy site left frontal parietal, with local mass effect. Subdural air is seen in the anterior left frontal lobe and to a lesser extent in the right frontal lobe.

Further Workup

- Laboratory
  - Routine labs
  - ABG
  - AED levels
  - LFTs
  - Tox screen especially in ER setting
  - Lumbar puncture as needed to r/o meningitis
- Imaging
  - CT to r/o hemorrhage
  - MRI if appropriate when stabilized
- Consultant
  - Neurology

Pathophysiology

Animal models and clinical evidence strongly support that focal motor status epilepticus (epilepsia partialis continua) originates from the motor cortex. The motor cortex, more than any other cortical area, has very strong surrounding inhibition and tight afferent-efferent relationships. This unique organization gives rise to nonspreading and precisely localized tremors/seizures. This is in contrast with the limbic cortex, which has diffuse connections that spread excitation to other regions, leading to rapidly generalized seizures.

Epilepsia partialis continua may be caused by focal lesions, such as: cortical dysplasias, traumatic lesions, hematomas, infections/abscess, vascular lesions, autoimmune encephalitis, or multiple sclerosis. Systemic and metabolic causes include: diabetic ketoacidosis, hyperosmotic hyperglycemia, hepatic and uremic encephalopathy, hyponatremia, or drug induced (e.g. penicillin and cefotaxime).

Treatment Protocol

- One status protocol
  - ABC's, labs
  - Treatment
    - thiamine 100mg
    - dextrose 50cc D50
    - vit B6 100mg (neonate)
    - ativan 2mg/min (max .1mg/kg) with 1 minute in between doses
    - fosphenytoin (20mg/kg at 150mg/min)
    - depakote (20mg/kg)
    - Intubate if above fails
    - pentobarb: load 10mg/kg over 30 min and maintenance of about 2mg/kg/hr for burst suppression
- Cell death can start as soon as 20 minutes after status begins.
  - obtain diagnosis

Surgical Technique (Figure 97-2)

For refractory focal continuous motor seizures (epilepsia partialis continua), multiple subpial transections can be performed. Once the area to be transected has been electrocorticographically mapped, a small pinhole-sized nick is made in the pia with the point of a No. 11 blade in an area of the cortex that is relatively avascular. An attempt is made to reach as deep into the sulcus as possible, but access is often limited by the presence of

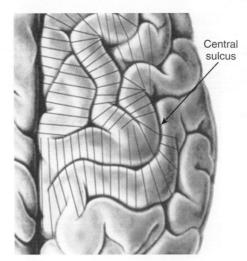

Central
sulcus

FIGURE 97-2 Central sulcus.

large vessels. The instrument is introduced through the pial opening and then swept forward, dipping in an arc-like fashion underneath the gyrus. The blade of the blunt hook is maintained in a strictly vertical orientation to avoid undercutting the cortex. The position of the blade is aligned with the flat side of the instrument handle to help maintain the correct orientation. The tip is raised at the far edge of the gyrus so that it is visible beneath and just elevates, but does not penetrate, the pia. The blade is then gently drawn straight back across the gyrus in the same plane as its forward movement, keeping its tip visible through the pia until the gyrus is transected. Care is taken not to snag any cortical vessels, especially from the opposite sulcus, in the hook of the blade. After the blade is removed, there is often some bleeding from the capillaries on the surface at the point of original insertion. This is usually easily controlled by application of a very small piece of thrombin-soaked Gelfoam. The next transection is made parallel to the first and 5 mm away. Transections are repeated as often as necessary to include the entire area of electrical abnormality and may encompass several gyri. The capillary bleeding associated with each traverse of the instrument results in a fine red line. The bleeding does not seem to cause damage, and the line is a useful reference against which to gauge the location of the next transection.

Complication Avoidance and Management

- No claim is made that horizontal or tangential connections are functionally irrelevant – only that the price of severing them is small compared with that of ablation. Moreover, in many patients the net result, including elimination of seizures, yields an improvement of function of the transected tissue. For example, preoperatively, four of the patients with Wernicke's area/angular gyrus transection and three of those with Broca's area transection suffered severe aphasic symptoms for many hours each day. The minimal postoperative language deficit, such as minimal decrease in fluency, was regarded as preferable in every case. The patients with epileptogenic lesions of the motor cortex who were not already afflicted with some degree of permanent hemiparesis were, nevertheless, functionally disabled by frequent clonic seizures. All of these individuals considered that the operation had improved their ability to utilize the involved hand and arm despite the diminution in fine movement skills.

KEY PAPERS

Cockerell OC, et al. Clinical and physiological features of epilepsia partialis continua: cases ascertained in the UK. *Brain*. 1996;119(2):393-407.

Morrell F, Whisler WW, Bleck TP. Multiple subpial transection: a new approach to the surgical treatment of focal epilepsy. *J Neurosurg*. 1989;70(2):231-239.

Thomas JE, Reagan TJ, Klass DW. Epilepsia partialis continua: a review of 32 cases. *Arch Neurol*. 1977; 34(5):266-275.

Case 98

Neurosarcoidosis

Ramsis Benjamin, MD

Presentation

A 49-year-old accountant began to experience difficulty fixating on the proper line when analyzing pages of numerical columns, worse with the left eye. Four months earlier, she developed a skin rash after a penetrating trauma to the left hip. Soon afterward left facial weakness was noted by her family physician when she complained of drooling. Bell's palsy was entertained. This was followed by headaches for 3 days before developing generalized tonic-clonic seizures. Peripheral smears and serum analysis offered no assistance in establishing a diagnosis.

- PMH:
  - Left meralgia paresthetica – 10 years earlier
  - Left carpal tunnel syndrome – 10 years earlier
  - Sudden onset vertigo and unsteady gait, Dx: labyrinthitis, 5 years earlier
- Exam:
  - Corrected visual acuity 20/50 O.U. with bilateral papilledema
  - Left facial asymmetry involving forehead, cheek, and chin
  - Sensation intact to cold, vibration, pinprick, and light touch
  - Symmetric strength
  - 3+/4 DTR in patellae with bilateral Babinski
- Cerebrospinal fluid: opening pressure 22.5 cm H_2O
- WBC 6/mm^3 (96% lymph); RBC 1/mm^3; glucose 59 mg/dL; and protein 55 mg/dL

Clinical Examination

Foreign body reaction

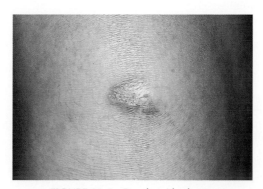

FIGURE 98-1 Papule with plaque.

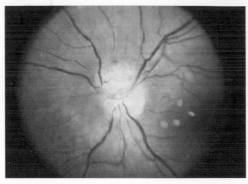

FIGURE 98-2   Vascularized mass superior to the optic disc and several "punched out" lesions with blurred disc margins superiorly.

Initial Imaging

Cranial MRI (Figure 98-3) shows (A) peri fourth ventricular enhancement and (B) left optic chiasm enhancement.

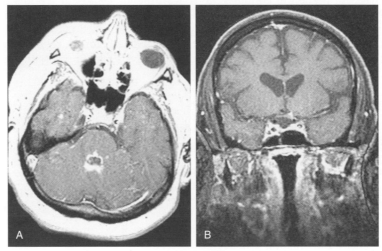

FIGURE 98-3

Differential Diagnosis

- Infection
  - Neuroborreliosis
  - Tuberculous meningitis
  - Neurosyphilis
- Cancer
  - Primary B-cell lymphoma
  - Gliomatosis cerebri
  - Metastatic carcinomatosis
- Vasculitide
  - CNS lupus erythematous
- Others
  - Multiple sclerosis (chronic relapsing-remitting form)
  - Idiopathic hypertrophic pachymeningitis
  - Bickerstaff syndrome
  - Heerfordt's syndrome
  - Pseudotumor cerebri

Further Workup

- Laboratory
  - ESR, CRP
  - ANA, RF
  - Serum/urine calcium
  - Serum γ–globulin
  - Serum angiotensin-converting enzyme (ACE)
- CSF analysis
  - Cell count, oligoclonal band, IgG index
  - ACE (questionable value)
  - VDRL
  - Borrelia
- Pulmonary function study
- Additional imaging
  - CT of the chest and abdomen, with contrast
- Gallium scan
- Consultants
  - Neurology
  - Ophthalmology
  - Pulmonary: bronchoalveolar lavage for lymphocytes

Pathophysiology

Sarcoidosis (the great mimicker) occurs worldwide, particularly in the higher latitudes. Although it preferentially involves the lungs and the draining mediastinal lymph nodes (hilar adenopathy and lymphadenopathy), it can also affect the eyes (uveitis, "candle wax drippings" and "punched out" lesions), skin, spleen, and in 5%–15% of the cases, central and peripheral nervous system. Sarcoidosis-related optic neuritis is considered a neuroophthalmic emergency due to rapidly occurring amaurosis if treatment is delayed.

Neurologic manifestations include cranial neuropathies (50% with facial paresis), aseptic meningitis (10%–20%), seizures (<20%), and hydrocephalus (10%). Myopathy and neuropathy account for 10%–25% of chronic cases of systemic sarcoidosis. Other symptoms include brain mass, pituitary/hypothalamic dysfunction, and cognitive impairment. A combination of a basal meningitis, multiple cranial nerve palsies, diabetes insipidus and hydrocephalous should definitely arouse suspicion. Chest radiograph is abnormal in 80% and serum angiotensin-converting enzyme levels are elevated in about half of all patients. CSF might be entirely normal one third of the time.

Sarcoidosis is a T-helper 1 (T_H1) lymphocyte-mediated noncaseating granulomatous disease. Microglial antigen-presenting cells (APCs) use their surface MHC II and B7 molecules to present antigen to the CD4 of T-cell receptors, costimulated by CD28. This interaction allows the resting T-cell (T_H0) to differentiate into a T_H1 cell, which forms granulomas in response to various interleukins, interferon-γ (IFN-γ), tumor necrosis factor-α (TNF-α), and granulocyte-macrophage colony stimulating factor (GM-CSF; Figure 98-4).

In two thirds of all patients, the disease is self-limited and monophasic; it may convert to chronic remitting and relapsing in others, mimicking multiple sclerosis.

Treatment Options

- Medical management: Immunosuppression and Chemotherapy
  - Steroids: methylprednisolone 1 g/d, or prednisone 1 mg/kg per day
  - Azathioprine (2–3 mg/kg per day)
  - Mycophenolate mofetil (500 mg bid)
  - Cyclophosphamide or methotrexate
  - Infliximab, a chimeric monoclonal antibody (attenuates TNF-α bioactivity)
  - Radiotherapy (of unclear benefit)
  - Secondary conditions: anti-seizure agents; neuroendocrine support

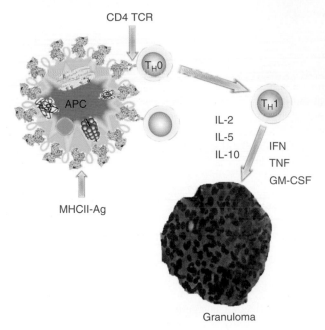

FIGURE 98-4   Pathophysiology of sarcoidosis.

- Surgical
  - Insertion of ventriculoperitoneal shunt for hydrocephalus. Note that ventricular compliance is very low and suspicion for shunt failure should be heightened even with minimal changes in ventricular size.
  - Conventional or neuroendoscopic biopsy of the enhanced lesions if no other lymph node or pulmonary mass can be identified. Definitive diagnosis requires tissue confirmation.
  - Debulking of expanding mass lesions
  - Spinal cord decompression

Surgical resection of neurosarcoidosis should be considered after all other options have been exhausted, and when corticosteroids and immunotherapeutic agents have failed. Asymptomatic ventricular enlargement does not require treatment.

KEY PAPERS

Nozaki K, Judson MA. Neurosarcoidosis. *Curr Treat Options Neurol.* 2013;15:492-504.
Spiegel DR, Morris K, Rayamajhi U. Neurosarcoidosis and the complexity in its differential diagnoses: a review. *Innov Clin Neurosci.* 2012;9(4):10-16.

Case 99

Transverse Myelitis

Audrey Kohar, DO ● Neal Prakash, MD, PhD

Presentation

A thin 50-year-old female has severe spasms on her right side and incontinence. The patient reports that her symptoms started a few years ago when she initially had weakness and numbness of her right arm. Her symptoms quickly progressed to right-sided hemiparesis, left-sided numbness, neck pain radiating to the spinal occipital area, walking difficulties, and urinary incontinence.

- PMH:
  - Lupus, myocardial infarction 4 years ago, DM II, depression, hypertension, COPD
- Exam:
  - CN II through XII intact bilaterally
  - Tender to palpation at thoracic midline spine
  - R UE/LE motor strength 4/5 proximally and 2/5 distally
  - L UE/LE motor strength 5/5
  - Sensory deficit (pinprick) diminished below the neck bilaterally
  - Temperature sensation diminished on the left
  - R DTRs hyperreflexive, Babinski + on R
  - Lhermitte's positive bilaterally
  - Weak rectal tone

Differential Diagnosis

- Neoplastic
  - Metastasis (h/o cancer)
- Vascular
  - Spinal hematoma
- Infectious
  - Spinal abscess
  - Acute disseminated encephalomyelitis
  - HIV/AIDS-related myelopathy
  - CMV
- Autoimmune
  - MS
  - SLE
  - Sjögren syndrome
  - Behçet disease
  - RA
  - Scleroderma and systemic sclerosis
  - Primary biliary sclerosis
  - Periarteritis nodosa
- Other
  - Vitamin B12 deficiency (h/o alcoholism)
  - Folate deficiency
  - Radiation myelopathy
  - Disseminated encephalomyelitis (acute)

Initial Imaging

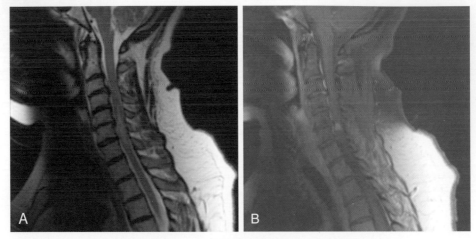

FIGURE 99-1

Imaging Description and Differential

- Cervical spine MRI in Figure 99-1A shows a sagittal T2-weighted image with hyperintensity in the spinal cord indicating spinal cord inflammation. Multiple disc protrusions at levels C2–C3 and C4–C5. No apparent involvement of other segments of the spine.
- Cervical spine MRI in Figure 99-1B shows a sagittal T1 image reflecting a 1 cm enhancing mass involving the right lateral aspect of the spinal cord with surrounding edema.
- Differential: Possible spinal cord tumor causing Brown-Sequard syndrome that eventually led to bladder incontinence.

Further Workup

- Laboratory
  - Routine labs
  - ESR, CRP
  - CSF analysis for IgG and pleocytosis to support inflammatory etiology (one of the criteria for diagnosis): moderate pleocytosis (50–100 lymphocytes/mm^3), elevated protein ($\approx$100 mg/100 mL) without (or transient) oligoclonal bands (OCB), and sometimes increased IgG index, 14-3-3 protein, interleukin-6, non-specific enolase, myelin basic protein, and S-100 protein.
  - Laboratory studies (serology and cultures) for viral and other infectious causes
  - Autoimmune serology to rule out Devic's syndrome
- Imaging
  - CT for evaluation of spine and brain to rule out neoplastic syndromes
  - MRI, with and without contrast, to identify spinal cord inflammation (one of the criteria for diagnosis). T2 hyperintensity in 50% of cases.
  - MRI to rule out compressive lesions and identify intramedullary cord lesion, if present
- Consultants
  - Medical oncology
  - Neurosurgery for compressive lesions or spinal cord biopsies if there is concern for neoplastic disease

Pathophysiology

Transverse myelitis is a mixed inflammatory disorder that can affect neurons, axons, and oligodendrocytes and myelin. TM is basically a heterogeneous collection of acute and subacute infectious and noninfectious inflammatory spinal cord syndromes. There is evidence of perivascular infiltration by monocytes and lymphocytes in the lesions.

Transverse myelitis is mostly triggered by infectious agents: syphilis, measles, Lyme disease, varicella zoster virus, herpes simplex, cytomegalovirus, Epstein-Barr virus, influenza, echovirus, human immunodeficiency virus (HIV), hepatitis A, rubella, and mycoplasma, either directly or as a postinfectious autoimmune process. It may also be induced by various vaccinations or be idiopathic. The latter may occasionally represent one (or the initial) attack of MS or neuromyelitis optica. In MS, transverse myelitis is usually partial and does not affect the whole extent of the spinal cord segment.

Treatment Options

- Medical
  - Short course IV methylprednisolone (1 g daily for 3 to 5 days) with an optional oral prednisone taper are indicated to reduce general inflammation
  - Antiviral or antimicrobial therapies, if there are underlying infectious causes
- Interventional
  - Plasmapheresis as a treatment option for patients who do not response well to corticosteroids (5–7 exchanges over 10 to 14 days)
  - Immunomodulatory or immunosuppressive therapy only indicated if TM poses significant risk of relapse
  - Symptomatic treatment started early: spasticity – baclofen, tizanidine, benzodiazepines; fatigue – amantadine, methylphenidate, 4-aminopyridine; pain – physical stretching, gabapentin, carbamazepine, phenytoin, amitriptyline, and oral or intrathecal baclofen
  - Spinal cord biopsy reserved for progressive neurologic dysfunction despite therapy

Surgical Technique
Spinal Cord Biopsy

Percutaneous technique: Cord biopsies are usually performed by a laminectomy with direct target visualization. Needle based techniques supplemented by myelography are an option. A safe path to the target lesion is chosen with CT or MRI imaging and the entry site on the skin surface is marked with indelible ink marker, prepped, and draped in a sterile fashion. A 1-cm wheal is raised at the skin entry site with a 25 gauge needle and local anesthetic agent. A No. 11 blade scalpel is used to make a dermatotomy incision at the skin entry site. A stylet bearing thin needle is then advanced with image guidance to administer local anesthetic into the deeper soft tissue. If vertebra is entered, infiltration of the anesthetic agent into the periosteum is helpful in decreasing discomfort.

The position of the needle tip relative to the lesion is adjusted and confirmed by means of image guidance. When the needle tip is in satisfactory position, the needle hub is removed and the needle then serves as a stiff guide wire. A guiding cannula is inserted over the hubless needle and advanced to the desired level under image guidance. Aspiration or core needles are then passed through this guiding cannula to obtain specimens.

Complication Avoidance and Management

- TM has high relapse tendencies early on (approximately 60% in the first year), and immunosuppressive therapy is recommended
- A high percentage of patients may be seropositive for neuromyelitis optica
- Complications of spinal cord biopsy may result in active hemorrhage, hematoma, vascular injury, neural injury (results in transient or permanent paralysis), pneumothorax, and infection. Incidences of reported complications in percutaneous skeletal biopsy are few and estimated to be less than 0.2%

KEY PAPERS

Orlando Ortiz A, Zoarski GH, Brook AL. Image-guided percutaneous spine biopsy. In: Mathis JM, Golovac S, eds. *Image-Guided Spine Interventions*. New York: Springer; 2010.

Sa MA. Acute transverse myelitis: a practical reappraisal. *Autoimmun Rev.* 2009;9:128-131.

Wingerchuk D, Weinshenker B. Acute disseminated encephalomyelitis, transverse myelitis, and neuromyelitis optica. *Continuum (Minneap Minn).* 2013;19(4):944-967.

Case 100

Giant Cell Arteritis

Ramsis Benjamin, MD

Presentation

A 60 year-old active woman has been experiencing progressive posterior headaches for 3 months. It was attributed to cervical spondylosis based on X-ray films. Acetaminophen provided no relief, and hydrocodone and cyclobenzaprine proved ineffective as well. For 3 days, her vision became blurry while watching television, as the headaches encompassed the entire cranium, unassociated with nausea or photosensitivity.

- PMH:
  - Coronary artery disease
  - Bilateral catarectomy
  - Left rotator cuff repair
  - Hypertension
- Exam:
  - BP 155/85
  - Supple neck, and tenderness in bilateral suboccipital region
  - VA 20/30 O.D.; light perception O.S.; anisocoria with sluggish left pupil
  - Left temporal artery palpable and tender (Figure 100-1)
  - Strength and sensation are preserved
  - Stretch reflexes and gait are normal
- Laboratory
  - WBC 9/μL, platelets 434,000/μL
  - C-reactive protein (CRP) level 7 mg/L (normal <2.5 mg/L); ESR 72 mm/hr

Clinical Examination

Left temporal artery

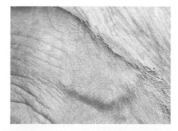

FIGURE 100-1   Prominent left temporal artery.

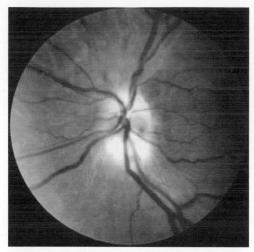

Figure 100-2   Funduscopy: blurred disc margins; Anterior Ischemic Optic Neuropathy involving posterior ciliary and ophthalmic arteries.

Initial Imaging

- 3 Tesla axial MRI + gadolinium

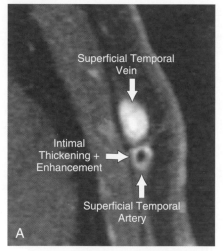

FIGURE 100-3A

- Color-coded Doppler study

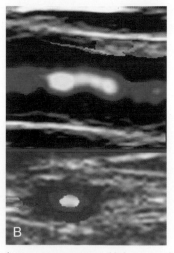

FIGURE 100-3B   Longitudinal and transverse sections of left temporal artery: hypoechoic, circumferential wall thickening (black halo) around the lumen.

Differential Diagnosis

- Ophthalmologic
  - Anterior and posterior ischemic optic neuropathy
  - Retrobulbar and bulbar neuritis
- Endocrine
  - Pituitary apoplexy
- Vasculitis
  - Polymyalgia rheumatic (~25% develop temporal arteritis)
  - Polyarteritis nodosa
- Vascular
  - Ophthalmic/carotid aneurysm
  - Hyperviscosity state
- Others
  - Amyloidosis
  - Ocular sarcoidosis
  - Postherpetic neuralgia
  - Trigeminal neuralgia

Further Workup

- Laboratory
  - CBC, ESR, and CRP
  - ANA, RF, and p-ANCA
- Additional imaging
  - CT or MR angiogram: circle of Willis and extracranial vessels
  - CT of chest and abdomen (aortic aneurysm in 10%–20%)
- Biopsy
  - Unilateral biopsy: false negative 15%
  - Lesion skips portions of the artery: 3–5 cm Bx is typically needed
  - Symptomatic side first; if negative frozen sections, contralateral side is biopsied next
  - Ultrasound may be useful to localize the best site for biopsy.
- Consultants
  - Neurology
  - Rheumatology
  - Ophthalmology

Epidemiology

Giant cell arteritis (GCA), temporal arteritis, and Horton's disease are synonymous. The disease affects aorta and its branches. Branches of the external carotid artery are more affected because intracranial vessels lack an internal elastic lamina. Clinical features include new onset of headache, trismus, scalp tenderness, and visual obscuration. Female predominate by a ratio of 3:1, with a mean age of 70 years at diagnosis. The combination of ESR (>50 mm) and CRP (>2.5 mg/dL) detect GCA with 97% accuracy. IL-6 levels >6 pg/mL also indicate the presence of the disease. A normal temporal artery by physical examination occurs in half of all patients who have high ESR by Westergren method. Anemia and elevated alkaline phosphatase are seen in 25%. Presence of thrombocytosis may be more diagnostic than ESR. GCA is also often associated with polymyalgia rheumatica which is characterized by myalgia of the hip and shoulder girdles accompanied by morning stiffness.

Pathophysiology

The exact etiology of the disease remains unknown. HLA-DR1, HLA-DRB1*04, HLA-DR3, HLA-DR4, and HLA-DR5 have been implicated as MHC antigens. Polymorphisms exist for IL-13, NOS2, VEGF, and Toll-like receptor 4 (TLR-4) genes. Certain infectious agents bind to specific TLRs, such as TLR-4 (LPS) or TLR-5 (flagellin). In susceptible individuals, dendritic cells (DCs) become activated and mature within the vessel wall, where they initiate an innate immune response by secreting high amounts of proinflammatory cytokines IL-2, IL-6, IL-12, IL-17, IL-18, and IL-23. As a result, IFNγ is upregulated in T-cells, which induce amplification of the immune response through positive feedback loops. The proinflammatory environment causes infiltration of the arterial wall adventitia by activated monocytes and neutrophils.

Treatment Options

- Surgical Biopsy
  - No epinephrine. Doppler available
  - Technique: on affected side obtain 3-5cms with incision parallel to STA. Note that STA is in the loose tissue beneath the superficial temporal fascia and above the temporalis fascia.
- Medical
  - If visual symptoms exist, begin Solu-Medrol 1 g/d for 3 days, followed by oral prednisone:
    Month 1   Prednisone 1 mg/kg per day in bid doses for weeks 1 and 2
      Week 3: consolidate to 40–60 mg/d
      Week 4: 40–60 mg/d
    Month 2   Reduce 2.5–5 mg/wk to reach 30 mg/d by month's end
    Month 3   Reduce 2.5–5 mg/wk to reach 20 mg/d by month's end
    Month 4   Reduce 2.5–5 mg/wk to reach 10 mg/d
    Month 5+   Reduce 1 mg/month
  - ESR and hematocrit normalizes after 4 weeks of treatment; if not, another diagnosis in patients with negative biopsy needs to be investigated
  - If prednisone is not tolerated, methotrexate (MTX) at 7.5 mg/wk is started and escalated to 2.5 mg/wk until it reaches 15–20 mg per week; prednisone is slowly tapered off.
  - If MTX fails, azathioprine (125 mg/d) or cyclophosphamide is tried.
  - In refractory patients with ESR >80 after 1 month of treatment and proven biopsy, cyclophosphamide 2 mg/kg per day p.o. daily for 6–12 months can be administered; CBC is checked q week ×2, then bimonthly ×2, then monthly. If WBC drops below 4000 c/mm^3, the dose is halved, and stopped if WBC <3000 c/mm^3; GCSF should be given 48 hours after cyclophosphamide; earlier use may harm stem cells. The risk of hemorrhagic cystitis is reduced if the patient drinks six glasses of water a day. After 6–12 months, cyclophosphamide is tapered off 50 mg every 1–2 months.
  - Tumor necrosis factor-α (TNFα) receptor chimeric monoclonal antibody: infliximab 5 mg/kg per 4–6 weeks; etanercept may paradoxically induce GCA
  - Human recombinant anti-TNFα monoclonal antibody: adalimumab (equivocal at this time)
- Supportive
  - To prevent osteoporosis, calcium 1500 mg + vitamin D 400 IU are added
  - Proton inhibitor for GI protection while on prednisone
  - MRI every 3–6 months for the first year
  - Aspirin 81 mg/d to prevent stroke

KEY PAPERS

Bley TA, Uhl M, Carew J, et al. Diagnostic value of high-resolution MR imaging in giant cell arteritis. *AJNR.* 2007;28:1722-1727.

Fraser AJ, Weyand CM, Newman NJ, et al. The treatment of giant cell arteritis. *Rev Neurol Dis.* 2008;5(3): 140-152.

Glossary

A1c: Glycosylated hemoglobin (hemoglobin A1c)
PO: "Per os," by mouth/orally
3D MIP: Three-dimensional maximum intensity projection
A/V: Audiovisual
AAD: Atlanto-axial dislocation
ABC: Airway, breathing, circulation
ABG: Arterial blood gas
AC: Anterior commissure
ACA: Anterior cerebral artery
ACDF: Anterior cervical discectomy and fusion
ACE: Angiotensin-converting enzyme
Ach A: Anterior choroidal artery
ACoA: Anterior communicating artery
ACTH: Adrenocorticotropic hormone
ADC: Apparent diffusion coefficient
ADEM: Acute Disseminated Encephalomyelitis
ADL: Adrenoleukodystrophy or Activities of daily living
AEDS: Antiepileptic drugs
AICA: Anterior inferior cerebellar artery
AIDP: Acute inflammatory demyelinating polyneuropathy
AIDS: Acquired immune deficiency syndrome
AIN: Acute interstitial nephritis
AION: Anterior Ischemic Optic Neuropathy
AKI: Acute kidney injury
ALIF: Anterior Lumbar Interbody Fusion
ALL: Anterior longitudinal ligament; acute lymphocytic leukemia
ALS: Amyotropic lateral sclerosis
ALT: Amino alanine transferase
AMSAN: Acute motor sensory axonal neuropathy
ANA: Antinuclear antibodies
AO: Anaplastic oligodendroglioma
AOx3: Alert and oriented to person, time, and place
APC: Antigen presenting cell
AQP4: Aquaporin-4
ARUBA: Randomized trial of unruptured brain arteriovenous malformation
AS: Ankylosing spondylitis
AST: Aspartate amino transferase
AT/RT: Atypical teratoid/Rhabdoid tumor
ATL: Anterior temporal lobectomy
ATLS: Advanced trauma life support
ATP: Acute thrombocytopenic purpura; adenosine triphosphate
ATRT: Atypical teratoid rhabdoid tumor
AVF: Arteriovenous fistula
AVM: Arteriovenous malformation

b/l: Bilateral
BA: Basilar artery
BAER: Brainstem auditory evoked response

BBB: Blood-brain barrier
Bcl-2: B-cell lymphoma 2
BDI: Basion-dens interval
BFFE: Balance fast field echo
bhCG: Beta-human chorionic gonadotropin
BID: Twice daily
BLE: Bilateral (or both) lower extremities
BMP: Bone morphogenic protein
Botox: Botulinum toxin
BP: Blood pressure
BPH: Benign prostatic hypertrophy
BUE: Bilateral (or both) upper extremities
Bx: Biopsy

CADASIL: Cerebral autosomal dominant arteriopathy with subcortical infarcts and leukoencephalopathy
CBC: Complete blood count
CCA: Common carotid artery
CES: Cauda Equina Syndrome
CIDP: Chronic inflammatory demyelinating polyneuropathy
CK: Creatine kinase
CLIPPERS: Chronic lymphocytic inflammation with pontine perivascular enhancement responsive to steroids
CM: Centromedian nucleus
CMA: Cingulate motor area
CMAP: Compound muscle action potentials
CMP: Comprehensive metabolic panel
CMT: Charcot-Marie-Tooth
CMV: Cytomegalovirus
CN II: Cranial nerve II (optic)
CN III: Cranial nerve III (oculomotor)
CNS: Central nervous system
Coag: Coagulation factors
COPD: Chronic obstructive pulmonary disease
CPA: Cerebellopontine angle
CPK: Creatine phosphokinase
CPN: Common peroneal nerve
CRH: Corticotropin-releasing hormone
CRP: C-reactive protein
CSF: Cerebrospinal fluid
CT: Computed tomography
CTA: Computed tomographic angiogram
CUSA: Cavitron ultrasonic surgical aspirator
CVJ: Craniovertebral junction
CXR: Chest x-ray

dAVF: Dural arteriovenous fistula
DBS: Deep brain stimulation
DC: Dendritic cell
DCE-MRI: Dynamic contrast-enhanced magnetic resonance imaging
DDD: Degenerative disc disease
DDx: Differential diagnosis
DHEAS: Dehydroepiandrosterone Sulfate
DIC: Disseminated intravascular coagulation
DIP: Distal interphalangeal
DIS: Dissemination in time
DIT: Dissemination in space
DM: Diabetes mellitus

DMARD: Disease-modifying antirheumatic drug
DMSO: Dimethyl sulfoxide
DNA: Deoxyribonucleic acid
DPN: Deep peroneal nerve
DREZ: Dorsal root entry zone
DRG: Dorsal root ganglion
DSA: Digital subtraction angiogram
DSC-MRI: Dynamic susceptibility contrast magnetic resonance imaging
DTI: Diffusion tensor imaging
DTR: Deep tendon reflex
DVT: Deep venous thrombosis
DWI: Diffusion weighted imaging

EBV: Epstein-Barr virus
ECA: Extracranial carotid artery
ECG: Electrocardiogram
ECHO: Echocardiogram
ECST: European Carotid Surgery Trial
ED/ER: Emergency department/emergency room
EEA: Expanded endonasal approach
EEG: Electroencephalogram
EGFR: Epidermal growth factor
EHL: Extensor hallucis longus
EMG: Electromyography
ENT: Ear nose throat
EOMI: Extraocular movements intact
ESR: Erythrocyte sedimentation rate
ETV: Endoscopic third ventriculostomy
EVD: Extra ventricular drain

FCU: Flexor carpi ulnaris
FDG PET: Fludeoxyglucose positron emission tomography
FDI: First dorsal interosseous
FDS: Flexor digitorum superficialis
FG: Fusiform gyrus
FLAIR: Fluid-attenuated inversion recovery
FMD: Fibromuscular dysplasia
fMRI: Functional magnetic resonance imaging
FSH: Follicle stimulating hormone
FT4: Free thyroxine

GABA: Gamma-Aminobutyric acid
GAD: Glutamic acid decarboxylase
GBM: Glioblastoma Multiforme
GBS: Guillain-Barre syndrome
GCA: Giant cell arteritis
GCS: Glasgow coma scale
GERD: Gastroesophageal reflux disease
GH: Growth hormone
GM-CSF: Granulocyte-macrophage colony stimulating factor
GPe: Globus pallidus externa
GPi: Globus pallidus
GSPN: Greater superficial petrosal nerve
GSW: Gunshot wound
GTR: Gross total resection

h/o: History of
HAART: Highly active antiretroviral therapy

HAND: HIV-associated neurocognitive disorder
HC: Hippocampus
HEENT: Head, eye, ear, nose, and throat
HH: Hypothalamic hamartoma
HIV: Human immunodeficiency virus
HPL: Human placental lactogen
HR: Heart rate
HSP: Hereditary spastic paraplegia
HSV: Herpes simplex virus
HTN: Hypertension
H-V: Horizontal-vertical

IAC: Internal auditory canal
ICA: Internal carotid artery; Internal cerebral artery
ICH: Intracerebral hemorrhage
ICP: Intracranial pressure
ICU: Intensive care unit
IDDS: Implantable drug delivery systems
IFN: Interferon
IG: Immunoglobulin
IGF: Insulin-like growth factor
IIC: Idiopathic intracranial hypertension
IL: Interleukin
iNPH: Idiopathic normal pressure hydrocephalus
INR: International normalized ratio
IPH: Infratentorial cerebellar hemorrhage
IRIS: Immune reconstitution inflammatory syndrome
ISUIA: International study of unruptured intracranial aneurysms
IT: Intrathecal
ITG: Inferior temporal gyrus
ITP: Idiopathic thrombocytopenic purpura
IU: International units
IV: Intravenous
IVC: Inferior vena cava
IVDA: Intravenous drug abuse®
IVH: Intraventricular hemorrhage
IVIG: Intravenous immunoglobulin

JC: John Cunningham/Jamestown Canyon virus

K: Potassium
KFT: Kidney function test
KPS: _____

LDH: Lactate dehydrogenase
LE: Lower extremity
LFT: Liver function test
LGG: Low grade glioma
LH: Luteinizing hormone
LLE: Lower left extremity
LMN: Lower motor neuron
LOS: Lipooligosaccharides
LP: Lumbar puncture
LPS: Lipopolysaccharide
LSR: Lateral spread reflex

MAG: Myelin-associated glycoprotein
MAPK: Mitogen-activated protein kinase

MAPs: Mean arterial pressure
MCA: Middle cerebral artery
M-CMTC: Macrocephaly-capillary malformation
MCP: Metacarpophalangeal
MEP: Motor evoked potential
MGMT: Methylguanine-DNA methyltransferase
MHC: Major histocompatibility complex
ML: Medial lemniscus
MLF: Medial longitudinal fasciculus
MMD: Moyamoya disease
MPNST: Malignant peripheral nerve sheath tumor
MRA: Magnetic resonance angiography
MRC: Medical Research Council
MRI: Magnetic resonance imaging
MRV: Magnetic resonance venography
MS: Multiple Sclerosis
MTG: Middle temporal gyrus
MTS: Mesial temporal sclerosis
MTX: Methotrexate
MuSK: Muscle-specific kinase
MVD: Microvascular decompression

Na: Sodium
NASCET: North American Symptomatic Carotid Endarterectomy Trial
NB: _____
NBCA: N-butyl-cyanoacrylate
NCS: Nerve conduction studies
NCV: Nerve conduction velocity
NF2: Neurofibromatosis 2
NIF: Negative inspiratory force
NIHSS: National institute of health stroke scale
NK Cell: Natural killer cell
NMO: Neuromyelitis optica
NNRTI: Non-nucleoside reverse transcriptase inhibitor
NPH: Normal pressure hydrocephalus
NRTI: Nucleoside reverse transcriptase inhibitor
NSAID: Non-steroidal anti-inflammatory drugs
NSCLC: Non-small cell lung carcinoma
NVC: Neurovascular compression

OCB: Oligoclonal bands
OCT: Optical coherence tomography
OD: Right eye (oculus dexter)
ONSF: Optic nerve sheath fenestration
OPLL: Ossification of the posterior longitudinal ligament
ORIF: Open fracture reduction and internal fixation
OS: Overall survival; Left eye (oculus sinister)

PA: Posterior-anterior
PaCO$_2$: Partial pressure of carbon dioxide
p-ANCA: Perinuclear anti-neutrophil cytoplasmic antibodies
PC: Posterior commissure
PCA: Posterior cerebral artery; Posterior cricoarytenoid
PCOM: Posterior communicating
PCR: Polymerase chain reaction
PERRLA: Pupils are equal, round and reactive to light and accomodation.
PFS: Progression free survival rate
PHG: Parahippocampal gyrus

PI: Protease inhibitor
PICA: Posterior-inferior communicating artery
PICU: Pediatric intensive care unit
PIP: Proximal interphalangeal
PLIF: Posterior Lumbar Interbody Fusion
PLL: Posterior longitudinal ligament
PMC: Pre-motor cortex
PMH: Past medical history
PML: Progressive multifocal leukoencephalopathy
PNST: Peripheral nerve sheath tumor
PPN: Pedunculopontine nucleus
PPRF: Paramedian pontine reticular formation
PRL: Prolactin
PROCESS Trial: Prospective, randomized, controlled multicenter study of patients with failed back surgery syndrome
PSA: Prostate-specific antigen
PSH: _____
PT: Prothrombin time; Physical therapy
PTEN: Phosphatase and tensin homolog
PTFE: Polytetrafluoroethylene
PTT: Partial thromboplastin time

qHS: Every bedtime (quaque hora somni)

RA: Rheumatoid arthritis
RBC: Red blood cell count
RCT: Randomized controlled study
RF: Rheumatoid factor; Radiofrequency
RLE: Right lower extremity
RLL: Right lower lobe
RR: Resting rate
RT: Reverse transcriptase

s/p: Status post
SAH: Subarachnoid hemorrhage
Sat: Slide agglutination test
SBP: Systolic blood pressure
SCA: Superior cerebellar artery
SCLC: Small cell lung cancer
SCM: Sternocleidomastoid
SCS: Spinal cord stimulation
SDAVF: Spinal dural arteriovenous fistula
SDH: Subdural hematoma
SDS: Speech discrimination score
SelAH: Selective amygdalohippocampectomy
SHH: Sonic hedgehog
SLE: Systemic lupus erythematosus
SLIC: Subaxial Cervical Spine Injury Classification System
SM scale: Spetzler-Martin scale
SMA: Supplementary motor area
SNc: Substantia nigra
SOD1: Superoxide dismutase 1
SPEP: Serum protein electrophoresis
SPN: Superficial peroneal nerve
SRS: Stereotactic radiosurgery
SRT: Speech reception threshold
SSEP: Somatosensory evoked potential
STAT3: Signal transducer and activator of transcription-3

STG: Superior temporal gyrus
STIR MRI: Short inversion time inversion recovery magnetic resonance imaging
STITCH trial: Surgical treatment for ischemic heart failure
STN: Subthalamic nucleus

T: Temperature
T2WI: T2-weighted image
TCL: Transverse carpal ligament
TDH: Thoracic disc herniation
TEG: Thromboelastographic
TENS: Transcutaneous Electrical Nerve Stimulation
TES-MEP: Transcranial electrical motor evoked potential
TFESI: Transforaminal epidural steroid injection
Th cell: T-helper cell
TIA: Transient ischemic attack
TICI: Thrombolysis in cerebral infarction
TLIF: Transforaminal Lumbar Interbody Fusion
TLR: Toll-like receptor
TM: Transverse myelitis
TMZ: Temozolomide
TN: Trigeminal neuralgia
TNF: Tumor necrosis factor
tPA: Recombinant tissue plasminogen activator
Treg cell: T-regulatory cell
TSH: Thyroid stimulating hormone
TTE: Transthoracic echocardiogram
Tx: Treatment

UE: Upper extremity
UMN: Upper motor neuron
UPDRS: Unified Parkinson's disease rating scale
UTI: Urinary tract infection

VA: Visual acuity
VA/VL: Ventral anterior/ventral lateral
VC: Vital Capacity
VDRL: Venereal disease research laboratory test
VEGF: Vascular endothelial growth factor
vHL: Von Hippel-Lindau disease
VILIP-1: Visinin-like protein 1
VNS: Vagal nerve stimulator
VPS: Ventriculo-peritoneal shunt

WBC: White blood cell count
WBRT: Whole brain radiation therapy
WHO: World health organization
WNT: Wingless
WNV: West nile virus

XRT: Radiation therapy

APPENDIX **A**

Neuropathology

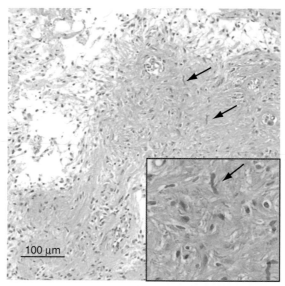

FIGURE A1-1 Hematoxylin and eosin (H&E) stain of a pilocytic astrocytoma. Arrows are pointing at Rosenthal fibers, which are characteristic of this tumor. Inset is a higher magnification of the image. *(Reprinted with permission from Ellenbogen RG, Abdulrauf SI, Sekhar LN. Principles of Neurological Surgery. 3rd ed. Elsevier. 2012.)*

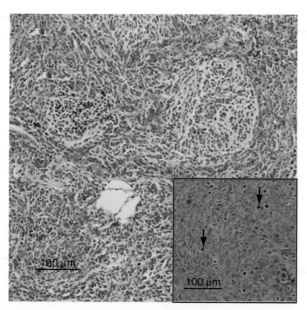

FIGURE A1-2 H&E stain showing a highly cellular small blue cell tumor. Note the numerous mitotic figures present in the magnified inset (arrows). *(Reprinted with permission from Ellenbogen RG, Abdulrauf SI, Sekhar LN. Principles of Neurological Surgery. 3rd ed. Elsevier. 2012.)*

542 Appendices

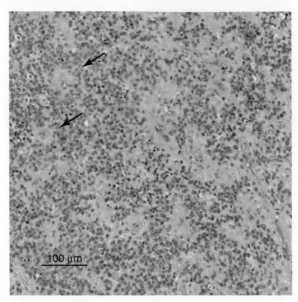

FIGURE A1-3 H&E photomicrograph staining showing typical perivascular rosettes (black arrows). *(Reprinted with permission from Ellenbogen RG, Abdulrauf SI, Sekhar LN. Principles of Neurological Surgery. 3rd ed. Elsevier. 2012.)*

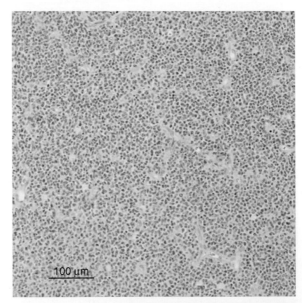

FIGURE A1-4 H&E histopathologic stain showing small blue cells intermixed with large spindle-shaped rhabdoid cells. *(Reprinted with permission from Ellenbogen RG, Abdulrauf SI, Sekhar LN. Principles of Neurological Surgery. 3rd ed. Elsevier. 2012.)*

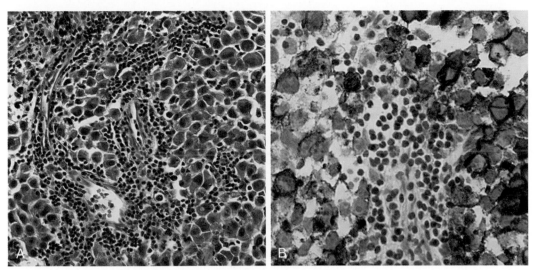

FIGURE A1-5   Histopathological features of a germinoma with typical lymphocytic infiltrates along fibrovascular septae (H&E, ×200) **(A)** and immunohistochemistry staining of the cytoplasm and cytoplasmic membrane with placental alkaline phosphatase (PLAP) (×400) **(B)**. *(Courtesy of O. Koperek, Neuropathological Institute, Medical University of Vienna.) (Reprinted with permission from Ellenbogen RG, Abdulrauf SI, Sekhar LN.* Principles of Neurological Surgery. *3rd ed. Elsevier. 2012.)*

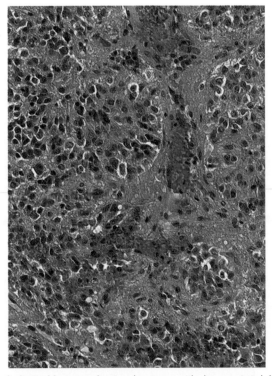

FIGURE A1-6   Histopathological features of a pinealocytoma with characteristic lobular pattern mimicking the structure of the normal pineal gland (H&E, ×200). *(Courtesy of O. Koperek, Neuropathological Institute, Medical University of Vienna.) (Reprinted with permission from Ellenbogen RG, Abdulrauf SI, Sekhar LN.* Principles of Neurological Surgery. *3rd ed. Elsevier. 2012.)*

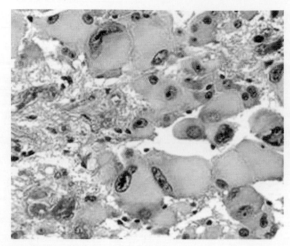

FIGURE A1-7   Subependymal giant cell astrocytomas form clusters composed of spindle cells and large dysmorphic, eosinophilic tumor cells with mixed glioneuronal appearance. *(Reprinted with permission from Winn HR. Youmans Neurological Surgery. 6th ed. Elsevier. 2011.)*

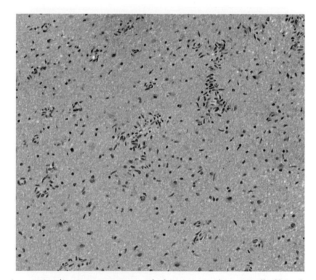

FIGURE A1-8   Angiocentric gliomas are composed of monomorphic, spindled bipolar cells, which assemble around blood vessels in a monolayered or multilayered fashion. *(Reprinted with permission from Winn HR. Youmans Neurological Surgery. 6th ed. Elsevier. 2011.)*

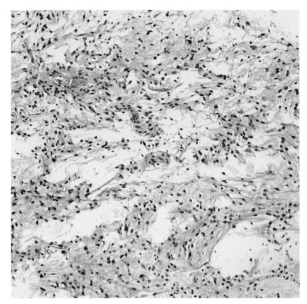

FIGURE A1-9   Pilomyxoid astrocytomas demonstrate a prominent mucoid matrix with small to intermediate-sized astroglial tumor cells, which tend to be angiocentric. *(Reprinted with permission from Winn HR. Youmans Neurological Surgery. 6th ed. Elsevier. 2011.)*

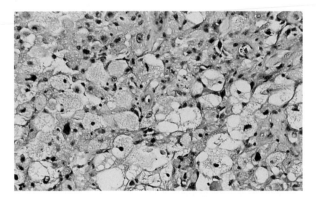

FIGURE A1-10   Pleomorphic xanthoastrocytomas exhibit a high degree of pleomorphism with intermixed spindle cells and astrocytes containing lipid droplets. *(Reprinted with permission from Winn HR. Youmans Neurological Surgery. 6th ed. Elsevier. 2011.)*

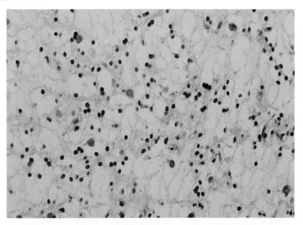

FIGURE A1-11   Dysembryoplastic neuroepithelial tumors form mucin-rich cortical nodules and are composed of oligodendroglioma-like cells intermingled with "floating neurons." *(Reprinted with permission from Winn HR. Youmans Neurological Surgery. 6th ed. Elsevier. 2011.)*

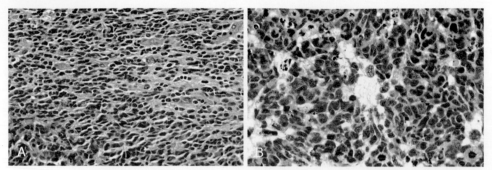

FIGURE A1-12   Medulloblastoma. **(A)** Dense reticulin fiber network surrounding a densely packed small cell tumor. **(B)** H&E stain demonstrates classic Homer Wright pseudorosettes with multiple mitotic figures. *(Reprinted with permission from Winn HR. Youmans Neurological Surgery. 6th ed. Elsevier. 2011.)*

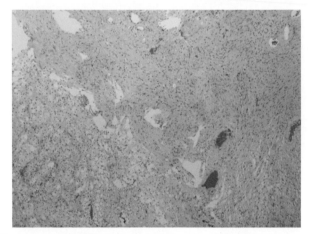

FIGURE A1-13   Microscopic H&E stain demonstrating the two main histologic patterns of schwannomas, Antoni A and B. The *right* side has spindle-shaped cells with rod-shaped nuclei and dense reticulin arranged in fascicles consistent with Antoni A areas. The *left* side has stellate cells and smaller hyperchromatic nuclei, less reticulin, prominent cytoplasmic processes, and a large myxoid stroma consistent with Antoni B areas. *(Reprinted with permission from Winn HR. Youmans Neurological Surgery. 6th ed. Elsevier. 2011.)*

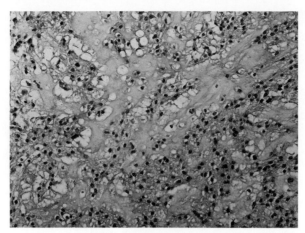

FIGURE A1-14   Histology of chordoma (H&E, ×200). Note the clusters of epithelial cells with mucinous matrix interspersed. Vacuolated cells are a common feature of chordomas. *(Reprinted with permission from Winn HR. Youmans Neurological Surgery. 6th ed. Elsevier. 2011.)*

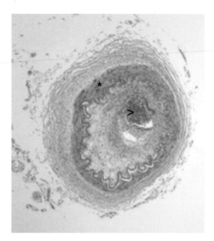

FIGURE A1-15   Studies of vessels in the ICA distribution demonstrate hyperproliferation (asterisk) of vessel wall components and abundant intraluminal thrombus (>), with resultant narrowing and occlusion of the lumen. The right ICA is particularly narrow, as seen in both the gross specimen and microscopic analysis. The images highlight how the vessel occlusion is a combination of both hyperplasia of smooth muscle cells and luminal thrombosis. *(Reprinted with permission from Winn HR. Youmans Neurological Surgery. 6th ed. Elsevier. 2011.)*

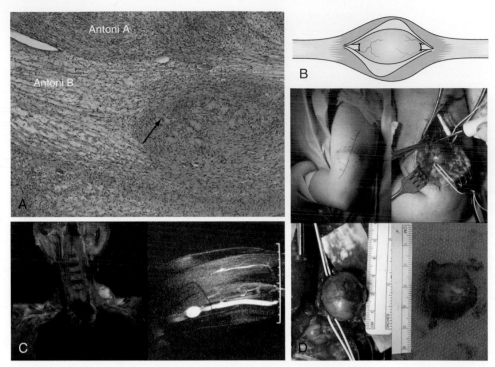

FIGURE A1-16   **(A)** Pathology slide of a peripheral nerve schwannoma. The compact array of spindle cells represents the Antoni type A tissue. The less compact array is the Antoni type B tissue. The palisading cells of the Verocay body are indicated by an arrow. **(B)** Artist depiction of a schwannoma. A single fascicle is seen at the proximal and distal portions of the tumor. **(C)** MRI of schwannomas. A hyperintense mass is seen in the left cervical area and ulnar nerve. **(D)** Intraoperative photographs. The tumor and involved nerve fascicles are exposed. The nerve fascicles are encircled with vasoloops. After the fascicles are identified as nonfunctional, the lesion is removed as a single mass. *(Reprinted with permission from Winn HR.* Youmans Neurological Surgery. *6th ed. Elsevier. 2011.)*

APPENDIX B

Neurology

TABLE A2-1

CLASSIFICATION OF DYSPHASIAS

Lesion	Deficit	Aphasia Type
Temporal	Retained repetition and fluency; no comprehension; no naming	Transcortical sensory
Wernicke's	Retained fluency; no comprehension, repetition, or naming	Wernicke's
Parietal	Retained comprehension and fluency; no repetition	Conduction
Broca's	Retained comprehension; no fluency, repetition, or naming	Broca's
Frontal	Retained comprehension and repetition; no fluency or naming	Transcortical motor

(Reprinted with permission from Ellenbogen RG, Abdulrauf SI, Sekhar LN. Principles of Neurological Surgery. 3rd ed. Elsevier; 2012.)

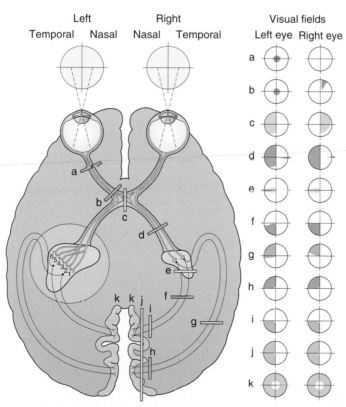

FIGURE A2-1 Characteristic defects of the visual field produced by lesions at various points along the visual pathways.

TYPICAL CEREBROSPINAL FLUID FINDINGS IN VARIOUS DISORDERS

Condition	Pressure	Red Blood Cells/mm³	White Blood Cells/mm³	Differential	Glucose (mg/dL)	Protein (mg/dL)
Normal	Normal	0	0–5	Mononuclear	45–80	15–45
Bacterial meningitis	↑	0	500–100,000	Neutrophils	Low	↑
Tuberculous meningitis	↑	0	50–500	Mononuclear	Low	↑
Viral meningitis	Normal to ↑	0	5–500	Mononuclear	Normal	15–100
Subarachnoid hemorrhage	Normal to ↑	10,000–500,000	↑ in proportion to red blood cells	Mononuclear and neutrophils	Normal	↑
Multiple sclerosis	Normal	0	0–50	Mononuclear	Normal	20–100
Guillain-Barré syndrome	Normal	0	0–50	Mononuclear	Normal	20–500
Brain tumors	Normal to ↑	0	0–100	Mononuclear	Normal	Variable (↑ in acoustic schwannoma)

(Reprinted with permission from Ellenbogen RG, Abdulrauf SI, Sekhar LN. Principles of Neurological Surgery. 3rd ed. Elsevier; 2012.)

ASIA IMPAIRMENT SCALE		
ASIA Grade	Complete or incomplete	Description
A	Complete	No motor or sensory function is preserved in the sacral segments S4-S5
B	Incomplete	Sensory but not motor function is preserved below the neurological level and includes the sacral segments S4-S5
C	Incomplete	Motor function is preserved below the neurological level, and more than half of the key muscles below the neurological level have a muscle grade less than 3
D	Incomplete	Motor function is preserved below the neurological level, and at least half of key muscles below the neurological level have a muscle grade of 3 or more
E	Normal	Motor and sensory function are normal

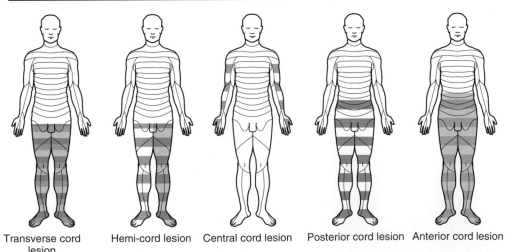

Transverse cord lesion   Hemi-cord lesion   Central cord lesion   Posterior cord lesion   Anterior cord lesion

■ Loss of vibration and position sense   ■ Loss of pain and temperature sense   ■ Loss of motor power

FIGURE A2-2 The ASIA impairment scale (*top*) and the spinal cord syndromes (*bottom*) are outlined. Central cord syndrome is representative of a small lesion. If the central cord lesion is large, one would expect involvement of the motor and vibration/position sense systems (see text for further explanation). Motor power is graded according to the following scale: 0 = total paralysis, 1 = palpable or visible contraction, 2 = active movement, full range of motion, and gravity eliminated, 3 = active movement, full range of motion, and against gravity, 4 = active movement, full range of motion, against gravity, and provides some resistance, 5 = active movement, full range of motion, against gravity, and provides normal resistance, NT = not testable because the patient is unable to reliably exert effort, or the muscle is unavailable for testing because of factors such as immobilization, pain on effort, or contracture. Sensory testing is graded according to the following scale: 0 = absent, 1 = impaired, 2 = normal, and NT = not testable. *(Reprinted with permission from Ellenbogen RG, Abdulrauf SI, Sekhar LN. Principles of Neurological Surgery. 3rd ed. Elsevier; 2012.)*

TABLE A2-3

HOUSE AND BRACKMANN FACIAL NERVE GRADING SYSTEM

Grade	Description/Deficit	Characteristics
I	Normal	Normal facial function
II	Slight	*Gross:* slight weakness noted on close inspection; slight synkinesis *At rest:* normal tone and symmetry *Motion:* *Forehead:* moderate to good movement *Eye:* complete closure with minimal effort *Mouth:* slight asymmetry
III	Moderate	*Gross:* obvious, but not disfiguring asymmetry Synkinesis noticeable, but not severe *At rest:* normal tone and symmetry *Motion:* *Forehead:* slight to moderate movement *Eye:* complete closure with effort *Mouth:* slight weakness with maximal effort
IV	Moderately severe	*Gross:* disfiguring asymmetry and/or obvious facial weakness *At rest:* normal tone and symmetry *Motion:* *Forehead:* no movement *Eye:* incomplete closure *Mouth:* asymmetrical with maximal effort
V	Severe	*Gross:* barely perceptible motion *At rest:* asymmetrical appearance *Motion:* *Forehead:* no movement *Eye:* incomplete closure *Mouth:* trace movement
VI	Total	No facial function

(Adapted from House JW, Brackmann DE. Facial nerve grading system. Otolaryngol Head Neck Surg. 1985;93(2):146-147.)

TABLE A2-4

MOST FREQUENT TUMORS OF THE PINEAL REGION: TYPICAL CHARACTERISTICS

Tumor Feature	Germinoma	Teratoma	Pinealoblastoma	Pinealocytoma	Glioma	Meningioma
Age	Child	Child	Child	Adult	Child	Adult
Sex predilection	Male	Male	None	None	None	None
Pineal versus parapineal	Pineal	Pineal	Pineal	Pineal	Parapineal (usually)	Parapineal (usually)
Signal intensity (heterogeneous versus homogeneous)	Homogeneous (but often hemorrhagic)	Strikingly heterogeneous	Homogeneous (unless hemorrhagic)	Homogeneous	Homogeneous (usually)	Homogeneous
Hemorrhage	Common	Typical	Common	Common	Rare	Rare
Calcification	Rare	Typical	Common	Common	Uncommon	Common
Brain edema or invasion	Common	Variable	Common	Uncommon	Primarily midbrain neoplasm	Occasional
Tendency to metastasize	Yes	Variable	Yes	No	Variable	No
Enhancement	Dense	Variable	Dense	Dense	Variable	Dense
Prognosis with 10-year survival rate, if available	Good with additional therapy: ~85% to >35%	Variable	Poor	Variable	Variable	Excellent

(Reprinted with permission from Ellenbogen RG, Abdulrauf SI, Sekhar LN. Principles of Neurological Surgery. 3rd ed. Elsevier; 2012.)

TABLE A2-5

DIFFERENTIAL DIAGNOSIS OF FACIAL PAIN

Condition/ Factor	Trigeminal Neuralgia	Atypical Facial Pain	Migrainous Facial Pain	Acute Herpes Zoster
Age and gender	>50 years, 60% F	30–50 years, 75% F	Typically, age range of 40–50 years; M = F	>70 years, F > M
Site	V2 or V3 most common alone or in combination, but limited to distribution of trigeminal nerve (intraoral or extraoral); unilateral	Deep nonmuscular areas of face, maxillary or whole face, unilateral or bilateral; does not follow nerve distribution	Anywhere in face; deep eye pain, sinus pain, or toothache	Herpetic lesions in the distribution of trigeminal nerve; V1 most common; most severe in eyebrow; facial or deep ear pain often precedes vesicular eruption
Character	Sudden severe, brief lancinating, and electric shock-like; no allodynia	Throbbing, deep, diffuse, nagging, aching, burning, and cramping; allodynia in some patients	Throbbing or pulsatile; lacrimation or conjunctival injection (cluster headache); no allodynia	Burning, tingling in quality; itching and dysesthesia; allodynia in some patients
Severity	Severe	Moderate to severe	Moderate	Severity varies
Duration	Seconds to minutes	Seconds to minutes or continuous	15 minutes to several hours	Continuous pain may precede vesicular eruption
Periodicity	Pain-free between attacks; long periods of no pain	Continuous background pain or dysesthesia; complete pain remission less likely; interferes with sleep	Often nocturnal or early morning	Continuous pain until vesicles heal; may develop as postherpetic neuralgia
Provoking factors	Non-noxious stimulation of discrete trigger zones in face or in buccal mucosa; hot/ cold fluids in mouth or chewing	Stress; fatigue	Alcohol, hormone replacement therapy; seasonal; cold, warm	Skin stimulation by clothing or touch

(Reprinted with permission from Ellenbogen RG, Abdulrauf SI, Sekhar LN. Principles of Neurological Surgery. 3rd ed. Elsevier; 2012.)

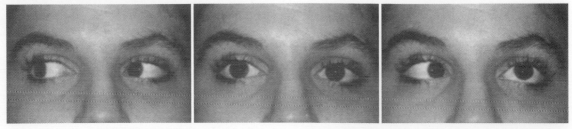

FIGURE A2-3 Abducens palsy in a 20-year-old woman with a traumatic left sixth cranial nerve palsy. Ocular versions are relatively normal on right gaze, but the marked weakness of the left lateral rectus muscle is evident on left gaze. *(Reprinted with permission from Winn HR.* Youmans Neurological Surgery. *6th ed. Elsevier; 2011.)*

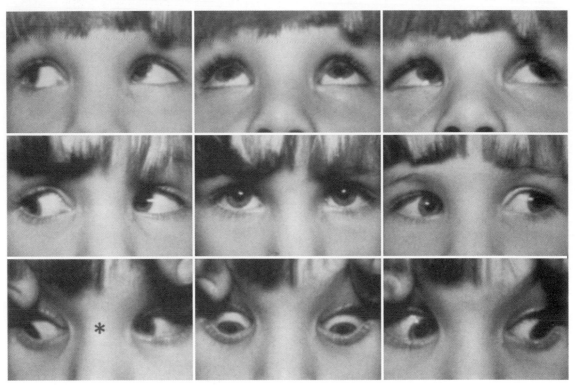

FIGURE A2-4 Superior oblique (trochlear nerve) palsy. This composite of the nine diagnostic positions of gaze demonstrates a left superior oblique palsy. The greatest deviation occurs when the patient looks down and to the right (asterisk). In this adducted position, the left superior oblique becomes the major depressor of the left eye, and its weakness is identified as a left hypertropia. *(Reprinted with permission from Winn HR.* Youmans Neurological Surgery. *6th ed. Elsevier; 2011.)*

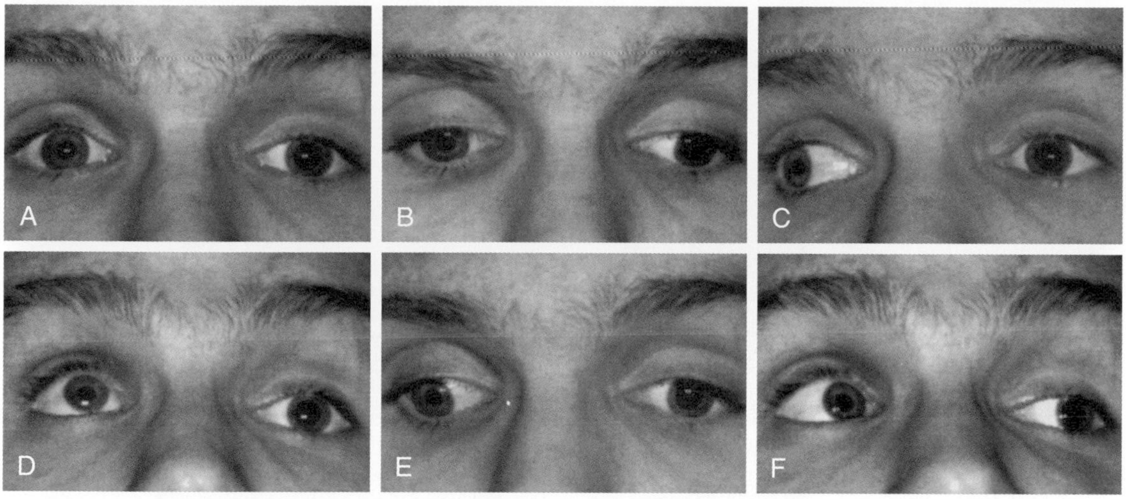

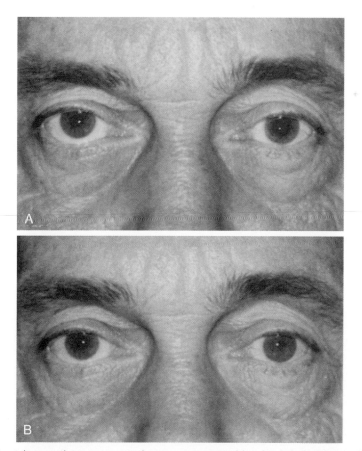

FIGURE A2-5 Oculomotor nerve palsy. In this patient, injury to the left third cranial nerve resulted from closed head trauma. Although motility is only partially affected, the left pupil is fixed and dilated **(A)**. In the primary position, a left ptosis (with compensatory right lid retraction) is seen, with the left eye in a "down-and-out" position **(A** and **B)**. The affected eye does not adduct **(C)**, elevate **(D)**, or depress **(E)** well. Notice that abduction (abducens nerve) is intact **(F)**. *(Reprinted with permission from Winn HR. Youmans Neurological Surgery. 6th ed. Elsevier; 2011.)*

FIGURE A2-6 Adie's pupil. **(A)** Anisocoria that was most noticeable in bright light developed in a 56-year-old asymptomatic individual. **(B)** Clinical suspicion of a left Adie pupil was confirmed with 0.125% pilocarpine. Thirty minutes after drops were placed in both eyes, left pupillary sphincter supersensitivity was evident. *(Reprinted with permission from Winn HR. Youmans Neurological Surgery. 6th ed. Elsevier; 2011.)*

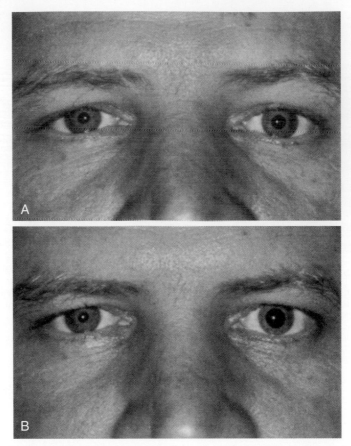

FIGURE A2-7 Horner's syndrome in a 37-year-old man with a history of right-sided cluster headaches being evaluated for right oculosympathetic paresis. **(A)** Right ptosis and miosis. **(B)** Forty minutes after bilateral instillation of 10% cocaine eyedrops, the left pupil dilates, but the right does not, thus confirming the diagnosis of oculosympathetic paresis. Paredrine (hydroxyamphetamine hydrobromide) testing (not shown) gave a similar result, which implicated the third-order neuron (postganglionic) lesion. *(Reprinted with permission from Winn HR. Youmans Neurological Surgery. 6th ed. Elsevier; 2011.)*

APPENDIX C

Neuroradiology

APPEARANCE OF HEMORRHAGE ON MAGNETIC RESONANCE IMAGING

Stage	Age of Bleed	Composition	T1	T2
Hyperacute	<12 hours	Intracellular oxyhemoglobin	Isointense	Hyperintense
Acute	12 hours to 2 days	Intracellular deoxyhemoglobin	Isointense	Hypointense
Early subacute	2–7 days	Intracellular methemoglobin	Hyperintense	Hypointense
Late subacute	8 days to 1 month	Extracellular methemoglobin	Hyperintense	Hyperintense
Chronic	Months to years	Hemosiderin	Hypointense	Hypointense

(Reprinted with permission from Ellenbogen RG, Abdulrauf SI, Sekhar LN. Principles of Neurological Surgery. 3rd ed. Elsevier; 2012.)

TABLE A3-2

STRUCTURES VISUALIZED DURING DIGITAL SUBTRACTION ANGIOGRAPHY

	Structures Seen in Study Phase (Seconds Elapsed)				
Feature	Early Arterial: 1–2 sec	Late Arterial: 2–3 sec	Capillary: 3–4 sec	Early Venous: 5–6 sec	Late Venous: 6–7 sec
Normal structures opacified	Main arteries	Arterial branches	Arterioles	Venules and veins	Veins and sinuses
AVM	Feeding arteries	Nidus	Draining veins and sinuses		
AVF	Feeding arteries	Draining veins and sinuses			

(Reprinted with permission from Ellenbogen RG, Abdulrauf SI, Sekhar LN. Principles of Neurological Surgery. 3rd ed. Elsevier; 2012.)

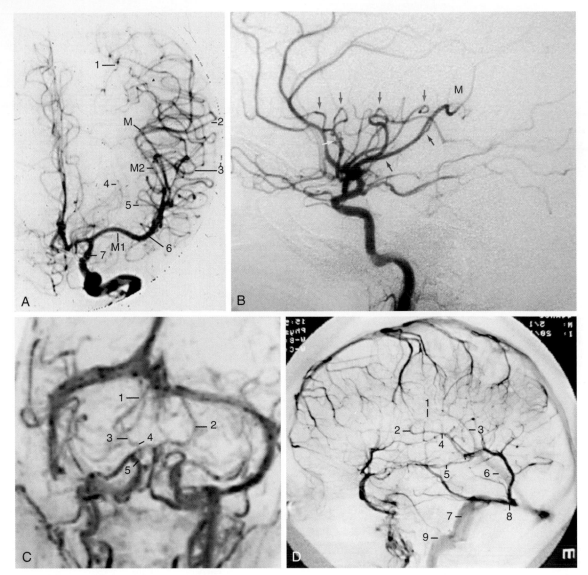

FIGURE A3-1 **(A)** Frontal view of a right carotid angiogram. *1*, intraparietal sulcus; *2*, M3 branches on the planum temporale; *3*, M3 branches in the central sulcus region; *4*, lateral lenticulostriate arteries; *5*, M3 branches in the anterior limiting sulcus of the insula; *6*, genu of the middle cerebral artery; *7*, internal carotid artery (supraclinoid segment); *M*, "M point" or "sylvian point." **(B)** Lateral view of a carotid angiogram. The *blue arrows* indicate the superior limiting sulcus of the insula, the *red arrows* indicate the inferior limiting sulcus of the insula, and the *yellow arrow* indicates the anterior limiting sulcus of the insula. **(C)** Frontal view of a venous magnetic resonance angiogram to display the basal vein. *1*, "thigh" (posterior mesencephalic segment); *2*, "knee" (junction between the anterior and posterior peduncular segments); *3*, "leg" (anterior peduncular segment); *4*, "ankle" (junction between the striate and peduncular segments); *5*, "foot" (striate segment). **(D)** Lateral view of a venous angiogram. *1*, thalamostriate vein; *2*, "venous angle;" *3*, inferior sagittal sinus; *4*, internal cerebral vein; *5*, basal vein; *6*, straight sinus; *7*, sigmoid sinus; *8*, transverse sinus and the "vein of Labbé complex;" *9*, bulb of the jugular vein. *(Reprinted with permission from Winn HR. Youmans Neurological Surgery. 6th ed. Elsevier; 2011.)*

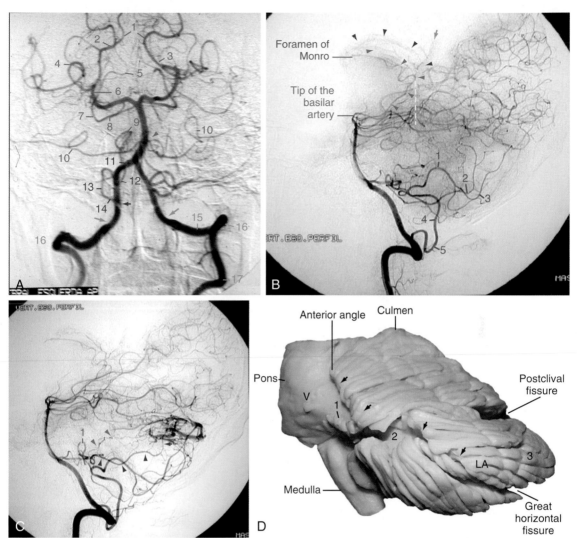

FIGURE A3-2   **(A)** Frontal view of a vertebrobasilar angiogram. *1*, collicular or quadrigeminal point; *2*, P3 segment; *3*, beginning of the P2A segment; *4*, collateral sulcus; *5*, beginning of the cerebellomesencephalic segment of the superior cerebellar artery (SCA); *6*, P2A segment; *7*, lateral pontomesencephalic segment of the SCA; *8*, anterior pontomesencephalic segment of the SCA; *9*, supratonsillar segment of the posterior inferior cerebellar artery (PICA, cranial loop); *10*, meatal loop of the anterior inferior cerebellar artery (AICA); *11*, posterior medullary segment of the PICA; *12*, caudal loop of the PICA; *13*, lateral medullary segment of the PICA; *14*, anterior medullary segment of the PICA; *15*, extradural vertebral artery behind the lateral mass of C1; *16*, vertebral artery in the foramen transversarium of C1; *17*, vertebral artery in the foramen transversarium of C2. The *blue arrowhead* indicates the origin of the AICA from the basilar artery, the *red arrowhead* indicates the origin of the PICA from the vertebral artery, and the *green arrows* indicate the probable transition between the extradural and intradural segments of the vertebral artery. Note the constriction in the vertebral artery. **(B)** Lateral view of the late arterial phase of a vertebrobasilar angiogram. *1*, "cranial loop" of the PICA; *2*, vermian division of the PICA (pyramidal loop); *3*, hemispheric branch of the PICA; *4*, posterior medullary segment of the PICA; *5*, "caudal loop" of the PICA. The *red arrowheads* indicate the posterior choroidal arteries in the lateral ventricle (indicate the location of the posterior wall of the pulvinar of the thalamus), the *green arrow* indicates the posterior pericallosal artery, and the *blue arrowheads* indicate the medial posterior choroidal artery (MPChA). The most posterior point of the trajectory of the MPChA indicates the posterior limit of the quadrigeminal plate and consequently the posterior limit of the brainstem in the lateral view (*yellow dashed line*). For the anatomic location of the lateral posterior choroidal artery and MPChA. Note that the foramen of Monro is located above the tip of the basilar artery (in the same coronal plane). **(C)** Lateral view of the arterial phase of a vertebrobasilar angiogram. *1*, "meatal loop" of the AICA. The *blue arrowheads* indicate small branches to the lateral recess of the fourth ventricle through the foramen of Luschka, and the *red arrowheads* indicate the main trunk of the AICA in the great horizontal fissure, which supplies an arteriovenous malformation located in the superior semilunar lobule. **(D)** Lateral view of the cerebellum. *1*, flocculus; *2*, petrosal fissure or great horizontal fissure; *3*, superior semilunar lobule; *LA*, lateral angle. The *arrows* indicate the anterolateral margin. *(Reprinted with permission from Winn HR. Youmans Neurological Surgery. 6th ed. Elsevier; 2011.)*

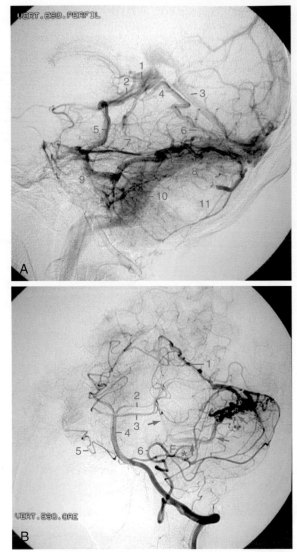

FIGURE A3-3 **(A)** Lateral view of the venous phase of a vertebrobasilar angiogram. *1*, vein of Galen; *2*, cerebellomesencephalic fissure; *3*, straight sinus; *4*, culmen; *5*, vein running on the middle cerebral peduncle that continues with a vein in the petrosal fissure (vein of the great horizontal fissure); *6*, vein running on the tentorial surface of the cerebellum (superior hemispheric vein) toward the vein of Galen; *7*, superior petrosal sinus; *8*, transverse sinus; *9*, vein running in the petrosal fissure or great horizontal fissure (vein of the great horizontal fissure); *10*, sigmoid sinus; *11*, suboccipital surface of the cerebellum; *, a superior hemispheric vein draining an arteriovenous malformation that runs on the tentorial surface, descends toward the petrosal surface, and joins the vein of the great horizontal fissure. **(B)** Left anterior oblique view of a vertebrobasilar angiogram. *1*, vein running on the tentorial surface toward the vein of Galen (superior hemispheric vein); *2*, posterior cerebral artery; *3*, superior cerebellar artery; *4*, basilar artery; *5*, meatal loop of the anterior inferior cerebellar artery (AICA); *6*, posterior inferior cerebellar artery (PICA). The *arrows* indicate the vein that originates from the tentorial surface (superior hemispheric vein) and descends toward the petrosal surface to join the vein in the great horizontal fissure. **(C)** Approximate location of the flocculus; it was estimated by the location meatal loop of the AICA. *(Reprinted with permission from Winn HR. Youmans Neurological Surgery. 6th ed. Elsevier; 2011.)*

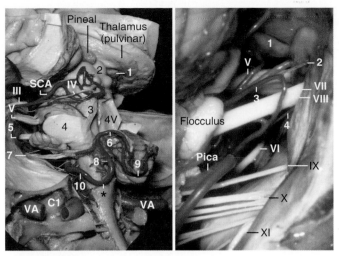

FIGURE A3-4   *Right*, retromastoid view of the cerebellopontine angle. *1*, superior petrosal vein; *2*, subarcuate artery (AICA); *3*, AICA; *4*, internal auditory artery. *(Reprinted with permission from Winn HR. Youmans Neurological Surgery. 6th ed. Elsevier; 2011.)*

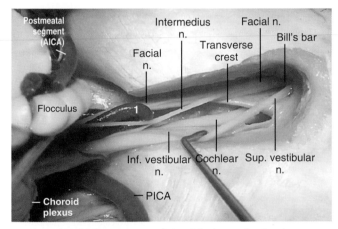

FIGURE A3-5   Posterior view of the contents of the right internal acoustic meatus. *1*, AICA (meatal segment). *(Reprinted with permission from Winn HR. Youmans Neurological Surgery. 6th ed. Elsevier; 2011.)*

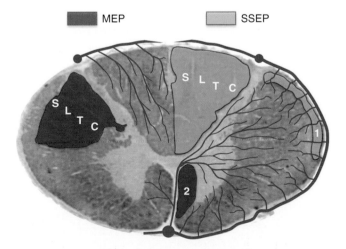

FIGURE A3-6   Schematic diagram of the functional tracts monitored by motor-evoked potential (MEP) and somatosensory-evoked potential (SSEP) recordings illustrating the complementary coverage of these two modalities. The anterior and lateral corticospinal tracts are primarily supplied by the anterior spinal and sulcal arteries. The dorsal columns are primarily supplied by the posterior spinal artery. The spinocerebellar tracts are supplied by penetrating branches of the arterial vasocorona. *1*, spinocerebellar tract; *2*, anterior cortical spinal tract; *C*, cervical; *L*, lumbar; *S*, sacral; *T*, thoracic. *(Reprinted with permission from Winn HR. Youmans Neurological Surgery. 6th ed. Elsevier; 2011.)*

TABLE A3-3

COMPARISON OF THE MAJOR MODALITIES USED FOR TYPICAL INTRAOPERATIVE MONITORING

Modality	SSEP	MEP/CMAP	EMG
Stimulation	Peripheral sensory nerves	Transcranial scalp electrodes	Free-running: none Triggered: bipolar stimulation of a specific structure
Recording	Cortical and cervicomedullary junction	Extremity muscles (e.g., thenar muscles and tibialis anterior)	Myotome specific
Alert threshold	50% reduction in amplitude 10% increase in latency	Disappearance of signal (all-or-none phenomenon)	Sustained activity (>2 sec)
Advantages	Specific and sensitive to sensory deficits Continuous monitoring; no interruption in surgical maneuvers	Specific and sensitive to motor deficits' large signal amplitude; instantaneous feedback	Allows surgical correlation with specific nerve roots; continuous monitoring; instantaneous feedback
Disadvantages	False-negative results for motor deficits; low signal amplitude; multitrace averaging required; delayed response (seconds to minutes)	Total intravenous anesthesia; intermittent monitoring; interruption in surgery required	No neuromuscular blockade; monitors only nerve roots

CMAP, compound muscle action potential; *EMG*, electromyography; *MEPs*, motor-evoked potential; *SSEP*, somatosensory-evoked potential.
(Reprinted with permission from Winn HR. Youmans Neurological Surgery. 6th ed. Elsevier; 2011.)

Spinal Fracture Grading

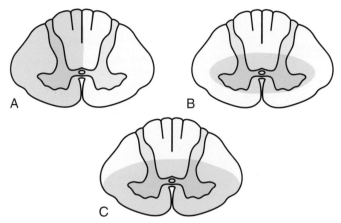

FIGURE A4-1 Spinal cord injury syndromes. **(A)** Hemicord syndrome (Brown-Sequard) is manifested as loss of contralateral pain and temperature sensation with preserved light touch (anterior spinothalamic tract) and ipsilateral loss of motor function and proprioception caudal to the lesion. **(B)** Central cord syndrome is caused by compression of the cord dorsoventrally with central hemorrhage and venous infarction. Clinical manifestations include motor weakness, more pronounced in the upper extremities (central gray matter), and variable sensory loss below the lesion combined with sphincter dysfunction. **(C)** Anterior cord syndrome is caused by injury to, or compression of, the anterior spinal artery with loss of motor function and pain and temperature sensation caudal to the lesion and preservation of joint position, vibratory sensation, and two-point discrimination. *(Reprinted with permission from Winn HR. Youmans Neurological Surgery. 6th ed. Elsevier; 2011.)*

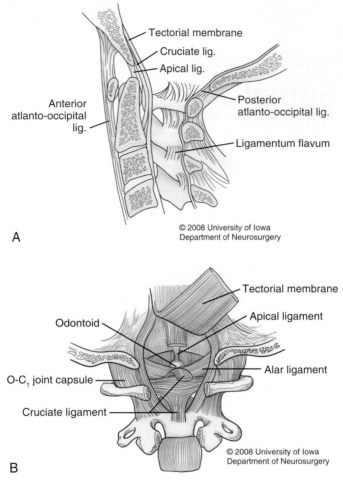

FIGURE A4-2 Lateral (**A**) and posterior (**B**) views of the craniovertebral junction. Note that the cruciate ligament is composed of horizontal fibers (i.e., the transverse ligament) and vertical fibers. The tectorial membrane, the rostral extent of the posterior longitudinal ligament, has been reflected in (**B**) to allow visualization of more ventral structures. *(Reprinted with permission from Winn HR. Youmans Neurological Surgery. 6th ed. Elsevier; 2011.)*

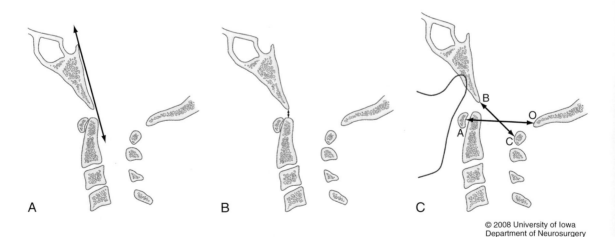

FIGURE A4-3 Schematic diagrams depicting various criteria developed to assess the craniovertebral junction. Wackenheim's line (**A**) is drawn as a caudal extension of the clivus and should tangentially intersect the tip of the dens in a normal individual. A normal dens-basion interval (**B**) should not exceed 5 mm in an adult and 10 mm in infants. (**C**) The distance between the basion, *B*, and inner surface of the posterior arch of C1, *C*, divided by the distance from the opisthion, *O*, to the inner surface of the anterior arch of C1, *A*, defines the Powers ratio. The mean value in normal subjects is 0.77. *(Reprinted with permission from Winn HR. Youmans Neurological Surgery. 6th ed. Elsevier; 2011.)*

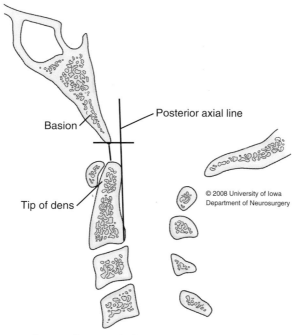

Basion

Posterior axial line

Tip of dens

© 2008 University of Iowa
Department of Neurosurgery

FIGURE A4-4   Schematic diagram depicting the basion–posterior axial line (BAI), and the basion–dental interval (BDI). *(Reprinted with permission from Winn HR.* Youmans Neurological Surgery. *6th ed. Elsevier; 2011.)*

TABLE A4-1

CLASSIFICATION SYSTEMS OF ATLANTO-AXIAL ROTATORY SUBLUXATION

White and Panjabi	Fielding	Description	Treatment
Bilateral anterior	II: if 3–5 mm, III: if >5 mm	Anterior displacement of C1 on C2	If small, probably stable; trial of conservative management or C1-C2 fusion if neurologic symptoms
Bilateral posterior	IV	Posterior displacement of C1 on C2	Unstable, C1-C2 fusion
Unilateral anterior	II: if 3–5 mm, III: if >5 mm	Anterior displacement of C1 on C2	If small, probably stable; trial of conservative management or C1-C2 fusion if neurologic symptoms
Unilateral posterior	I	No anterior displacement of C1 on C2; lateral masses in different positions	Probably stable, attempt reduction; fusion of C1-C2 if neurologic symptoms require
Unilateral combined anterior and posterior	I	No anterior displacement of C1 on C2; lateral masses in different positions	Probably stable, attempt reduction; fusion of C1-C2 if neurologic symptoms require

(Data from Fielding JW, Hawkins RJ: Atlanto-axial rotatory fixation (fixed rotatory subluxation of the atlanto-axial joint). J Bone Joint Surg Am. *1977;59:37-44; White AA, Panjabi MM: Clinical Biomechanics of the Spine. Philadelphia: JB Lippincott; 1978.)*

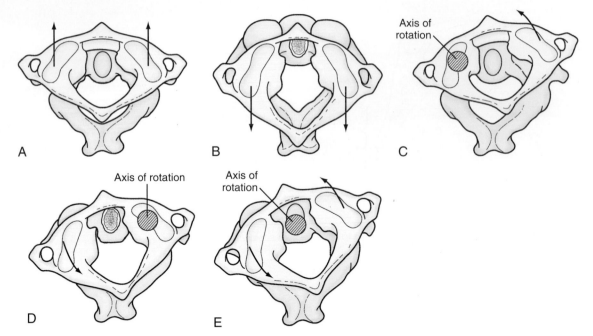

FIGURE A4-5   White and Panjabi classification of atlanto-axial rotatory subluxation. **(A)** Bilateral anterior. **(B)** Bilateral posterior. **(C)** Unilateral anterior. **(D)** Unilateral posterior. **(E)** Unilateral combined anterior and posterior. *(Adapted from White AA, Panjabi MM. Clinical Biomechanics of the Spine. Philadelphia: JB Lippincott; 1978.)*

TABLE A4-2

ATLANTO-OCCIPITO DISLOCATION

Atlanto-Occipito Dislocation	Condyle to C1 mass lat mass interval: >4 mm abnormal

TABLE A4-3

CONDYLAR FRACTURES

Anderson and Montesano Classification System

Type I	Comminuted from axial load
Type II	Extension of skull base
Type III	Avulsion of alar ligament (tip of dens to condyles)

TABLE A4-4

Atlanto-Axial Subluxation	Look at ADI (atlanto dens interval), evaluates TAL, >3.5 mm is abnormal

TABLE A4-5

JEFFERSON

Jefferson Fracture Classification

Type I	Single arch fracture
Type II	Anterior and posterior arch fractures
Type III	Arch fractures and involvement of lateral mass; with disruption of transverse atlantal ligament (TAL)

TABLE A4-6	
ODONTOID	
Odontoid Fracture Classification	
Type I	Through tip (above transverse ligament, which extends medial C1 lat mass to opposite C1 lat mass)
Type II	Through base of neck
Type IIA	Like Type II, but with large bone chips at fracture line
Type III	Through C2 body

TABLE A4-7	
HANGMAN	
Hangman Fracture Classification	
Type I	C2 pars fracture; no displacement
Type II	Angulation >11 mm and subluxation >3 mm
Type IIA	Severe angulation; vertical fracture line, but no subluxation (possible disc disruption)
Type III	High degree of angulation and subluxation; disc and facet capsules disrupted

Screw placement

C1

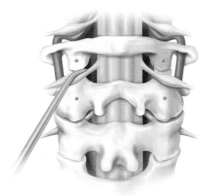

FIGURE A4-6 Curettes are used to define the bony margins of the inferior portion of the posterior ring of C1 out to the lateral masses of C1. Surgifoam is used to stop bleeding from the nearby vertebral venous plexus. The C1-C2 joint must be exposed and denuded of soft tissue to provide a surface for bone grafting. The starting point for C1 lateral mass screws and C2 pars/pedicle screws is shown. *(Reprinted with permission from Jandial R, McCormick P, and Black PM.* Core Techniques in Operative Neurosurgery. *Elsevier; 2011.)*

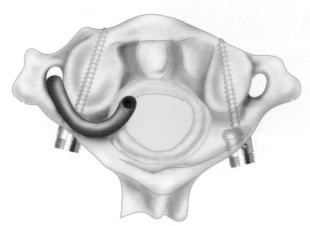

FIGURE A4-7 We perform C1-C2 fixation using lateral fluoroscopic guidance. Gentle caudal retraction on the C2 dorsal root ganglion is required to expose the C1 lateral mass screw entry point, which lies halfway between the junction of the C1 posterior arch and the inferior posterior part of the C1 lateral mass. A No. 4 Penfield dissector can be used to feel the medial border of the C1 lateral mass. A high-speed burr is used to mark the entry point. We recommend drilling some of the posterior ring of C1 that lies above the C1 lateral mass screw entry point to allow adequate room for the polyaxial head of the C1 screw. The pilot hole is drilled with the hand-held drill in a 5- to 10-degree medial trajectory along a plane parallel to the plane of the C1 posterior arch. We recommend checking the pilot hole with a blunt 1.0-mm probe and then tapping the hole. A 3.5-mm-diameter polyaxial screw whose length typically measures 18 to 30 mm is placed. *(Reprinted with permission from Jandial R, McCormick P, and Black PM.* Core Techniques in Operative Neurosurgery. *Elsevier; 2011.)*

C2

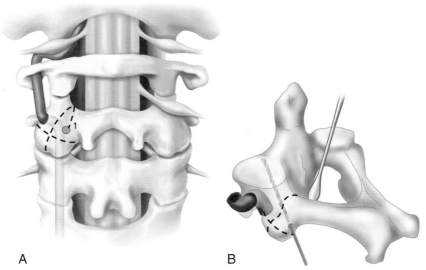

A   B

FIGURE A4-8 A No. 4 Penfield dissector is used to feel the medial border of the C2 pars interarticularis. The atlanto-axial membrane is detached using a blunt dissector to expose the upper surface of the C2 pedicle. The inferior articular process of C2 is divided into quadrants. The C2 pedicle screw starting point lies in the superomedial quadrant of the inferior articular process of C2 (approximately 1.75 mm caudal to the lateral mass–pars interarticularis transition zone). The pilot hole is again prepared with a high-speed bit, and the pilot hole is drilled in a trajectory oriented 20 degrees medial and 20 degrees cephalad with lateral fluoroscopic guidance. The hole is checked with a probe and tapped. A 3.5-mm screw is placed. Typical screw lengths are 30 to 35 mm. *(Reprinted with permission from Jandial R, McCormick P, and Black PM.* Core Techniques in Operative Neurosurgery. *Elsevier; 2011.)*

Lat mass

FIGURE A4-9 The appropriate starting point can be determined by creating an imaginary "X" over the lateral mass. The superior and inferior boundaries are the facet joints, and the medial and lateral boundaries of the lateral mass serve as the other boundaries. The ideal starting point is 1 mm medial to the middle of the imaginary "X". *(Reprinted with permission from Jandial R, McCormick P, and Black PM. Core Techniques in Operative Neurosurgery. Elsevier; 2011.)*

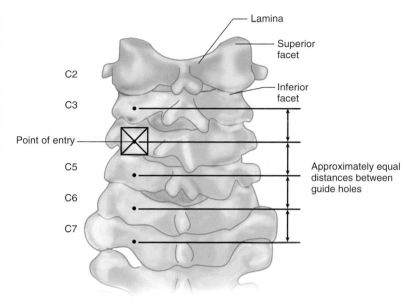

FIGURE A4-10 An up-and-out technique is used for hand drill trajectory. A medial-to-lateral trajectory at 30 degrees avoids injury to the vertebral artery, and a cephalad-caudal trajectory at 20 degrees avoids injury to the nerve root. *(Reprinted with permission from Jandial R, McCormick P, and Black PM. Core Techniques in Operative Neurosurgery. Elsevier; 2011.)*

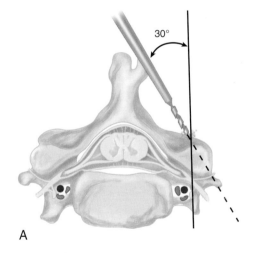

A

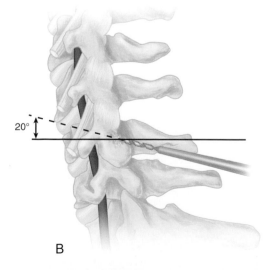

B

Thoracic pedicle screws

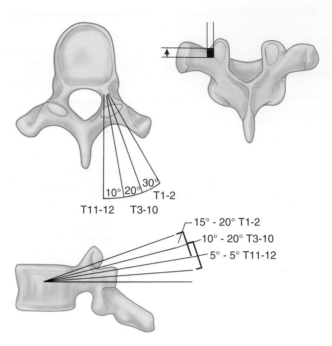

FIGURE A4-11 Thoracic pedicle screws should be placed using established landmarks and trajectories. *(Reprinted with permission from Jandial R, McCormick P, and Black PM.* Core Techniques in Operative Neurosurgery. *Elsevier; 2011.)*

Peripheral Nerve Exam

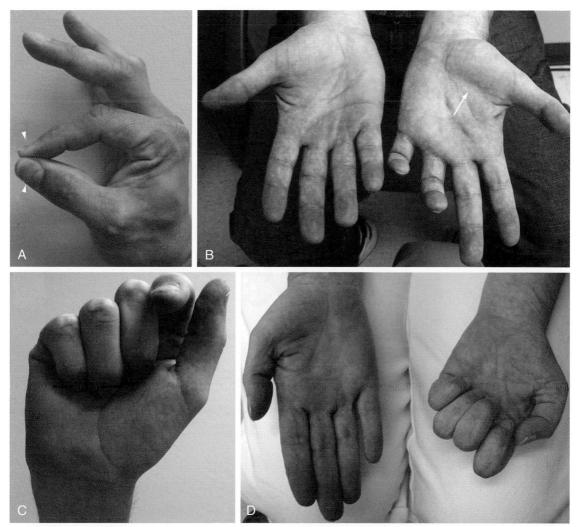

FIGURE A5-1   Nerve palsies affecting the hand. **(A)** Anterior interosseous nerve palsy with an inability to oppose the tips of the thumb and index finger (*arrowheads*). **(B)** This patient has a left-sided ulnar clawhand. Atrophy of the adductor pollicis is also evident (*arrow*). **(C)** This patient has a complete median nerve palsy preventing him from fully flexing his thumb and index finger (i.e., a Benedictine sign) when he attempts to make a tight fist. **(D)** A left-sided simian hand is present, as a result of a lower trunk injury, affecting both the median and ulnar nerves. *(Reprinted with permission from Winn HR. Youmans Neurological Surgery. 6th ed. Elsevier; 2011.)*

Peripheral Nerve Exam

APPENDIX F

Neurocutaneous Disorders

TABLE A6-1

NF1	NF1 gene (ch 17q) Autosomal dominant Diagnosis: see next box ≫	Diagnosis: *Must have two or more of the following:* • Six or more café au lait macules (0.5 cm in children or 1.5 cm in adults) • Two or more cutaneous/subcutaneous neurofibromas, or one plexiform neurofibroma • Axillary or groin freckling • Optic pathway glioma • Two or more Lisch nodules (iris hamartomas seen on slit lamp examination) • Bony dysplasia (sphenoid wing dysplasia and bowing of long bone pseudarthrosis) • First degree relative with NF1
NF2	NF2 gene (ch 22q12) Autosomal dominant Diagnosis: see next box ≫	Diagnosis: • Bilateral vestibular schwannomas – none • Family history – unilateral vestibular schwannoma or two NF2-associated lesions* • Unilateral vestibular schwannoma – two NF2-associated lesions associated with the disorder* • Multiple meningiomas – unilateral vestibular schwannoma or two other NF2-associated lesions*
VHL	VHL gene (ch 3) CNS hemangioblastomas Pheochromocytomas Retinal hemangioblastomas	
Schwannomatosis	Ch 22 Autosomal dominant Lack of vestibular nerve involvement No ocular symptoms No h/o NF2	
Sturge-Weber Syndrome	Port wine nevus in V1 Leptomeningeal angiomatosis (tram-track calcifications) Seizures Glaucoma	
Tuberous Sclerosis	TSC 1 (ch 9) and TSC 2 (ch 16) Tubers SEGA Retinal hamartoma	

*Meningioma, glioma, neurofibroma, schwannoma, or cataract.

Neuromuscular Disorders

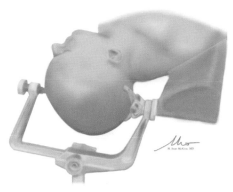

FIGURE A7-1 Positioning for pterional craniotomy. The ipsilateral shoulder is elevated with a shoulder roll, head flexed slightly, and rotated approximately 45 degrees toward the contralateral shoulder. The degree of rotation is adjusted on the basis of the surgical target. Ideal positioning should place the malar eminence at the highest point of the surgical field. *(Reprinted with permission from Winn HR. Youmans Neurological Surgery. 6th ed. Elsevier; 2011.)*

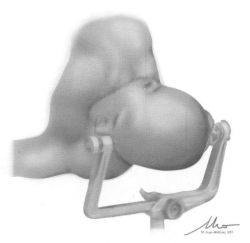

FIGURE A7-2 Lateral decubitus positioning for subtemporal or temporal approach. Once the head is positioned with the sagittal plane parallel to the ground, it is tilted slightly toward the floor, a maneuver that allows the temporal lobe to fall away from the middle cranial fossa. This position can also be used for a lateral suboccipital craniotomy by rotating the face toward the floor, allowing the operative site to be the highest point on the surgical field. *(Reprinted with permission from Winn HR. Youmans Neurological Surgery. 6th ed. Elsevier; 2011.)*

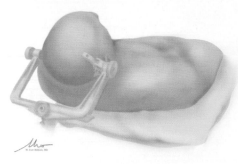

FIGURE A7-3 Positioning for anterior parasagittal or subfrontal approach. This is achieved through a standard supine position. The degree of flexion or extension of the head depends on the surgical target. For the subfrontal approach, the neck is extended past a perpendicular plane with the floor, allowing the frontal lobe to fall away from the anterior cranial fossa. For the anterior parasagittal approach, the head is flexed until the desired surgical site is comfortably within the surgeon's operative field. This positioning may occasionally be modified to accommodate a posterior parasagittal approach and entails shifting the pins in front of the external auditory meatus. This also requires a higher degree of flexion than in the anterior parasagittal approach. If too much flexion is needed, it may be necessary to perform the procedure from a prone position. *(Reprinted with permission from Winn HR. Youmans Neurological Surgery. 6th ed. Elsevier; 2011.)*

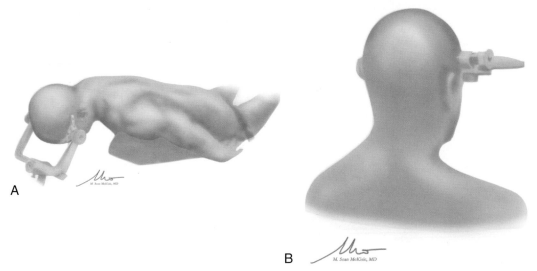

A

B

FIGURE A7-4 **(A)** Prone positioning for midline suboccipital approach. This is typically performed from the Concorde position. The head is flexed and elevated, making sure to keep two fingerbreadths between the chin and the chest. **(B)** Seated positioning for midline suboccipital approach. *(Reprinted with permission from Winn HR. Youmans Neurological Surgery. 6th ed. Elsevier; 2011.)*

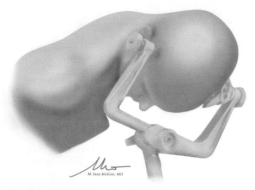

FIGURE A7-5 Positioning for lateral suboccipital approach. This position is similar to that for the midline suboccipital approach; however, the head is rotated so that the ipsilateral mastoid process is brought into the operative field. This head positioning may also be achieved from the lateral position. *(Reprinted with permission from Winn HR. Youmans Neurological Surgery. 6th ed. Elsevier; 2011.)*

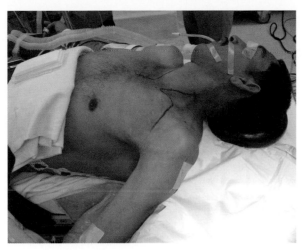

FIGURE A7-6 **(A)** A patient positioned for a full brachial plexus exploration. The incisions for a supracla-vicular and infraclavicular exposure are marked. **(B)** The lower trunk (LT) is retracted inferiorly to demonstrate the proximal aspect of the cervical rib (asterisk). Note the swollen appearance of the lower trunk secondary to compression by the cervical rib. The upper (UT) and middle (MT) trunks and the phrenic nerve (PN) are also visualized. *(Reprinted with permission from Winn HR. Youmans Neurological Surgery. 6th ed. Elsevier; 2011.)*

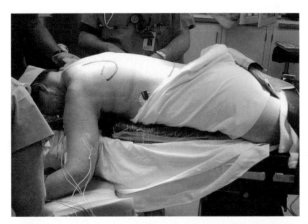

FIGURE A7-7 A patient positioned for a posterior subscapular approach to the brachial plexus. This patient had previous radiation treatments to the anterior neck, making a traditional approach to the plexus not feasible. *(Reprinted with permission from Winn HR. Youmans Neurological Surgery. 6th ed. Elsevier; 2011.)*

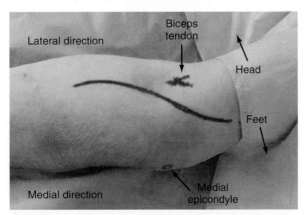

FIGURE A7-8 The incision for exposure of the anterior interosseous nerve. *(Reprinted with permission from Winn HR. Youmans Neurological Surgery. 6th ed. Elsevier. 2011.)*

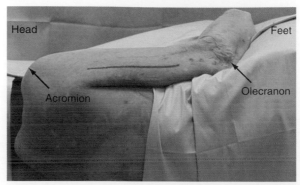

FIGURE A7-9   A patient in the lateral decubitus position for exposure of the radial nerve. Note that in this position, the surgeon may move from the posterior aspect of the patient to the anterior aspect of the patient to reach the radial nerve distal to the spiral groove. *(Reprinted with permission from Winn HR. Youmans Neurological Surgery. 6th ed. Elsevier; 2011.)*

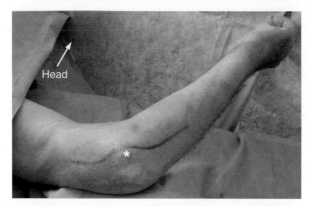

FIGURE A7-10   A patient positioned with an incision drawn for an ulnar nerve exposure. The *asterisk* marks the palpated olecranon. *(Reprinted with permission from Winn HR. Youmans Neurological Surgery. 6th ed. Elsevier; 2011.)*

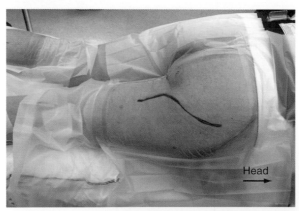

FIGURE A7-11   A patient positioned with an incision drawn for a sciatic nerve exposure. The patient is in the prone position on abdominal bolsters. The incision may be extended distally as needed. *(Reprinted with permission from Winn HR. Youmans Neurological Surgery. 6th ed. Elsevier; 2011.)*

Index

Page numbers followed by "*f*" indicate figures, "*t*" indicate tables, and "*b*" indicate boxes.